COMMIT TO BE FIT:
NOW AND FOREVER
Second Edition

Steve Frierman
Hofstra University

American Press
Boston, Massachusetts
www.americanpresspublishsers.com

Dedication

I am dedicating this book to my family, friends and especially my students who are always there to listen to me over and over again. Writing this book has instilled in me the importance of "practicing what you preach" and hopefully you will all be inspired by what I have written as you "commit to be fit now and forever."

Acknowledgements

Once again, I learned that for me the writing and the research is the easy part. In fact, I thoroughly enjoyed going to the library to just write (and play a few games in between). It's the picture taking, the formatting and the editing that's the hard part and at times it felt like a never-ending process. Fortunately, I had several people that were always there for me to guide and support me through this challenging and incredibly worthwhile process.

Thank you to all of my students who graciously volunteered to participate in the picture taking process. I bet you didn't know how many times I was going to ask you to take more pictures. Matthew—your patience in teaching me how to use PDF will not be forgotten. Jeremy—you've become positively addicted to exercise which is a great thing—for me. It enabled me to watch you exercise and take hundreds of pictures. Josh—for letting me share my thoughts with you during the writing process. Just keep shaking your head. Grace—for your gracious hospitality allowing me to use your exercise facility and you, too. Chris—for your mastery of exercise form. Lincoln—for your unconditional love and support during our long brainstorming walks. Melanie—for just being such a special person and demonstrating in your runs the true meaning of dedication and perseverance. Finally, Mom Wolf—for listening to me share my ideas with you and then you asking me, are you done yet? Is it finished? Yes, mom, I am. It's all done and thank you!!

Preface

They say that time stands still when you're having fun. Well, I've spent the last three years reading, writing and revising the second edition of this book and it feels like just yesterday when I first started. The sole purpose of this edition is to invite you to "commit to be fit." Oh sure, we all have our moments in life when we reflect back and think "I should have joined the gym" and "I know I could have gotten up a little earlier to go for a run" or "Why didn't I ask him/her to work out with me?"

The simple fact is that some of us get started and then stop. Others never really get started and then there's the few of us who just keep on going because we've learned that exercise, fitness and wellness are more than just what we should do. It's who we've become. Ironically, we all know that exercise and living healthy makes us feel so much better, yet we often hold onto to our barriers as a means to rationalize why we aren't exercising even though we know we should.

Many years ago, I used to be like that. Inherently, I knew what to do. I knew how to do it. I knew where to go to exercise and even what times worked best for me. Yet, I often got stopped and then it dawned on me. How could I tell people what to do in terms of exercise and eating healthy if I wasn't doing it myself. Then I realized that regardless of my education and background or how fit I used to be, I was just like everyone else. I got stopped. First, it was the new job, then the two boys, then the tenure process, then the conference and the articles and then and then and then.

We'll I'm proud to say that it was the barriers that stopped me that helped me to get started and write this book. Moreover, I have learned so much from the students that I have taught about what works and does not work that I have and continue to apply it to my own life each and every day. It's been about 14 years now that I have exercised an average of 4-6 times per week and actually love it. It's true that I may not always like the first few minutes of the run or the first few sets of lifting or even the twenty minutes it takes me to change into exercise clothes, put on my compression sleeves, knee pads and of course my 1970's style bandana. However, I am so fortunate to have made the commitment to exercise that finding the time is no longer an issue. As I've told many students and clients over the years," how can we not find the time for something that makes us feel better, improves our mood, gives us more energy, increases our daily productivity and enhance our overall quality of life." I've been told by a few people in my personal life that I see things black and white and when it comes to exercise and living healthy, I agree. It is black and white. Make the commitment to do it and you will feel better mentally, physically, emotionally and spirituality because you know you are doing something that is good for yourself and in many cases good for the people in your life, too.

So, now it's your turn to learn what stops you from exercising and living a healthy lifestyle and what motivates you to overcome your barriers so that you can commit to be fit, now and forever. Below is an outline of each chapter. Don't let me stop you. Get started.

WHAT'S IN EACH CHAPTER

Chapter 1 introduces you to the barriers that stop you from exercising, being more physically active and living a healthier lifestyle. You will learn what really motivates you to be more physically active and fit as you prepare yourself to get started exercising.

Chapter 2, reveals the variety of motives individuals have to exercise and determine what really motivates you to exercise, be more physically active and fit today and for the rest of your life.

Chapter 3 will enlighten you on the purposes of setting goals and then introduce you to two of the most effective ways to set goals: (1) The SMAART Principle and the (2) Stairway to Success. You will identify some of the problems that occur when you set goals and then apply several strategies designed to minimize and ultimately prevent these problems from occurring. This will help you to improve three crucial factors related to long-term exercise participation: (1) enjoyment; (2) performance and (3) commitment to continue.

Chapter 4 includes 8 basic principles of lifetime fitness that map out the guidelines for how to exercise properly and improve your health-related fitness. This will help you to explore how to apply each principle into your workouts to create an exercise program that is safe, productive and fun.

Chapter 5 addresses seven important questions that will help you determine your true desire to exercise. By answering these questions, you will begin to learn exactly how committed you are toward exercise as you begin to create a "Plan" for how to fit exercise into your life and make it fun.

Chapter 6 introduces you to cardiorespiratory endurance (CRE). Learn the benefits of CRE and why it is so important to living healthy. Discover how to formally and informally assess your CRE and then develop a personalized CRE exercise prescription based on two important factors: (1) your present level of CRE fitness and (2) your commitment to improve your CRE.

Learn how to set SMAART goals to improve your CRE and then evaluate the success of you CRE program. Identify ways to spice up your workouts to create new and inviting challenges that increase your enjoyment and motivation to work on your CRE. Finally, become familiar with exercising properly and preventing injuries.

Chapter 7 distinguishes muscular strength and muscular endurance and introduces you to the wealth of benefits of working on your muscular fitness (MF). Learn how to assess your muscular fitness (MF) and then develop an exercise prescription tailored for you. Become familiar with two different muscular fitness programs, designed for three different levels of muscular fitness (low-moderate-high) and identified by your level of commitment to exercise from one to five days per week. Learn how to set SMAART goals to improve your MF and then evaluate the success of you MF program. Identify ways to spice up your workouts to create new and inviting challenges that increase your enjoyment and motivation to work on your MF. Finally, become familiar with exercising properly and preventing injuries.

Chapter 8 focuses on flexibility where you will learn what flexibility is, the benefits of being flexible and how to assess your level of flexibility. You will be introduced to five different flexibility techniques: (1) static; (2) passive static; (3) ballistic; (4) PNF and (5) dynamic. Explore the benefits and limitations of each technique as you develop your own flexibility exercise prescription and determine when you should stretch, what flexibility techniques you should practice before, during and after exercise. Learn how to set SMAART goals to improve your flexibility and then evaluate the success of your flexibility program. Identify ways to spice up your workouts to create new and inviting challenges that increase your enjoyment and motivation to work on your flexibility. Finally, become familiar with stretching properly in order to prevent injuries.

Chapter 9 introduces you to a variety of different ways to assess body composition. You will learn the differences between being underweight, overweight, overfat, obese and extremely obese. Discover strategies to improve body composition and determine how committed you are to improving your own body composition. Finally, recognize myths about improving body composition.

Chapter 10 will help you distinguish between poor vs. healthy eating. Understand why people eat poorly and what motivates them to eat this way. Compare the old and new food guide pyramids with the healthy plate. Learn the roles of the six basic nutrients. Discover just exactly how committed you are to eating healthier and improving your nutritional habits. Set SMAART goals to improve your nutritional habits and evaluate your success over time.

Chapter 11 introduces you to four different cognitive strategies (association, dissociation, positive self-talk and imagery) as you learn how and when to use each during exercise. Evaluate the effectiveness of using cognitive strategies to enhancing exercise enjoyment, performance and motivation.

Chapter 12 will help you discover what stress is and identify the stressors in your life. You will learn how to take control of your stressors by practicing five different stress management techniques (1) progressive muscle relaxation; (2) relaxation response; (3) yogic breathing; (4) time out; and (5) exercise. Learn how to incorporate each of these stress management techniques into your daily life as you begin to transform negative stress (distress) into positive stress (eustress).

Chapter 13 is a new chapter that reviews the research on smoking and smoking-related illness. Learn why people smoke, the consequences associated with smoking from costs to illness and how to stop smoking.

So there you have it! *Thirteen exciting and invigorating chapters* just waiting for you to read and apply in your life. My goal for you is that after reading this book you will have a high level of commitment to exercise and you will transform "working out" and "living healthy" from something you know you should do to something that has become part of you. So commit to be fit: now and forever (what a catchy title)!!

Contents

8 DEVELOPING AN EXERCISE PRESCRIPTION FOR FLEXIBILITY 157

9 BODY COMPOSITION 199

10   IMPROVING YOUR NUTRITION BY EATING AND DRINKING HEALTHY 231

13 IT'S TIME TO STOP SMOKING

Chapter 1

What's Stopping You?

In this chapter you will:

- Identify what stops you from being more physically active
- Determine what really motivates you to be more physically active
- Prepare yourself to get started exercising

Each year more and more people are recognizing the importance of living a healthy life-style. Factors such as medical doctors recommending and prescribing physical activity and exercise to treat and promote mental and physical health, healthier lifestyles and longevity, business corporations making monetary contributions to local exercise facilities for employee membership and an increase in exercise programs in both public and private sectors have increased the knowledge about the importance of exercising, eating properly and living healthier in youth, adult, and elderly populations.

Unfortunately, knowledge about the importance of exercise and how to exercise properly has not been enough to keep most people physically active and exercising for long periods of time. Over the years, research has discovered that only 20% of the North American population exercises enough to achieve cardiovascular benefits. Approximately 40% are active to a lesser degree, with some receiving health-related benefits, and at least 40% are completely sedentary. Further research has demonstrated that over half the population in North America who begin an exercise program quit within the first six months (Wankel, 1987). More recently, the U.S. Department of Health and Human Services (USDHHS) reported that only one of the 13 physical activity and fitness objectives proposed by the federal government's Healthy People 2000 document was actually met (USDHHS, 2004).

THE QUESTION IS WHY?

Why is that most people know how to live healthy and for the most part be more physically active and eat right, yet choose not to. Although at one time it was thought that a lack of activity was due to a complete lack of motivation, today researchers have discovered a variety of reasons, referred to as "barriers," that interfere with the motivation to become more physically active and exercise on a regular basis. In this chapter, you will identify the barriers that stop you from being more physically active and discover what motivates you to become more physically active and fit. So let's get started.

WHAT'S STOPPING YOU?

If you want to be more physically active, fit and live a healthier lifestyle than you currently are and you are not doing it now then clearly something is stopping you. In order to get started exercising again, you must first examine what is stopping you. Take a few moments and answer the following questions:

1. When was the last time you were physically active?
2. How long did you keep it up for (days, weeks, months)?
3. When did you stop?
4. Why do you think you stopped?

If you are like most people, your answer(s) to question 4 will probably parallel at least one or more of these 8 common reasons: (1) I don't have time; (2) I don't enjoy it; (3) I don't get the results I wanted; (4) I don't have a good place to exercise; (5) I don't have anyone to show me how to exercise correctly; (6) I don't reach my own goals; (7) I injured myself and just never got back to it; (8) My significant others do not support my efforts to exercise.

While many individuals are confronted with these exercise barriers, only about 20% have been able to overcome them and stay physically active for a lifetime. The rest of the population gets stopped and allow these barriers to take control of your lives.

Everyone who is involved in exercise at any capacity, whether it is contemplating when to start exercising or deciding what exercises to do, how long to do it for, what time of the day works best, where to exercise or whom to exercise with has been confronted with barriers that could stop them from exercising. Imagine for a moment if you actually knew what might stop you from exercising before you actually quit. Now imagine if you had access to strategies that could remove these barriers and teach you how to fit exercise into your life without stopping. Well, don't fret—by the time you complete this book, you will be there—exercising on a regular basis and loving every minute of it. So let's find out what may be stopping you.

IDENTIFYING YOUR EXERCISE BARRIERS

No time—This is the most popular reason people give for not exercising (Lox, Martin Ginis, & Petruzzello, 2006; Gettman, Pollock, & Ward, 1983). While phrases like "I would if I had the time" or "I'm so busy" imply that you would exercise if only the time was right or there was more time in the day, this is really more of a perception than a reality (Willis & Campbell, 1992). In fact, if you take a closer look into your daily schedule, how much time do you make to watch television, talk on the phone, text your friends, play video games, read the newspaper, e-mail and surf the web? If you have time for any of that, then you certainly have time to exercise. The question becomes not whether or not you have time to exercise, but do you really want to make the time to exercise?

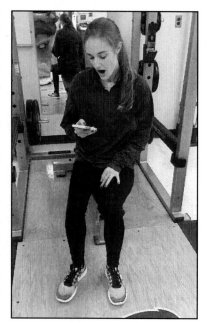

Ironically, research has shown that people who exercise regularly accomplish more in their day than people who don't (Thayer, 2001; Shaw, Bonen, & McAbe, 1991). Now take a few moments and think about a time in your life when you exercised regularly and compare it with a time that you were less physically active. Do you notice a difference in the amount of energy that you had? What about your productivity at school or work? Did you feel more energetic and productive because you chose not to exercise or because you did exercise? Did you ever not have the time to do what you wanted because of exercising?

If you are like most people then you probably noticed you felt more invigorated and full of energy after exercising and tired and lethargic during the times in your life that you weren't exercising. Scientists have explained that when we exercise, our endorphins (which are a morphine-like substance) are released from the pituitary gland in the brain and induce feelings of euphoria and well-being. This gives you more energy to be productive and accomplish more in a day than if you didn't exercise.

Once you choose to make exercise a priority in your life, you will find the time. Oh sure, sometimes you may have to modify your exercise schedule, but you will inevitably find the time for the things that provide you the most benefits (e.g. better health, more energy, greater productivity at work and school, having fun, happier moods, less stress) that lead to a higher quality of life.

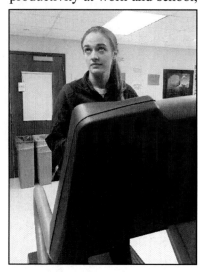

So the next time you tell yourself that you can't exercise because you don't have the time—think again. Do you really not have the time or do you not want to make the time? Remember, there are 1440 minutes in every day and all you need is about 2% (20-30 minutes) of that each to reap the wealth of benefits associated with exercising and living healthy.

No fun—Another popular reason people give for not exercising is that it is "no fun." To put it simply, if you don't enjoy exercising, then why would you want to find the time to do it? While many people give reasons to exercise such as: "I want to lose weight"; "I want to tone my muscles"; or "My doctor said I had to" the bottom line is if you're not having fun exercising, you're not going to do it over the long term (Franklin, 1986; Emmons & Diener, 1986). You may make the initial effort to get started, but before long, you will start focusing on all the reasons not to exercise. Later in the book, you will identify the things in your life that you perceive to be fun and then learn how to incorporate these activities into your exercise routine.

Lack of results—If you start working out and don't achieve the results that you are seeking, you are probably going to quit exercising. After all, why put in "hard time" if you are not getting what you want out of it. Problems such as setting unrealistic goals (e.g., lose 10 lbs in the next two weeks), being misinformed by exercise infomercials (e.g., turn fat into muscle), overemphasizing physiological factors (e.g., washboard abs; increasing muscular size in a few short workouts) and exercising improperly are just a few of the reasons why people sense a lack of accomplishment, become impatient and look to quit exercising. Unfortunately, nothing that you truly have a passion to achieve is possible without hard work and dedication. So before you start your workout, you should make sure that the results you want are challenging, realistic and 100% within your control. (Chapter 3 entitled "BE SMAART" helps you set important goals that are focused on getting the results that you want both in the short and long term).

Inconvenient Location/Convenience—Having to travel far distances, inaccessible transportation, lack of facilities, and poor or lack of equipment are just a few of the more popular reasons why people fail to engage in regular physical activity (Lox, Martin-Gillis, & Petruzzello, 2006). Research has demonstrated that proximity and convenience to the exercise facility were two of the most important factors in exercise participation for both corporate and community exercise programs (Teraslinna, Partanen, Koskela, & Oja, 1969; Cox, 1984; Goodrick, Hartung, Warren, & Hoepfel, 1984). In fact, the easier the facility is to get to, the better your chances of using it. So for those of you who have extra space in your house, why not see about getting some exercise equipment. For those of you who work in large corporations, consider asking your boss about having an exercise facility in or near the office. Research has found that effectively run corporate fitness programs have increased employee productivity, improved efficiency, concentration, creativity, and decision making time, increased morale, reduced mental errors and worker absenteeism, decreased health care, disability, and worker compensation costs, and reduced employee turnover (Genesis Personal fitness: Your 1st step is to begin http://www.genesispersonal/fitness.com/CorporateFitness.htm) Just tell your boss that a fit worker is a more productive worker. Finally, for those of you in college, how about taking an activity class and/or using the campus recreational or fitness facilities.

Poor exercise leader—Perhaps the most important determinant of an individual's continued participation in an exercise program is the quality of leadership (Franklin, 1988, Weinberg & Gould, 2007). A good exercise leader is someone who has a positive influence on exercisers and can contribute to increases in their fitness, self-efficacy, enjoyment, and motivation to exercise. A good exercise leader should be energetic and enthusiastic and be able to identify and meet the needs of their exercisers. He/she should have a formal education in the exercise sciences (e.g., exercise physiology, exercise psychology, health-related fitness, counseling, personal training) and have expertise in creating a safe exercise environment, developing proper exercise prescriptions and motivating clients to exercise on their own. In contrast, the poor exercise leader is someone who can have a negative social influence on exercisers and may ultimately cause them to drop out of a fitness program (Lox, Martin-Ginis, & Petruzzello, 2006; Bray, Gyurcsik,, Culos-Reed, Dawson, & Martin, 2001). He/she often uses criticism and blame rather than praise and encouragement and does not individualize instruction or interact positively with participants (Fox, Rejeski, & Gauvin, 2000).

Today, many exercise facilities are hiring individuals without the appropriate education. In some cases, people who call themselves certified personal trainers have no college education, no internship experience, and in fact, have only taken a written exam to become a "certified" personal trainer. Unfortunately, "certified" does not always mean "qualified." Ask yourself how someone with so little training can help a client who has arthritis, osteoporosis, a heart condition, low self-esteem, poor time management skills or a general lack of motivation to exercise. Some of the managers of exercise facilities who hire these people are only interested in gaining more memberships each year and care little about the people who are signed up and have stopped coming. When was the last time you received a call from the gym inquiring why you haven't been attending in a while?

Setting unrealistic goals—When beginning an exercise program, people sometimes set goals that are unrealistic and difficult, if not impossible to achieve (e.g., losing 10 lbs in the next week; turning fat into muscle; going from 0 days of exercise per week to 5). Many times, individuals look to change their entire lives around to fit exercise in rather than learning how to fit exercise into their lives the way it presently exists. Unfortunately, this does not work for very long. When the goals are not met, exercise is often stopped, thus forgoing all of the other important health benefits that might have been gained from exercise. In fact, after a short while you probably realized that this new change in your schedule (e.g., getting up early to exercise; going to the gym right after work), while commendable in its intentions, simply did not fit into your lifestyle. You wind up missing a few scheduled workouts and before you know it, you are back to where you started—not exercising at all. In order to have goals that work, you must set goals that are within your reach. They must be challenging, yet attainable. They must be measurable and modifiable, so that the focus of your workout centers on strategies and effort to reach these desired goals. Most important, they must excite you to get started exercising and motivate you to continue in the long-term. (In chapter 3, you will become SMAART and learn more about how to set goals that work for you).

Injury—A major cause of inactivity is injury. Clearly, exercise should be avoided when an injured body part is required for activity in order to allow time to heal. However, once the individual has been given a clean bill of health to begin exercising, that does not mean he/she is ready to start exercising again especially when the focus may be on the amount of fitness lost rather than being able to getting started again. Here's an example of how an injury temporarily stopped Lincoln from exercising and how he got back into his regular exercise routine.

Several years ago Lincoln, a regular exerciser since high school, needed to have surgery. He spent two weeks in the hospital and his doctor told him that he couldn't exercise for 8-10 weeks. After the recuperation period was over, he got approval to start slowly, so he decided to go for a "little walk." Having always been used to running at least 3-5 miles, Lincoln thought the walk would be a breeze. Well, it wasn't. It took Lincoln 20 minutes to walk about a mile and when he finished his heart rate was sky high and he became depressed. Even though his physical injuries had healed, Lincoln was upset that his fitness level had dropped so low. Consequently, Lincoln considered stopping exercise altogether, but deep down he knew that exercise was the best thing for him and so he decided to continue and just start slowly by combining walking with jogging and eventually running. For the first time in Lincoln's life, exercise was not a self-induced competition. Instead, it became fun. Rather than compare how fit he used to be prior to his injury, Lincoln was just happy to be exercising pain free. He began to set goals for himself to improve his present level of fitness (e.g., jogging 1-2 minutes longer each week; adding a day to his exercise routine). After six months of physical activity and exercise, Lincoln accomplished more than he ever could have imagined. Not only did he make significant improvements in his fitness, he was also enjoying and looking forward to exercising on a regular basis. (In Chapters' 6-8 you will learn how to develop health-related fitness programs that address you physical as well as your mental and emotional needs).

Lack of support from significant other—How would you feel if you started to exercise and began to look and feel better and nobody in your life noticed? Whether you choose to exercise alone or with a partner, it is so important to have support from a significant other, someone with whom you can share the experience of exercise and the benefits that have been gained from being more physically active. When you don't get that support, it can decrease your level of motivation to exercise and make you want to quit. In fact, research has consistently demonstrated that getting support from spouses, parents and significant others increased physical activity and exercise compliance rates for a variety of populations including mothers with young children (Miller, Trost, & Brown, 2002), cardiac rehabilitation patients (Erling & Oldridge, 1985) and children participating in competitive and recreational sports, structured exercise, and active leisure (USDHHS, 1996). Once you identify what support you need, you can then identify the people in your life that can provide you with this type of support (e.g., parents, spouses, friends, teachers) and thus enhance your overall exercise experience.

Boring—One of the drawbacks of exercise is that it can be boring. Whether it's sitting on the exercise bike for 30 minutes or doing the same exercises over and over again, exercise can seem a bit monotonous and boring. When you focus on how boring the exercise is, chances are you will lose the motivation to continue. However, there are many strategies that can be incorporated to not only decrease boredom, but to make exercise fun and exciting for you. Chapters' 3 (goal setting) and 11 (cognitive strategies), are specifically designed to teach you how to have fun while exercising. I bet you can't wait!

In conclusion, there are a variety of barriers that stop people from starting and or continuing to exercise on a life time basis. The first step in transforming exercise from something you know you should or have to do to something that you genuinely want to do is to identify the barriers that stop you. Once you have completed this, then it is on to Chapter 2 where you will identify your motives for getting stated and hopefully continue exercise "now and forever." Catchy phrase—don't you think?

REVIEW QUESTIONS

1. List at least five possible reasons for not exercising.

2. Which of the reasons you listed above have you used for not exercising?

3. Is finding time really a problem for you with exercising? If so, explain why?

4. Explain why exercise may be perceived as "NO FUN."

5. Why do you think some people do not get the results they want from exercising?

6. List two strategies that you can use to make your location to exercise more convenient.

7. If you were the owner of an exercise facility, what requirements would you have for your exercise leaders and why?

8. Explain why setting unrealistic exercise goals can decrease your desire to exercise on a regular basis.

LAB ASSIGNMENT 1.1

Are You Motivated To Exercise This Week?

1. How motivated are you to exercise this week?

1	2	3	4	5	6	7	8	9
not motivated							highly motivated	

2. Are you actually planning to exercise this week? If you answer "Yes" then move on to answer questions 3-6. If you answer "NO", then skip questions 3-6 and answer questions 7-13.

If "YES":

3. What exercises do you plan to do? _____

4. When do you plan to exercise? _____

5. Where do you plan to exercise? _____

6. For how long will you exercise? _____

If "NO":

7. Why have you decided that you will not exercise this week?

8. List all of the things that are stopping you from exercising this week.

9. List all of the reasons why you should not exercise this week.

10. List all of the reasons why you think you should exercise this week.

11. What can you do to motivate yourself to exercise at least one time this week?

12. Has your level of motivation to exercise increased? Please explain.

13. Do you still plan on not exercising this week?

At the end of the week, please answer the following:

14. For those who intended to exercise this week and did not, please answer the following:

    A. What really stopped you from exercising?

    B. What have you learned from this experience?

    C Do you plan on exercising next week?

    D. If yes, list what you plan to do.

    E. What are the chances that you follow your plan to exercise this week?

0%	10%	20%	30%	40%	50%	60%	70%	80%	90%	100%
No										Very strong
Chance										chance

    F. What are the chances you will not exercise this week?

0%	10%	20%	30%	40%	50%	60%	70%	80%	90%	100%
No										Very strong
Chance										chance

    G. List all of the possible barriers that might stop you from exercising next week.

    H. Take a few minutes to think about the possible solutions to overcome your exercise barriers and jot them down below.

    I. How confident are you that you will incorporate the solutions to your barriers in the upcoming weeks?

1	2	3	4	5	6	7	8	9
not							extremely	
confident							confident	

LAB ASSIGNMENT 1.2
(FOR EXERCISE SCIENCE MAJORS)

Applying Your Expertise

As a result of your background in exercise, you have been hired by a corporate exercise company to decrease the rate of exercise dropout in local exercise facilities.

1. Discuss five possible reasons why people drop out of exercise programs.

2. For each reason listed above, explain a strategy that can be incorporated to decrease exercise dropout and increase exercise compliance and adherence.

3. As an exercise specialist, describe at least three things that you would do to make sure you have met your clients' needs?

REFERENCES AND RECOMMENDED READINGS

Bray, S.R., Gyurcsik, N.C., Culos-Ree, S.N., Dawson, K.A., & Martin, K.A. (2001). An exploratory investigation of the relationship between proxy efficacy, self-efficacy and exercise attendance. *Journal of Health Psychology, 6,* 425-434.

Cox, M.H. (1984). Fitness and life-style programs for business and industry: Problems in recruitment and retention. *Journal of Cardiac Rehabilitation, 4,* 136-142.

Erling, J., & Oldridge, N.B. (1985). Effect of a spousal-support program on compliance with cardiac rehabilitation. *Medicine and Science in Sport and Exercise, 17,* 284.

Emmons, R. A., & Diener, E. (1986). A goal-affect analysis of everyday situational choices. *Journal of Research in Personality, 20,* 309-326.

Fox, L.D., Rejeski, W.J., & Gauvin, L. (2000). Effects of leadership style and group dynamics on enjoyment of physical activity. *American Journal of Health Promotion, 14,* 277-283.

Franklin, B.A. (1988). Program factors that influence exercise adherence: Practical adherence skills for the clinical staff. In R.K. Dishman (Ed.), *Exercise adherence: Its impact on public health* (pp. 237-258). Champaign, IL: Human Kinetics.

Franklin, B.A. (1986). Clinical components of a successful adult fitness program. *American Journal of Health Promotion. 1(1), 6-13.*

Frierman, S. (2005). What's stopping us?: The role of higher education in increasing lifetime physical activity. Presented at the 2005 NAKPEHE conference, Tucson, AZ.

Genesis Personal fitness (2006): Your 1st step is to begin http://www.genesispersonal/fitness. com/CorporateFitness.htm

Gettman, L.R., Pollock, M.L., & Ward, A. (1983). Adherence to unsupervised exercise. *The Physician and Sportsmedicine*, 11 (10), 56-66.

Goodrick, G.K., Hartung, G.H., Warren, D.R., & Hoepfel, J.A. (1984). Helping adults to stay physically fit: Preventing relapse following aerobic exercise training. *Journal of Physical Education, Recreation, and Dance, 55,(2), 48-49*

Lox, C.L., Martin Ginis, K.L., & Petruzzello, S.P. (2006). *The psychology of exercise: Integrating theory into practice*, 2nd edition , *10-11*. Holcomb Hathaway, Publishers, Inc.

Miller, Y.D., Trost, S.G., & Brown, W.J. (2002). Mediators of physical activity behavior change among women with young children. *American Journal of Preventative Medicine, 23 (2 Suppl), 98-103*

Shaw, S.M., Bonen, A., & McCabe, J.F. (1991). Do more constraints mean less leisure? Examining the relationship between constraints and participation. *Journal of Leisure Research, 23, 286-300.*

Teraslinna, P., Partanen, T., Koskela, A., & Oja, P. (1969). Characteristics affecting willingness of executives to participate in an activity program aimed at coronary heart disease prevention. *Journal of Sports Medicine and Physical Fitness*, 17, 224-229.

Thayer, R. E. (2001). *Calm energy: How people regulate mood with food and exercise.* New York: Oxford University Press

U.S. Department of Health and Human Services, (1996). *Physical activity and health: A report of the Surgeon General.* McLean, VA: International Medical Publishing.

Wankel, L. (1987). Enhancing motivation for involvement in voluntary exercise programs. in M.L. Maehr (Ed.),, *Advances in motivation and achievement: Enhancing motivation* (Vol. 5, 239-286). Greenwich, CT: JAI Press.

Weinberg, R. & Gould, D. (2005). Exercise behavior and adherence. *In Foundations of sport and exercise psychology (3rd edition,* 400-410. Human Kinetics: Champaign, Il.

Willis, J. & Campbell, L.F. (1992). Why people exercise: Motives for fitness. *In Exercise psychology pp. 3-7, 15-16.* Human Kinetics: Champaign, Il.

U.S. Department of Health and Human Services (2004). Healthy People 2010, Washington, D.C. U.S. Government Printing Office.

Chapter 2

Getting Started: What's My Motive?

In this chapter you will:

- Learn the variety of motives individuals have for exercising
- Determine what really motivates you to be more physically active and fit
- Get prepared to exercise

WHAT'S YOUR MOTIVE?

If you are like most people, you start to exercise, then stop, then start and stop again. It's a vicious cycle. In chapter 1, you identified what stops you from exercising and being more physically active. In this chapter, you will examine the various motives individuals have for wanting to exercise. Once you understand what motivates you to exercise and be more physically active, you can structure your workouts to meet your motives and enjoy exercising more.

In 1968, Gerald Kenyon developed a theoretical model that explained six motives people have for being more physically active (Kenyon, 1968a; Kenyon, 19868b). While other theories and models, like Health Belief Model and Social Cognitive Theory, have been more recently developed to explain what motivates people to be more physically active, it is Kenyon's work that serves as the foundation for much of what is presently used today both in theoretical development as well as practical application. Below are Kenyon's six categories of motives individuals have to be physical active and fit. Hopefully, one or more of these describes your motives for wanting to exercise. If so, then all you have to do is use exercise as the vehicle to help you satisfy these motives.

1. ***Physical Activity for Physical Fitness***—This motive focuses on being physically fit and improving the physical features of your body (e.g., toning and defining your muscles; losing weight, etc).

2. ***Physical Activity/Exercise to Experience Vertigo***—Vertigo involves the participation of risky and dangerous activities usually derived from speed or acceleration. Activities in this category include sky diving, skiing, mountain climbing, snow-boarding, kayaking, etc…

3. ***Physical Activity as a Social Experience***—This motive emphasizes the need to meet other people. Many people choose to
   exercise as a way of meeting individuals with similar interests or
   enhancing the quality of already existing relationships. Today,
   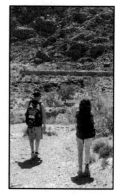
   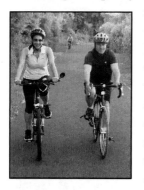
   many exercise facilities offer a variety of
   classes based on age, gender, fitness
   levels or other similarities (e.g., senior
   citizens; mothers-to-be, cyclists) hoping
   to motivate people to rely on each other
   and to want to work out together (e.g.,
   calling each other to set up a workout
   schedule; carpooling to the local exercise facility; signing up
   to take the same exercise class; encouraging and supporting
   each other).

4. ***Physical Activity/Exercise as Catharsis***—An important benefit
   of regular exercise is its ability to relieve stress and tension in
   your life. Since exercise forces you to concentrate on factors
   unrelated to your stress and tension in life (e.g., how your body
   feels, your heart rate and breathing, muscular tension, form), you
   become distracted from your stressors, and replace your
   negative emotions with positive energy.

5. ***Physical Activity/Exercise as an Aesthetic Experience***—This motive relates to physical activity and exercise as a form of art and an opportunity for individuals to express
   their beauty, grace, and symmetry through structured move-
   ment patterns (e.g., aerobic dance, synchronized swimming,
   gymnastics, yoga, ballet, cardio kickboxing, martial arts).
   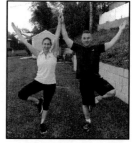

6. ***Physical Activity/Exercise as an Ascetic Experience***—Exercise is viewed as a means to be challenged through intense,
   vigorous training in order to accomplish important personal
   goals (e.g., running a marathon, climbing a mountain, learning
   how to swim in deep water).

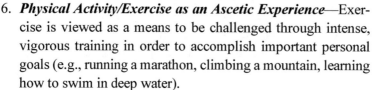

While Kenyon's motives have been and remain popular catalysts of individuals getting
started exercising, research has discovered that there are several other motives that people seek
to achieve through exercise. The first of these motives is for ***lifelong health***. Specifically, as
people get older, they sometimes realize they have not been living their lives in a healthy
manner and thus have increased their risks for lifestyle illness and disease (e.g., heart disease,
cancer, stroke, diabetes). Sometimes this ignites a wake-up call to start taking care of one's
health by exercising.

Another motive to be physically active and exercise is for ***psychological well-being***. When people exercise, they often feel good about themselves for the efforts expended as well as the outcome achieved. In fact, research has found that exercise has been related to positive mood states with individuals expressing an increase in positive mood states (happiness, vigor, self-esteem) and a decrease in negative mood states (anxiety, tension, depression) as a result of participating in a variety of different physical activities (walking, jogging, aerobic dance, weightlifting, yoga, swimming). Moreover, exercise is now being prescribed to treat and prevent individuals diagnosed with both acute and chronic mental and emotional disorders (depression, anxiety) as well as to improve positive mood states (happiness, vigor).

One final motive to exercise is *competition*. Many people thrive on competing vs. others and use exercise as a means to fulfill their need to compete by exercising with a partner and challenging each other to get to the next level by participating in exercise competitions (e.g., running races, weight lifting events, dance contest), taking exercise classes and competing for most improved or most fit, and hiring personal trainers to design exercise programs in order to achieve a level of fitness that has never been reached before.

So which one(s) of these motives work for you? Discovering what motivates you to want to exercise is an important first step in beginning an exercise program. It will help you to structure your program around your motives, thus increasing your exercise enjoyment and adherence in the long-term.

Now it is time to move on to Lab Assignment 2.1 which will help you to: (1) determine how motivated you are to start exercising this week; (2) identify any possible barriers that may stop you from exercising; and (3) help you to incorporate strategies to overcome these potential barriers. After that, it is on to Chapter 3, where you will learn how to set "SMAART' goals that are designed to increase your motivation and commitment to exercise as well as your overall level of fitness.

REVIEW QUESTIONS

1. List Kenyon's six motives to be physically active and provide an example of each.

2. Explain what you can do to achieve each of Kenyon's motives by exercising.

3. How can you use exercise as a means to fulfill the motive to live a healthy lifestyle?

4. What psychological benefits can be derived from being physically active and exercise?

5. Explain the motive to exercise for competition.

LAB ASSIGNMENT 2.1

1. Circle the motive(s) that you interest you the most your to be physically active and exercise this week, over the next month and for the next year.

Physical Fitness	Catharsis	Health
Vertigo	Aesthetic Experience	Psychological Benefits
Social Experience	Ascetic Experience	Competition

2. List and explain the actions you will take that will help you achieve your exercise motives.

3. Identify any barriers that may stop you from achieving your exercise motives this week, over the next month and for the next year.

4. What strategies can you use to overcome your exercise barriers this week, over the next month and for the next year?

After the week has been completed, answer the following questions:

5. Did you achieve your motive(s)?

   YES   NO

6. Explain why or why not.

7. How did it feel to exercise with a specific motive in mind?

8. Explain the actions you plan to take to fulfill your motives to exercise next week.

REFERENCES AND RECOMMENDED READINGS

Berger, B.G. (1996). Psychological benefits of an active lifestyle: What we know and what we need to know. *Quest, 48,* 330-353.

Berger, B.G. & Motl, R. (2001). Physical activity and quality of life. In R. Singer, H. Hausenblas, & C. Janelle, (Eds.), *Handbook of sport psychology*, (2nd edition., pp. 636-670). New York: Wiley.

Buckworth, J. & Dishman, R.K. (2002). Affect, mood, and emotion. In Exercise Psychology, pp 91-92, Human Kinetics, Champaign, IL

Dishman, R.K., Washburn, R.A., & Heath, G.W. (2004). *Physical activity epidemiology.* Champaign, IL, Human Kinetics.

Kenyon, G.S. (1968a). Conceptual model for characterizing physical activity. *Research Quarterly, 39*, 96-105.

Kenyon, G.S. (1988b). Six scales for assessing attitude toward physical activity. *Research Quarterly, 39*, 566-574.

National Heart, Lung, and Blood Institute. National Heart, Lung, and Blood Institute Report of the Task Force on Behavioral Research in Cardiovascular, Lung, and Blood Health and Disease. Bethesda, MD: Public Health Service, US Department of Health and Human Services; February, 1998.

Statistics Canada (2005). *Physical activity by age group and sex* (CANSIM, Catalogue No. 82-221-X). Ottawa, ON: Statistics Canada. Retrieved from http://www40.statscanca/101/cst01/health46.htm?sdi=physical%20activity

Stephens, T., Jacobs, D.R., & White, C.C. (1985). A descriptive epidemiology of leisure-time activity. *Public Health Reports*, 100 (2), 147-158.

Teraslinna, P., Partanen, T., Koskela, A., & Oja, P. (1969). Characteristics affecting willingness of executives to participate in an activity program aimed at coronary heart disease prevention. *Journal of Sports Medicine and Physical Fitness*, 17, 224-229.

Thayer, R.E. (2001). *Calm energy: How people regulate mood with food and exercise.* New York: Oxford University Press.

U.S. Department of Health and Human Services (2000). Healthy people 2010: Volume II, 2nd ed. Retrieved from http://www.healthypeople.gov/Document/html/uih_4.htm$physactiv.

U.S. Department of Health and Human Services (2004). Healthy People 2010, Washington, D.C. U.S. Government Printing Office.

Wankel, L.M. (1988). Exercise adherence and leisure activity: Patterns of involvement and interventions to facilitate regular activity. In R. Dishman (Ed.), Exercise adherence: Its impact on public health (pp.369-396). Champaign, IL: Human Kinetics Books.

Weinberg, R. & Gould, D. (2007). Exercise and psychological well-being. In *Foundations of sport and exercise psychology,* 4th edition, pps. 398-413. Human Kinetics: Champaign, Il.

Weinberg, R., & Gould, D. (2007). Exercise behavior and adherence. In *Foundations of sport and Exercise psychology* (4th edition, 431-433 Human Kinetics: Champaign, IL.

Willis, J.D. & Campbell, L.F. (1992). Why people exercise: Motives for Fitness. In *Exercise Psychology*, pps. 4-17, Human Kinetics: Champaign, IL.

Chapter 3

Setting Goals: "Be SMAART"

In this chapter, you will:

- learn what SMAART goals are and how to use them in your exercise program
- create staircase goals that help increase your short-term and long-term motivation to achieve success
- identify barriers that stop you from reaching your goals
- develop strategies to overcome goal setting barriers in order to increase your exercise motivation and performance

When you begin to exercise program, you usually have certain goals in mind. These goals can be the driving force towards increasing your motivation and commitment to exercise and improve your present level of fitness. It is important to note, however, that not all goals are equally effective. For example, if you set goals that are too easy and can be achieved without much effort (e.g., exercise once this month or take a two-minute walk once this week), then you are not going to see any positive results and quite possibly think that exercise is not working for you. Conversely, if you set goals that are too difficult or unrealistic, (e.g., run a marathon after a few weeks of training; increase exercise from one to five days per week over the next two weeks; lose ten pounds in a week), you may become frustrated when your goals are not achieved right away and then lose your motivation to continue exercising in the long-term. Finally, if you set goals that are too vague, (e.g., I want to get fit), the information you receive from your workouts may not be conclusive enough to determine whether or not you reached your goal. Thus, the problem is not so much getting people to set goals. It is getting them to set the right kind of goals-ones that provide direction and enhance motivation—and help people to learn to stick to and achieve their goals (Weinberg & Gould, 2006). This chapter introduces you to one of the most effective ways to establish and maintain high levels of motivation while exercising. Learn how to set goals that work for you rather than against you. The only criterion you need is to "Be SMAART."

SMAART GOALS

SMAART stands for: Specific, Measurable, Adjustable, Action-Oriented Realistic, and Time framed. Setting SMAART goals enables you to identify exactly what you want to accomplish, determine how close you are towards reaching your goal(s), decide whether or not you need to modify or change your goal, and identify exactly how long you think it will take to achieve your goal. Most important, the goals you set are completely within your control. Below are the definitions of each of the six components of the SMAART principle, along with examples of how to use SMAART goals to improve health-related fitness. In Chapters 6-9, you will learn how to use SMAART goals when designing your exercise programs for cardiorespiratory endurance, muscular fitness, flexibility, and eating healthy.

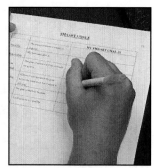

Specific—Specific goals are goals that state what you want to accomplish. Goals like losing weight, improving cardiorespiratory fitness (CRF) or getting stronger are all examples of specific goals because they state what you want to accomplish. Over the years, research has indicated that setting specific goals was more effective in increasing performance than setting no goals, vague goals or do-your-best-goals (Frierman, 1995; Gould, 2006; Hall, Weinberg, & Jackson, 1987; Weinberg, Bruya, Longino, & Jackson; Weinberg & Gould, 2003).

Measurable—In order for a goal to work, it must be measurable and put in numerical form. This way you know exactly how far along you are towards reaching what you want to accomplish. Although goals like getting fit and toning up specifically address why you decide to exercise, they are hard to measure since one day you may feel fit and toned and the very next day you may think you are not. Moreover, there is no way to measure tone. However, once you put your goal into numerical form, you can measure its effectiveness. For example, instead of saying that you want to tone up, set a goal for the number of abdominal reps you want to accomplish in today's workout (50) or the number of minutes you will run (25) without stopping. By setting measurable goals you will always be able to determine exactly how much you are progressing from one workout to the next. Most important, reaching these numerical goals will inevitably increase your motivation to continue exercising and make you feel better about yourself, too.

Adjustable—Setting a goal doesn't guarantee that you will reach it. For instance, if you set a goal to exercise three times in a week and you have taken the first five days off, you are not going to reach your goal. However, adjusting the goal (e.g., exercise one time in the next two days) allows you to stay on task and concentrate on accomplishing something worthwhile. Then when the week is over, you can focus on what you accomplished, exercising one time in the last two days, rather than on why you did not reach your original goal (taking six out of seven days off in the week).

Action-Oriented—To advance your goal(s) from actual words to accomplishment, you have to put it into action. In other words, once you set your goal, you should have a clear-cut plan of action that you will incorporate to help you reach your desired goal(s). For example, if you want to improve your muscular fitness, an action plan to help you reach you goal could be to go the gym three times per week and work two body parts per workout. If your goal is to eat healthier, then your action plan could be to replace fried food with grilled or baked foods, eat fruit instead of candy, and drink water instead of soda. If your goal is to become more aerobically fit, your action plan could be to jog three times per week at a particular time (for example 5:00 to 5:30 PM) at your local gym or school exercise facility. By creating an action plan you take the goal from mere thoughts to actions.

Realistic—In order for a goal to work, it must be realistic and within your reach of accomplishing. The best way to set realistic goals is to first identify your present level of fitness and put that into numerical terms. For instance, how many minutes can you exercise continuously? How long can you hold a stretch for? How many sets and repetitions can you do in a muscular fitness workout? How many days will you exercise in a week? Once you answer these questions, then you can set a goal that is slightly more challenging than what you currently do. For example, if you exercise 10 minutes without stopping, set a goal to do 11-12 minutes in your next workout. If you worked out two times this week, set a goal to go three times next week. If you held a stretch for five seconds, set a goal to hold for six or seven seconds. Finally, if you did 6 sets of muscular fitness exercises last week, then set a goal to accomplish 7 or 8 sets this week..

Time Frame—Time frame is the amount of time you give yourself to reach your goal(s). In order for a goal to motivate you on a day-to-day basis, you must select a time frame that boxes you in and directs your energy and attention to get started right away and work hard towards reaching your goal. For example, if your goal is to start exercising four times per week, and you give yourself ten years to reach your goal, the chances that you are going to get started exercising immediately are rather low. However, if you set a goal to exercise four times per week by the end of the month, you are immediately called into action. Each week you will have to decide the days and times that you will allocate for exercise. If you are progressing nicely (e.g., increasing frequency from two times to three times per week over the last two weeks), you will probably feel quite proud of yourself and have a high level of motivation to continue your quest towards reaching your goal of four times per week. However, if you are not progressing towards your goal (e.g., you went from three workouts in week two to two workouts in week three), you can immediately analyze what happened: Was it because you were lazy? Did you have a problem with time management? Once you find your answer, you can apply it to the next week and get right back into action (I will exercise on M, T, R, F from 4PM-5PM in the Fitness Center).

In addition to using SMAART goals, there are several other types of goals that you should consider when beginning an exercise program. Below is a description of the variety of goals that you can set which will enhance your motivation and commitment to exercise and improve your fitness, too.

Set short-term and long-term goals—*Short-terms* goals are goals that can be achieved within a short period of time usually ranging from one day to one or two weeks. They are designed to keep you focused on what you want to accomplish right away (e.g., today's work-out). Short-term goals provide instant feedback that assists you in determining your immediate level of progress. This regular progress check can help you to adjust your goals in the event that they become too easy or difficult. *Long-term goals* are more like dream goals. They define what you want to accomplish in the distant future and they provide the initial direction towards what you want to achieve, however, by, themselves they will not motivate you to exercise on a daily basis because they are too far in the future.

STAIRWAY TO SUCCESS

An effective way to understand the connection between short and long term-goals when starting an exercise program is to view them as a "***Stairway to Success***" (See Figure 3.1). The bottom of the stairs represents your baseline which is your present level of fitness and what you can do right now. The top of the stairs represents your long-term goal (what you want to accomplish in the distant future). Each step from the bottom up represents your short-term goals. When you achieve your first short-term goal, you then move to the next step up and set your next short-term goal and so on until you get to the top of the staircase and reach your long-term goal.

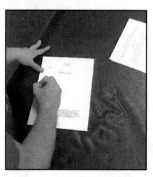

To get a clear picture of how to use the stairway to success, let's use "Archie" who has a long-term goal of running the marathon in 6 months and is presently running one mile without stopping. The bottom of the stairs represents the one mile that Archie can currently do (present level of fitness as of 1/15). The next step up is Archie's first short-term goal which is to be able to run two miles by 1/30. Each time Archie reaches his short-term goal, he moves one step up the stairway until he inevitably finds himself closer to his one-time long-term goal of running the marathon (top of the stairs) than to his original starting point of one mile. If at any time, Archie does not reach his short-term goal he can do the following: (1) give himself a little more time and set a new short-term target date; (2) put in another step in between the last goal he reached and the next goal he is striving to accomplish.

Set Positive Goals—Positive goals focus on what you want to accomplish rather than what you are trying to avoid. By setting positive goals (e.g., I want to exercise three times this week) rather than negative goals (e.g., I don't want to take more than two days off in a row), you will feel better about yourself and what you are striving to accomplish instead of what you don't want to occur.

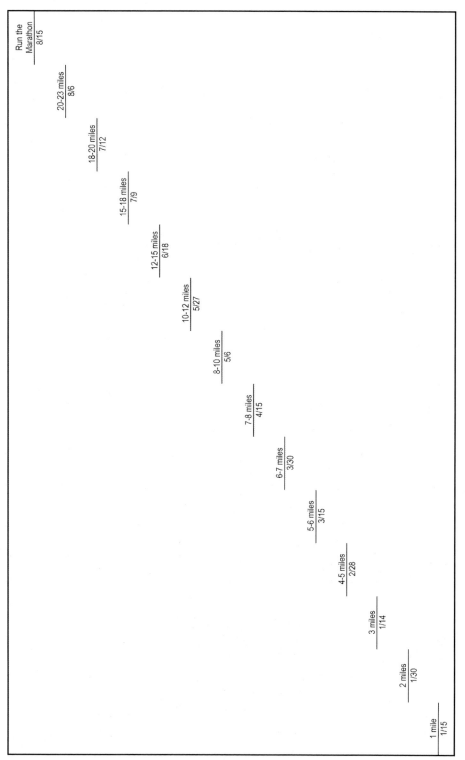

Figure 3.1—Archie's Stairway to Exercise Success

Once you have set your SMAART goals it is important that you **write them down** and keep them in a visible place (e.g., refrigerator door, car seat, desk, day planner, computer screensaver, cell phone. This will help you to keep your goals in mind and remind you on a daily basis exactly what you want to accomplish. (See Appendix 3A: Your Weekly Goal Sheet).

Have an Action Plan—An action plan consists of the strategies you create to reach your goals. For example, if you want to exercise three times this week, your action plan should consist of the days and times that you plan to exercise as well as the place where you would like to exercise. You may also include who you plan to exercise with as well as what exercise(s) you would like to do. This will help you to see how and where exercise fits into your daily life without having to make unrealistic changes. See Appendix 3B to use your action plan form to transform your goals from words into successful actions.

IDENTIFYING EXERCISE BARRIERS AND SOLUTIONS

Although goal setting can be a powerful motivational tool for exercising, simply setting a goal doesn't guarantee that you will reach it. Below are five common barriers that can stop you from reaching your exercise goals along with viable solutions to minimize or prevent these barriers from occurring.

Setting Too Many Goals—The more goals you set, the harder they are to achieve because it becomes more difficult to track the progress of each goal set and determine what strategies are working or not working for you. For example, say that you want to improve your health-related fitness and you set weekly goals to go to the gym 5×, complete 100 minutes of aerobic activity with 30 minutes of running, 40 minutes on the bike, 20 minutes on the elyptical and 10 minutes rowing. In addition, you want to do 20 sets of lifting and increase your weight 10% as well as stretch for 20 minutes combining both dynamic and static stretches into your routine. Finally, you want to eat healthier by adding fruits and drinking water to each meal and cutting out the candy and coffee you have grown accustomed to.

Solution: Set between one and two goals each week so you can stay focused on your goals and monitor your progress from one workout to the next, always knowing how much you need to do in order to reach your goal(s). So if you want to complete 100 minutes of aerobic activity, then just leave it at that. You do not need to set separate goals for each type of exercise that you plan to do in order to get to the 100 minutes.

Setting Outcome Goals—Outcome goals are goals that are based on winning or doing better than someone else. The focus centers more on comparing your performance to someone else's rather than improving. Moreover, outcome goals take the emphasis off your own individual accomplishment and on to how well you are doing compared to others (e.g., my goal is to stay on the bike longer than the person next to me). Consequently, you lose control over reaching your goal because no matter how much you may have improved from your previous workout, if your goal was to do better than someone else and you fail, then you don 't reach your goal and you wind up feeling frustrated and dissatisfied.

Solution: Set performance goals that focus on your own individual accomplishments. For example, set goals based on increasing time, distance, sets, reps, weights, days per week, etc. You can improve your most recent performance for what you have accomplished in your workouts with what you aspire to achieve in the next few workouts and set your goals based on that.

Setting Unrealistic Goals—Unrealistic goals occur when you strive to achieve something that is out of your control and/or not within your immediate reach. This is common when you take time off from exercise and then try to start where you left off without realizing that you have lost some of your fitness and can't perform at the level that you used to.

Solution: Set goals that are based on your present level of fitness and not on what you used to be able to do or what other people you know can or strive to accomplish. Your goals should be just one "step" above what you can already do. This will increase your desire to work hard since your goal is completely within your reach.

Failing to Modify Your Goal(s)—If you consistently fail to reach your goal(s) week after week, you need to assess what happened, otherwise you may begin to doubt your abilities to accomplish what you want and lose your motivation to exercise.

Solution: Modify your goal(s) so that they can be achieved. For example, if you set a goal to work on your flexibility for 20 minutes each of the last three weeks and the most you have accomplished has been 5 minutes then set a goal to do 6 minutes. In addition, incorporate a strategy for how you will increase your chances of reaching your goal (e.g., stretch before bed; stretch after lunch).

No Follow-Up and Evaluation—A big problem that many exercisers have is setting goals at the beginning of the week and then not using them in their workouts. As each day passes, the importance of the goals appears forgotten until the start of the new week when the individual realizes that he/she did not put his/her goals into action.

Solution: Develop a follow-up and evaluation plan and set up a time where you will examine it critically to determine the effectiveness of the goals you recently set. (Weinberg & Gould, 2003). This will help you to see if your goals motivated you to exercise, increased your performance, improved your self-efficacy and made exercise more fun for you.

In conclusion, goal setting is one of the most effective ways to increase your motivation to exercise. Setting "SMAART goals" allows you to identify exact what it is that you want to

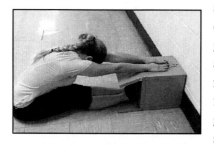

accomplish and then provide you with strategies that increase your chances for success. Setting stairway to success goals enables you to visualize your long-term dream goals and establish a clear pathway of success by focusing on reaching your short-term goals, one step at a time. Identifying your barriers that may stop you from reaching your goals can help you to create strategies that can develop and sustain high levels of motivation and keep you committed to being physically active and fit for a lifetime. So, just remember when it comes time for you to set your exercise goals, write them down and BE SMAART!

REVIEW QUESTIONS

1. What does SMAART stand for? Give an example for each of the six components of SMAART.

2. Explain the purpose(s) of setting Stairway to Success goals.

3. Describe the benefits of setting positive goals instead of negative goals.

4. What are the drawbacks of setting goals that are too easy or too hard?

5. Why is it important to have an action plan when setting exercise goals?

6. List and explain at least four barriers that can stop you from reaching your exercise goals.

7. What solutions can you employ to minimize and/or prevent the exercise barriers that you identified in question 6?

LAB ASSIGNMENT 3.1

1. List one to two SMAART goals that you would like to achieve over the next week and write them down in the space provided below.
   My exercise goal for this week is _____
   My exercise goal for this week is _____

2. For each goal listed above, develop your action plan for how you will reach your goal.
   Days of the week you plan to exercise _____
   Time of the day you plan to exercise _____
   Place where you plan to exercise_____
   What do you plan to do to reach your goal _____

3. Using your present level of fitness and recent exercise history (past 1-3 weeks), how realistic is/are the goal(s) that you have set for this week?

4. If you do not reach your goal(s) for this week, list the possible barriers that might stop you.
   A. _____
   B. _____
   C. _____
   D. _____

5. For each barrier listed above, create a solution that increases your chances of reaching your weekly exercise goals.

   A. _____

   B. _____

   C. _____

   D. _____

6. What were the numerical results of the goals that you set last week?

7. How did exercising with SMAART goals make you feel before, during and after your workouts?

8. What are your SMAART goals for next week?

LAB ASSIGNMENT 3.2

1. Using your "Stairway to Success" sheets located in Appendix 3C, select a long-term fitness goal that you would like to achieve over the next 10-20 weeks (Stairway 1) or 6 months (Stairway 2) and jot it down on the top of the stairway. Underneath your long-term goal, select the target date that you plan to reach your long-term goal by.

2. On the bottom step, write down your present level of fitness in numerical terminology and the actual date that you are starting to set your stairway goals.

3. Using the step just above the bottom, select your first short-term goal in numerical form and the date that you plan to be able to reach this goal by.

4. Each time you reach your short-term goal, continue to use the next step up the stairway and set your next short-term goal along with your target date which should be one to two weeks from the date you just reached your last short-term goal.

5. If you do not reach your short-term goal on the target date listed, you should select another short-term target date 1-7 days later than the original date listed. If you reach your goal by then, you should continue to climb up the stairway by setting another challenging short-term goal. Be sure to select a target date that is realistic to your present fitness accomplishments.

6. If you do not reach your goal by the second target date set, then you need to modify your goal by either adding a step in between your last goal reached and present goal not reached or crossing out the goal not reached and replacing it with a more realistic goal.

7. At the conclusion of the target date listed at the top of your stairway (10 weeks, 20 weeks, or six months, discuss the effects of using the stairway to success on the following:

    a. your motivation to exercise

    b. your level of confidence while exercising

    c. your level of enjoyment to exercise with stairway to success goals

    d. your level of effort and perseverance while exercising

    e. your ability to identify and handle exercise barriers

    f. your overall performance using the stairway to success

    g. if you plan to use stairway to success goals again; explain why or why not;

    h. who would you recommend stairway to success goals for and why?

REFERENCES AND RECOMMENDED READINGS

Frierman, S. (2001). Be SMART: How to use goal to succeed in fitness. Presented at the Nassau Zone AAHPERD, Hofstra University March 15, 2001.

Frierman, S. (1996). Going for Your Goal: How to motivate your players in the off-season. *American Football Quarterly, 2, 1,* 64-65.

Frierman, S. (1996). The importance of setting realistic goals. *American Football Quarterly Mind Zone Section, 2,* 3.

Frierman, S. (1995). The effect of individual, group, and competitive goals on muscular endurance performance. *Journal of Sport and Exercise Psychology,* 17, 51.

Frierman, S., Weinberg, R.S., & Jackson, A.J. (1990). The relationship between goal proximity and specificity in bowling: A field experiment. *The Sport Psychologist, 4,* 145-154

Gould, D. (2006). Goal setting for peak performance. In J.M. Williams, *Applied Sport Psychology: Personal Growth to Peak Performance,* 5th edition, McGraw-Hill.

Hall, H.K., Weinberg, R.S., & Jackson, A. (1987). Effects of goal specificity, goal difficulty, and information feedback on endurance performance. *Journal of Sport and Psychology,* 9, 43-54.

Kyllo, L.B., & Landers, D.M. (1995). Goal setting in sport and exercise: A research synthesis to resolve the controversy. *Journal of Sport and Exercise Psychology, 17,* 117-137.

Locke, E.A., & Latham, G.P. (1985). The application of goal setting to sports. *Journal of Sport Psychology, 7,* 205-222.

Locke, E.A., & Latham, G.P. (1990). *A theory of goal setting and task performance.* Prentice Hall, Englewood Cliffs, NJ.

Locke, E.A., Shaw, K.N., Saari, L.M., & Latham, G.P. (1981). Goal setting and task performance. *Psychological Bulletin, 90,* 125-152.

Weinberg, R.S., Bruya, L., Longino,, J., & Jackson, A. (1988). Effect of goal proximity and specificity on endurance performance of primary-grade children. *Journal of Sport and Psychology,* 10, 81-91.

Weinberg, R.S. & Gould, D. (2003). *Foundations of Sport and Exercise Psychology*, 3rd edition, pp. 330-348. Human Kinetics.

APPENDIX 3A
WEEKLY GOAL SHEET

Name _____   Date: _____

Below is a list of four categories that you can set your ***weekly*** goes in: (1) Cardiorespiratory Endurance; (2) Muscular Fitness; (3) Flexibility; and (4) Nutrition. Select 1-2 goals that represent the area(s) of fitness that you need to work on and are motivated to do so. Write down your goal(s) in the "Goal(s) Selected" column next to the category of goal that you have selected. Using the Seven-Day Chart below, record each day's workout next to the appropriate activity and under the actual day. After the week is up, add up your total workout performances and put them in the "Performance Results" column. If you achieved you weekly goal, mark an "A" across from your goal category in the "Achieved" column. If you did not reach your goal, mark an "NA" across from you goal category and under the "Not Achieved" column.

Category of Goals to Select From	Goal(s) Selected	Performance Results	Achieved = A	Not Achieved = NA
CRE Goals				
Frequency of Weekly Workouts				
Time in Minutes Exercised for Week				
Activity Selected				
Run/Walk				
Bicycle				
Elyptical				
Rowing				
Stairmaster				
Other				
Muscular Fitness Goals				
Frequency of Weekly Workouts				
Sets				
# of Exercises				
Increased Weight				
Flexibility Goals				
Frequency of Weekly Workouts				
Time in Minutes Exercised for Week				
# of Exercises Achieved				
Nutritional Goals for Week				
Fruits Consumed				
Vegetables Consumed				
Meals Planned				

	Day 1	Day 2	Day 3	Day 4	Day 5	Day 6	Day 7
CRE							
Run/Walk							
Bicycle							
Elyptical							
Rowing							
Stairmaster							
Other							
Muscular Fitness							
Sets							
Reps							
# of Exercises							
Increased Weight							
Flexibility							
Time							
Sets							
# of Exercises							
Nutrition							
Fruits Consumed							
Vegetables Consumed							
Meals Planned in Advance							

APPENDIX 3B
PLAN OF ACTION FORM

1. My goals for this week are:

   A. _____

   B. _____

2. In order to reach my goals, I will _____

   _____

   _____

3. I will exercise ___ times this week   1   2   3   4   5   6   7

4. I will exercise on the following days of the week: M   Tu   W   Th   F   Sat   Sun

5. For each of the day(s) I circled above, *I will exercise at the follow times and places*

DAYS	TIMES	PLACE
M		
T		
W		
R		
F		
Sa		
Su		

6. If I do not reach my goal(s) the barriers that will stop me are:

   a . _____

   b. _____

   c. _____

7. The strategies that I will use to stick to my goals and overcome my barriers are:

   a . _____

   b. _____

   c. _____

APPENDIX 3C
FOR LAB ASSIGNMENT 3.3

Stairway to Exercise Success

Stairway to Success for 10-20 weeks

If you would like to use the Stairway to Success over the next 10 weeks, use the top step for your long-term goal which is 10 weeks from the time you start. Write your present level of fitness on the bottom step and set your first short-term goal on the next step above. Each step from bottom to top represents a short-term goal of approximately one week. If you would like to use the Stairway to Success over the next 20 weeks, each step from bottom to top represents approximately two weeks.

If you would like to use the Stairway to Success over the next six months, use the top step for your long-term goal which is six months from the time you start. Write your present level of fitness on the bottom step and set your first short-term goal on the next step above.

Chapter 4

Principles of Health-Related Fitness

In this chapter you will:

- distinguish between health-related fitness and skill-related fitness
- learn and apply the eight principles of health-related fitness to meet your health-related fitness needs
- incorporate strategies to increase exercise enjoyment

PHYSICAL FITNESS: HEALTH RELATED VS. SKILL-RELATED

Physical fitness is the ability of the body to function at optimal efficiency (Robbins, Powers, & Burgess, 2002). Someone who is physically fit is able to complete the daily demands of life and still have energy left over for leisure and recreational activities. In addition, someone who is physically fit can exercise for long periods of time at moderate to high intensities without getting overly fatigued (e.g., being able to jog for thirty minutes without stopping, performing 15-20 sets of resistance training exercises or stretching one's joints past the normal range of motion without feeling tight or sore) (See Figure 4.1).

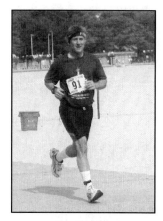

Cardio fitness

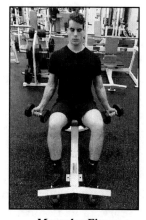

Muscular Fitness
Figure 1

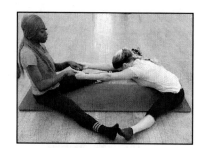

Flexibility fitness

Physical fitness involves two components: health-related and skill-related. Health-related fitness concentrates on areas that are related to health (cardiorespiratory endurance, muscular strength and endurance, flexibility, and body composition) while skill related fitness emphasizes components that are necessary to succeed in sport yet are not directly related to health (agility, balance, coordination, power, reaction time and speed). For example, you can have a high level of hand-eye coordination and excel in sports like archery, billiards or bowling, yet not be fit in one or more components of health-related fitness (e.g., difficulty exercising continuously for more than a few minutes; unable to lift moderately heavy objects; poor range of motion in lower joints—hamstrings, quadriceps). Conversely, you may possess a high level of health-related fitness and be able to lift moderate to high levels of weight, perform aerobic exercises for long periods of time (e.g., 40 minutes) and demonstrate an excellent range of motion in your joints (e.g., you can touch your toes; vertically interlock your fingers behind your back, rotate your trunk all the way across your body) yet not be very athletic in sports.

In order to create a fitness program that addresses your health-related concerns and works for you (e.g., improving your cardiorespiratory endurance, increasing your muscular fitness, becoming more flexible, establishing the appropriate body weight), there are eight principles of fitness that you need to learn so you can apply them into your exercise program. Each principle serves as a guideline and addresses important information about the following: (1) what you have to do in order to improve your health-related fitness; (2) exactly how much exercise you should be doing in order to improve; (3) what exercises you should do in order to improve specific components of health-related fitness (e.g., cardiorespiratory endurance, muscular fitness, flexibility, body composition); (4) why you should focus on yourself and not others; (5) what happens if you stop exercising for prolonged periods of time; (6) how much rest you need after exercise overload; (7) the importance of warming up before starting to exercise and why and how to warm up properly; and (8) the benefits of having fun while exercising.

In this section, you will be introduced to each of these eight principles of health-related fitness and learn the value of incorporating them into your fitness program. Examples of compliance and noncompliance with each principle so that you get a clear picture of how to utilize each in order to address your health-related fitness needs and exercise goals. In chapters' 6-8, you will learn how to apply each principle into your cardiovascular (chapter 6), muscular fitness (chapter 7) and flexibility (chapter 8) programs.

THE EIGHT PRINCIPLES OF HEALTH-RELATED FITNESS

1. ***Principle of Overload***—in order to improve a system, you must place it under more than its usual amount of healthy stress. In other words, you have to do more than what your body is used to doing. For example, if you are living a sedentary lifestyle and do little or no physical activity and you rode your bicycle for 20 minutes one day and took a 30-minute walk a few days later, both times increasing your heart rate from its'

normal resting state, you would be doing more than what your cardiovascular system is used to and thus overloading that system. If you went to the gym and lifted weights that created some muscular tension that you weren't used to experiencing that would be an example of overloading your muscular fitness. Finally, if you hadn't stretched in a while (too long to remember) and you decided to stretch your major muscle groups (e.g., quadriceps, hamstrings, neck, chest, and back) by holding each stretch at a position where you felt some tension for at least 10 seconds that would be an example of overloading your joints in order to improve your flexibility in those areas. In each example, you are creating a certain degree of work that your body is not used to causing what is referred to as exercise overload. By overloading your muscles your body begins to improve its functionality by getting stronger, improving resistance to fatigue, having more energy and feeling more flexible.

Compliance: Each week you do a little more than you did the previous week and increase any one or more of the following: (frequency-exercising more days per week; intensity-working harder; time-exercising longer, doing more exercises). When you gradually increase your exercise load over a period of time, you begin to see improvements. For example, in Week 1 Linda exercised for 20 minutes per day on two separate days. In Week 2, she exercised for 22 minutes per day on two separate days and in Week 3, she exercised three times for 23 minutes each day. By increasing time per workout in week 2 and then time and frequency of workouts in week 3, Linda has succeeded in meeting the overload principle because she has accomplished more in each week than she was doing in the previous week. Consequently, her level of fitness has improved.

Noncompliance: Regardless of your intentions to exercise more, when you do less work from one week to the next (e.g., fewer minutes, fewer days per week, fewer reps) or if you take a few weeks off from exercising, you are not overloading. For example, last week Linda walked two times for 20 minutes each at a 15 minute per mile pace with her heart rate ranging between 60% - 65% of her max heart rate. This week, Linda walked one time for 172minutes and her heart rate ranged from 40% - 45% of her max heart rate. As a result of Linda's decrease in frequency, time and intensity, she has not overloaded and thus her fitness level will not improve.

2. ***Principle of Progression***—in order to continuously improve, you must incorporate a systematic increase in the work that you do. Rather than deciding to do just a little more or work harder than your last workout, progression requires you to quantify exactly how much you plan to improve.

   Compliance: You incorporate systematic increases into your workouts. For instance, four weeks ago, Melissa exercised two days per week and her workouts consisted of: (1) walking for 20 minutes; (2) performing 10 sets of muscular fitness training; (3) stretching for six minutes and (4) being able to reach her ankles when performing the modified hurdler's stretch. In order to comply with the Principle of Progression, each week Melissa set short-term goals each week to: (1) increase her walking time two to three minutes; (2) complete one more set of muscular fitness training than the previous week; (3) stretch for one more minute than the previous week, and (4) increase her exercise frequency from 2-4 times per week over the next 3 weeks.

As a result of reaching her goals, after four weeks, Melissa is now able to walk for 30 minutes, complete 14 sets of muscular fitness training, stretch for 10 minutes and reach her toes when she does the modified hurdler's stretch. Most importantly, Melissa has now found the time to exercise four times per week.

By incorporating a systematic increase in your workout (e.g., adding a specified amount of time to your workouts, increasing the frequency), you are actually programming your improvement and thus guaranteeing success.

Noncompliance: You did not increase your workload (intensity, frequency, time) over the last few weeks. Perhaps you exercised one day instead of two, walked for 15 minutes instead of 20, and stretched for five minutes instead of six. Maybe you did absolutely nothing and did not exercise at all. While it is certainly better to do something than nothing, in order to improve your present level of physical fitness, you must incorporate some form of progression into your workouts. The first step is to determine what stopped you from progressing. The next step is to decide what part of your exercise regimen you are going to increase from last week. Will you add a day to workout, increase an extra minute or two, add a few reps, select a new exercise to perform or hold a stretch for 4 more seconds? Your answer to this question increases your chances of complying with the principle of progression and improving your present level of fitness.

3. ***Principle of Specificity***—in order to improve a particular area of fitness, or specific bio-energenic system, you must select the proper exercises. While this might sound easy, it is not uncommon for individuals to either select exercises that do not target the intended area of fitness (e.g., doing sit ups to decrease body fat; lifting weights to improve cardiovascular endurance) or select the right exercises, yet work them improperly (e.g., lifting light weight to improve muscular strength; performing static stretches to improve flexibility before actually warming up.; jogging for five minutes to improve cardiorespiratory fitness).

Compliance: Mike has 32 percent body fat and he has decided that the best way for him to decrease body fat is to begin working on improving his cardiovascular endurance and eat healthier than he has in the past. He has selected brisk walking and the stationary bicycle as the exercises he will do continuously for at least 15-30 minutes two-three times per week to improve his cardiorespiratory endurance. In addition, Mike has chosen to improve his nutritional habits and reduce his caloric intake by 200 calories by replacing two glasses of soda with water each day. By improving his cardiorespiratory endurance through walking and bicycling and decreasing his caloric intake by 200 calories per day, Mike has clearly satisfied the principle of specificity.

For those of you who want to improve your cardiorespiratory endurance, you should select activities that require oxygen and that you can do for moderate (at least 15 minutes) to long periods of time (45-60 minutes) (e.g., walking, jogging, bicycling, swimming, rollerblading) (see chapter 6). If your goal is to body shape, tone/define your muscles then you should select a series of resistance training exercises that address each of your major muscle groups (e.g., chest, back, shoulders, biceps, triceps, abdominals, legs) and perform 10-15 reps per set. (see chapter 7). If your goal is to become more flexible, then you should work on stretching and familiarize yourself with the proper procedures for warming up before stretching and the various flexibility techniques to consider (e.g., static, passive static, PNF) (see chapter 8). Finally, if your goal is to lose weight (like Mike), you should combine cardiorespiratory and resistance-training exercise with healthy eating (see chapter 9). Each of these examples demonstrates how to identify the system that you want to work on and select exercises that are specifically designed to improve those components of health-related fitness.

Noncompliance: Mike's goal is to lose body fat and he decided to lift heavy weights to increase muscular strength and burn off excessive body fat. While lifting weights will improve Mike's muscular fitness, he will not lose weight this way since muscle weighs more than fat does. In fact, there is a chance that Mike may even get weight, especially if he is working out with heavy weight (at least 70% of his max) and eating poorly.

4. *Individuality Principle*—everyone is different and progresses at their own rate; therefore, the only comparison that is meaningful is between where you start and where you get to at some point in the future. Comparing yourself to someone else is meaningless and it can be demoralizing because you cannot control someone else's level of fitness or progress.

   Compliance: You focus on your own health-related fitness needs and then you set SMAART goals (Chapter 3) that will help you to concentrate on yourself and improve at your own rate. You avoid trying to do what others are doing and instead set your attention on what is best for you. You determine how long, hard, and often you will exercise based on what your present health-related fitness needs are not what everyone else around you can or cannot do. Each new week, you can use your previous accomplishments to help you determine what, when and how much to increase. Doing so will inevitably create results that you will be proud of.

   Noncompliance: You base your level of improvement on whether you are doing more or better than others. While many people have a natural competitive instinct, deciding how fit you are and how much exercise you should do based on what others do is not the most productive way to exercise because you can only control what you do (e.g., what exercises you do; how hard you exercise; how long you exercise; your present level of fitness) and not what anyone else does or how fit they are. Consequently, there is a good chance that you will feel dissatisfied and frustrated if you do not accomplish as much as your competitor, regardless of how much you actually do and thus reduce your effort to improve your health-related fitness.

5. ***Principle of Reversibility***—Wouldn't it be great if exercising was like a blue-chip stock? You work out for a few weeks and then your fitness level improves more and more as the years go by, regardless of how little physical activity you engage in. Unfortunately, you cannot bank your fitness. Exercising for a few weeks will not increase your fitness years later unless you follow the principles of health-related fitness and continue to exercise on a regular basis. The principle of reversibility states that your body will adjust to the level of activity that it becomes used to. When you increase your level of physical activity or exercise, your body will begin to show improvements (e.g., you can exercise longer; stretch farther; lift more weights, improve body composition). However, when you decrease your level of physical activity or exercise, your body becomes de-conditioned and you will start to lose what you have gained. In other words, "if you don't use it, you lose it." In fact, the rate of loss will occur more rapidly than your rate of gain. However, not all levels of fitness reverse at the same rate. For example, cardiorespiratory and flexibility fitness reverse more quickly than muscular fitness. You can work as little as once per week on muscular fitness and still maintain your muscular strength and endurance. Conversely, you will have to work on your cardiorespiratory and flexibility more frequently (at least 3X per week). Otherwise your fitness gains will begin to reverse themselves. On the positive side, once you get back into exercising, you will regain what you lost more quickly than when you first started (provided you haven't taken too much time off).

Compliance: This is the one principle where compliance is not recommended since complying with the principle of reversibility means you are not physically active and losing what you have recently gained.

Noncompliance: To avoid losing what you have gained, stay active and plan your workouts in advance. Recognize possible barriers (Chapter 1) that may stop you from exercising regularly (every week), and continue to incorporate strategies that motivate you to exercise and overcome these barriers. During times when it is more difficult to "find time" to exercise (e.g., final exam week, paper due dates, deadlines at the office, prior family obligations), plan ahead and jot down the available times that you do have to exercise. Decide where you will work out and focus on all the benefits you will receive from sticking with your exercise program (e.g., more energy, greater self-esteem, feeling proud of yourself, decrease in stress, guilt, frustration, and self-focused anger, living your life rather than your life living you).

You are in danger with losing what you have gained when your barriers to exercise are greater or more intense than your motives or reasons to exercise. When you start believing that you really "do not have time" or that exercising is "no longer convenient" for you, you have put the principle of reversibility into motion.

6. ***Principle of Recuperation***—the body needs time to recuperate after exercise overload and if you don't give your body enough rest, your chances of injury increase, you are more prone to experiencing excessive soreness and you may become less motivated to exercise.

   Compliance: Just as you plan on which days to exercise, the principle of recuperation requires that you also plan your day(s) off. The lower your level of fitness, the more time your body may need to recuperate because it is not used to the overload from exercise. Once your fitness level improves and your body becomes used to the demands of exercise, you will recuperate more rapidly from exercise overload, and you can exercise for longer periods of time and more frequently per week if you choose to. Therefore, when you first start to exercise, plan on working 2-3X per week while taking 1-2 days off in between your workouts to recuperate. This will allow your body the necessary time it needs to repair itself and get you back stronger, more energetic and ready for your next weeks' workouts.

   Noncompliance: After a long period of not exercising, Brian decided to work on CRE seven days per week. He felt that more was better, especially since he had exercised regularly several years ago and achieved a high level of fitness. After exercising four days in a row for the first time in months, Brian began to experience muscular soreness as well as fatigue and he noticed a decrease in his exercise performance from what he achieved on the very first day. Brian then realized that he was overdoing it and needed to give his body 1-2 days of rest so he could recuperate from all the work he had been doing from the previous four days.

7. ***Principle of Warm Up***—before exercising, you need to get your body and mind warmed up and ready for exercise overload. You can warm up your body by increasing muscle temperature which will enhance elasticity and provide better blood flow to the working muscles. One of the most effective ways to accomplish this is to select the same or similar exercises that you plan to do in your workout only at a lower intensity (i.e., walking fast before you begin to jog; doing a set of light lifting before you start your muscular fitness workout). You can warm up your mind by training yourself how to think while exercising (e.g., listening to music, focusing on your breathing, and verbalizing positive statements that make you feel good about exercising (ie., I can do this; this is going to be a great workout; this feels great). In chapter 11, you will learn how to create cognitive strategies that will teach you how and what to think during cardiovascular, muscular fitness and flexibility exercises.

   Compliance: The first step is to learn how to warm up properly. For example, before lifting heavy weights, determine the exercises that you plan on using for your workout and warm up with them by lifting weights that are lighter than those you plan to use in your workout (e.g., using 30%-40% of your max for about 8-15 reps on a bench press for a chest workout). If the lighter weights feel too heavy, you can warm up by using no weight and simply moving that particular muscle group in the same motion that you would during the weight training exercise (See Figure 4.2). Before participating in cardiorespiratory exercise, warm up by engaging in that same or a similar activity at a lower intensity (e.g., walking briskly before jogging; jogging before running; pedaling slowly before bicycling at your normal pace). Finally, before working on flexibility you should warm up your body by engaging in large muscular activity for a few minutes (e.g., walking or jogging on the treadmill before stretching your leg muscles). Warming up properly decreases your chances of injury and prepares your mind and body for exercise overload.

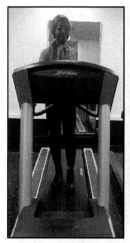
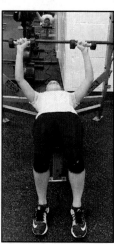
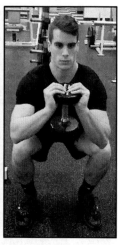

Warming up with CRE   *Warming up with Muscle fitness*   *Warming up with Lunges*
Figure 2

Noncompliance: Rather than walking briskly for the first five minutes, you immediately begin jogging or running at or near the speed you intend to maintain for the exercise duration. Rather than beginning a weight-lifting routine with light or no weights, you begin lifting weights that are at 70% of your max. This can increase your chances of getting injured and quite possibly reduce the overall productivity of your workout. Ouch!

8. ***Principle of Fun***—in order adhere to an exercise program, you must enjoy your workouts and perceive it as something you like to do otherwise you will find reasons not to exercise.

Compliance: Identify what you perceive as fun and incorporate that into your workouts. For example, if you like to listen to music, you can download songs onto your cell phone, iPad or iPod and use that while exercising. If you like to socialize and/or meet people with similar interests, then find a partner/friend to exercise with or sign up for an exercise class at your college or university, local gym or exercise facility, community center, library or continuing education program. If you like challenges, then try new exercises and set goals for yourself that take you to higher fitness levels that you want to attain. Consider entering competitions or races that challenge you to work hard (e.g., marathon, triathlon). Finally, if fun for you means being by yourself for a few minutes each day, then consider exercising alone and label that "My Own Quality Time."

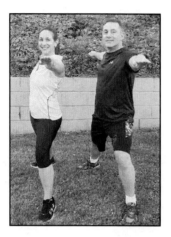 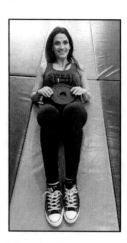

Having fun exercising

So start thinking about things that are fun and enjoyable for you that you can do while you exercise and incorporate them into your workouts so that you look forward to exercising (See Table 4.1 for a list of strategies to make exercise fun.)

Noncompliance: You focus on factors related to the desired outcome of your workout (e.g., lose weight, tone muscles) rather than enjoying the actual process of exercising. Your thoughts are more on getting the workout over with than liking what you are doing.

In conclusion, the principles of health-related fitness are designed to guide you to exercise properly so that you can reap all of the benefits associated with being physically fit and having a healthy lifestyle. Learning how to overload and meet your own individual exercise needs, selecting exercises that address the areas of fitness you need to work on, making sure you incorporate the right amount of rest, being able to fit exercise in to your weekly schedule, warming up properly, and making your workouts fun are essential components in developing and implementing a sound exercise program that is certain to reward you with not only getting fit, but staying fit for life.

Table 4.1
Activities to Help Make Exercising Fun

Please check the appropriate box to determine your level of interest in selecting these activities while you exercise to make exercise more fun for you.

	Not Interested	Somewhat Interested	Very Interested
Listening to Music			
Texting on your Cell Phone			
Talking on your Cell Phone			
Playing Hand-held Video Games			
Reading			
Playing Hand-held Video Games			
Watching TV			
Exercising with a Partner			
Taking an Exercise Class			
Exercising Outdoors—Parks, Beach, Lakes, Trail			
Competition Races, Fitness Challenges (e.g., Mud Run)			
Community Events—Walkathon			
Other			

REVIEW QUESTIONS

1. Define physical fitness and explain the difference between someone who is physically fit vs. someone who is not.

2. List and define the components of health-related and skill-related fitness.

3. Give an example of how to exercise each of the components of health-related fitness.

4. List and explain the purpose(s) of the principles of health-related fitness.

5. Define the overload principle and give an example of how you can overload during cardiorespiratory, muscular fitness and flexibility exercise.

6. Define the progression principle and explain the similarities and differences between overload and progression.

7. Give an example of how you plan to incorporate the principle of progression into your cardiorespiratory, muscular fitness and/or flexibility workouts.

8. Define the specificity principle and explain how you can incorporate the specificity principle into improving your cardiorespiratory endurance, muscular fitness and/or flexibility workouts.

9. What is the individuality principle? What advice would you give someone who was upset that his/her friend was progressing more rapidly than he/she was?

10. Explain the principle of reversibility. What suggestions can you offer to minimize or prevent reversibility from occurring in your exercise program over the next six months to one year?

11. Define the principle of recuperation. Give an example of how you can incorporate this principle in your cardiorespiratory and/or muscular fitness exercise programs.

12. Explain the warm up principle. Give an example of how you would warm up prior to engaging in cardiorespiratory, muscular fitness, or flexibility exercises.

13. Define the principle of fun and explain why having fun is important to your exercise. Give an example of how you can make exercise fun.

LAB ASSIGNMENT 4.1

For the next week you are invited to begin exercising on your own. Select an exercise(s) that you are motivated to do over the next week and answer the following questions.

1. List the exercise(s) that you plan to working on over the next week.

    _____   _____

    _____   _____

2. Explain how you will incorporate the overload principle for each exercise(s) you listed above (e.g., exercising more frequently, longer, or more vigorously than you did last week).

3. How do you plan to incorporate the principle of progression into the exercises that you selected to perform this week?

4. In order to satisfy the principle of specificity, list the exercises that you plan to do for:
    CRE _____
    MF _____
    Flexibility _____

5. Explain how you are going to determine your own individual progress for each of the 3 components of health-related fitness mentioned above (CRE, MF, flexibility)..

6. Have you ever experienced the principle of reversibility? If so, explain how you felt about yourself and your own fitness level during this period. What strategies are you using to prevent the principle of reversibility?

7. Explain how your prescribed exercise plan for this week includes the principle of recuperation. In other words, how do you plan to rest each system or body part that you have overloaded this week?

8. For each exercise that you plan to do this week, describe how you will warm up before overloading.

9. What strategies do you have in mind to make your exercises more fun for you this week?

REFERENCES AND SUGGESTED READINGS

ACSM Guidelines (2006). www.acsm.org

ACSM fitness book (2003). pp 9 3rd edition. Champaign IL: Human Kinetics.

Blair, S. (1995). Exercise prescription for health. *Quest*, 47, 338-353.

Blumenthal, J., Babyak, M., Moore, K., Craighead, W., Herman, S., Kharti, P., Waugh, R., Napolitano, M., Forman, L., Applebaum, M., Doraiswamy, M., & Krishman, R. (1999). Effects of exercise training on older patients with major depression. *Archives of Internal Medicine, 159,* 2349-2356.

Lox, C.L., Martin Ginis, K.A., & Petruzello, S.J. (2006). The Psychology of Exercise: Integrating Theory and Practice pp. 393-394. Holcomb Hathaway Publishers. Robbins, G., Powers, D., & Burgess, S. (2002). A wellness way of life. pp 50-110. McGraw-Hill. U.S. Surgeon General's Report. www.cdc.gov/needphp/sgr/adults.atm

Chapter 5

The Plan

In this chapter you will:

- answer seven important questions that will help you to develop your plan for exercising
- learn how to fit exercise into your life
- determine how to incorporate fun into your exercise workouts

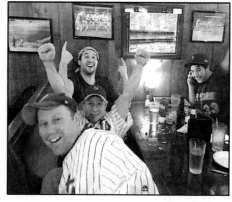

In chapter 2, you learned that people have a variety of motives for exercising (e. g., tone muscles, decrease stress, meet people with similar interests). When their motives are unfulfilled, they eventually decide there are other things that they would rather be doing and replace exercise with different activities (e.g., watching TV, playing video games, communicating with friends via e mail or cell phone; becoming attached to their i-pod). Imagine if you had a plan that helped you identify why you wanted to exercise, what you wanted to get from exercise, where you liked to exercise and how to incorporate fun into your exercise program. You would look forward to exercising more and probably find the time to get fit and stay fit, every week and every year for the rest of your life. This chapter invites you to first ask yourself and eventually answer seven important questions that will help you establish a "Plan" for fitting exercise into your daily life.!

SEVEN BASIC QUESTIONS TO GET STARTED EXERCISING

The Plan begins with these seven questions:

1. Why do you want to start exercising?
2. What do you want to get out of your exercise program?
3. With whom will you be exercising?
4. Where do you plan to exercise?
5. When will you start exercising? Time of day? Days of the week?

6. How many days per week will you exercise?

7. What do you like to do that is fun that can be done during exercise?

1. *Why do you want to start exercising?*

If you don't know why you want to start exercising, your chances of adhering to an exercise program in the long term are significantly reduced. That is why you should be clear about your choice to exercise. Is it because you want to lose weight and/or improve the way your body looks? Perhaps you want to get rid of the stress in your life or live healthy and reduce risk factors for lifestyle diseases. Maybe you want to meet new people with similar interests or perhaps your doctor has recommended that you start exercising. As long as you are clear as to why you want to start exercising, you can begin to view exercise as something that will meet your needs and give you exactly what you want. When you envision exercise as the vehicle to take you where you want to go, your motivation to find the time and get started exercising will increase. Once you have identified your motives (a.k.a reasons) to start exercising, the challenge becomes incorporating these motives into your exercise program so that you get what you want. Below are some common reasons why people want to start exercising along with strategies to structure an exercise program to meet these needs.

A. *Lose weight*—This is one of the more popular reasons adults decide to exercise. As you get older your metabolism naturally slows down and if your level of physical activity has decreased and you eat poorly, there is a good chance you are going to gain some "fat weight." Simply put, you gain weight when you are consuming more calories than what you expend. Through exercise and eating properly (e.g., fruits, vegetables, whole grains), you expend more calories to help get rid of the unwanted fat. For more information on eating properly, see Chapter 10.

B. *Improve the way your body looks*—Exercise is a terrific way to shape your body by strengthening and defining your muscles. In fact, there is no better way. As you will learn in the upcoming chapters, working on cardiorespiratory endurance (Chapter 6) will help get rid of unwanted fat and shape your lower body. Working on muscular fitness (Chapter 7) will help strengthen and tone your major muscles groups (e.g., chest, back, shoulders, legs, arms, abdominals) while also increasing body metabolism at rest. Finally, working on flexibility (Chapter 8) will help increase your range of motion and allow you to move freely and comfortably, prevent pain in your joints and lower back, and reduce the chances of soreness and injury.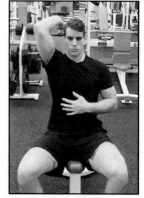

C. *Reduce stress*—Everyone has some degree of stress in their lives. When things do not go your way (e.g., bad job; lack of finances; difficulty in school; overworking yourself; relationship problems, family spats), the end result is often negative stress "distress."

However, experiencing stress is not really the problem. The problem is not knowing how to deal with your stress. One of the great things about exercise is that it can take your mind off of negative stress because it requires you to spend a certain amount of time thinking about what you are doing (e.g., correct form, pacing yourself, breathing correctly, reaching your exercising goals) and thus take your mind off of your stressors (the things that create stress for you. For example, Leslie recently graduated from school and she has begun a new job. Every morning she was required to meet with her boss and review her daily responsibilities (e.g., deadlines, expectations, work involved). Having grown up a perfectionist and always wanting to excel in everything she does, Leslie began to feel a 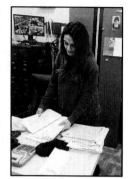 great deal of stress in her life. Fortunately for her, Leslie became friendly with one of her new colleagues, Andy, who invited her to the local gym after work. He suggested

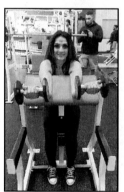 that they go to the gym together three times per week right after work and take an aerobics dance class together. After a few weeks, Leslie's work stress had disappeared. She began to enjoy exercising with Andy and going to the gym created a buffer to handle her daily work-stress. Moreover, after work she felt invigorated and excited about her day and all that she had accomplished at work as well as in the gym.

So whether you are working on your cardiorespiratory endurance, muscular fitness, and/or flexibility, the exercises you do will require you to associate and focus on what you are doing for at least some period of time during your workout (e.g., heart rate, pace and time during CRE activity; proper form and breathing while lifting weights; tension point and length of time holding a stretch for flexibility exercises). This will help you to take your mind off of your stressors and onto your exercise, thus decreasing your stress and making you feel better. In chapter 11, you will be introduced to cognitive strategies and learn how and when to program your thoughts while using associative and dissociative strategies. In chapter 12, you will learn more about the causes of your stress and how exercise can be used to transform negative stress (distress) into positive stress (eustress).

D. ***Live healthy and reduce risk factors for lifestyle diseases***—In recent years, there has been a dramatic increase in the number of studies examining exercise for the treatment of lifestyle illnesses/diseases (e.g., heart disease, cancer, diabetes, hypertension, arthritis, chronic anxiety and depression (Lox, Martin Gillis, & Petruzzello, 2006). The results have generally demonstrated that exercise is an essential component in living healthy, reducing risks and treating individuals who have been stricken with these

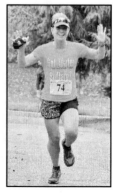

illness/diseases (Mayo Clinic, 2015, Matteo, (2016), Saxton, 2013); Woodward 2007; Long, 1984; Long & Haney, 1988; Long & Stavel, 1995; Landers & Petruzzello, 1994; Blair, 1995; Blumenthal, et al., 1999). For those of you who want to live a healthy lifestyle, exercise is more than just an option. It's a necessity and a significant part of our everyday lives. By working on health-related fitness (cardiorespiratory endurance, muscular fitness, flexibility, body composition), you decrease the chances of acquiring these lifestyle illnesses/diseases and enhance the quality and longevity of your lives.

E. ***Meet people with similar interests***—Many people join a gym or take an exercise class in order to meet others with similar interests. Although the desire to start exercising may have been with you for quite a while, the mere thought of doing it all by yourself (e.g., planning where and when to exercise, deciding what activities to participate in,

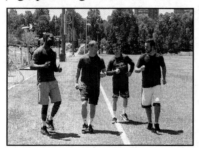

having nobody you know around to communicate with) can be enough to deflate your interests to get started. However, once you find someone with similar needs and interests, you may notice that you are more motivated to start exercising. In fact, research has found that people who exercise in groups had a higher adherence rate than individual exercise alone (Dishman & Buckworth, 1996). According to Weinberg & Gould (2003), group programs offer enjoyment, social support, an increased sense of personal commitment to continue, and an opportunity to compare progress and fitness levels with others. Being part of a group also fills the need for affiliation as well as a greater commitment to exercise when others are counting on you. Today, many companies have corporate fitness centers or memberships at local exercise facilities designed to get their employees to exercise because they know that a healthy worker is a more productive worker. In addition, individuals often seek co-workers to exercise with so that they can get the necessary support and encouragement needed to stick with exercising. Finally, fitness clubs offer a variety of programs or classes in order to attract individuals with similar exercise and health-related interests (e.g., weight loss, body sculpting, spinning; yoga, cardio kickboxing). By focusing on similarities, people often develop a connection and look forward to spending time and coordinating schedules together which can be a lot more motivating than getting yourself to go to the gym all by yourself.

F. ***My doctor told me I had to***—Many people begin an exercise program because their doctor(s) recommended it as a means to treat or prevent both physical and mental illness (e.g., heart problems, cancer, diabetes, obesity, arthritis, hypertension, anxiety, depression) or reduce already discovered warning signs for lifestyle illness (weight gain, high blood pressure, abnormal heart rate, chronic fatigue, uncontrollable mood swings). While the doctor's recommendation is an important factor in getting these individuals started exercising in the short-term, it is usually not a sufficient source of motivation to keep them exercising in the long-term (over six months). In fact, research has demonstrated that the average dropout rate for cardiac patients was between 44% and 48% (Franklin, 1988; Erling & Olridge, 1985). Moreover, it was Dishman who discovered way back in 1988 that 40% of the people who begin an exercise program will drop out within six months. Unfortunately, those dropout rates still exist today. Factors such as insurance running out, check-ups with the doctor decreasing over time, and a lack of knowledge of how to exercise properly by yourself have all contributed to the decline in exercise participation. The simple fact is that the only way exercise tends to continue in one's life is if the individual finds something that he/she enjoys from exercise (e.g., an exercise partner or group, an updated facility, seeing desired results).

2. *What do you want to get out of the program?*

Now that you have made the decision to start exercising, it is time to identify what you want to get out of your workouts. Whether your goal is losing weight or body shaping, meeting people with similar interests or reducing stress in your life, increasing your self-esteem or mastering fitness-oriented challenges, you should identify what you would like to get out of exercising so that you can make the choices that work best for you and give you what you want. You can start by making a list of all the activities/ exercises that you like and familiarize yourself with the benefits of each. Remember that the exercises you choose should work to improve one or more components of health-related fitness (cardiorespiratory endurance, muscular fitness, flexibility, appropriate body composition/eating healthy). In Chapters 6-9, you will develop a more comprehensive understanding of each component of health-related fitness. Table 5.1 displays a list of activities/exercises that you can choose to determine exactly what interests you and help you accomplish what you want.

Table 5.1

Activities/Exercises That Can Help to Improve Health-Related Fitness

Activities/Exercises	Components of Health-Related Fitness Being Emphasized
Aerobic Dance	Cardiorespiratory Endurance, Muscular Fitness
Bicycling	Cardiorespiratory Endurance
Calisthenics	Cardiorespiratory Endurance
Cardio-kickboxing	Cardiorespiratory Endurance
Circuit Training	Cardiorespiratory Endurance, Muscular Fitness
Cross-country skiing	Cardiorespiratory Endurance
Heavyhands	Cardiorespiratory Endurance, Muscular Fitness
Hiking	Cardiorespiratory Endurance
Ice Skating	Cardiorespiratory Endurance
Jogging/Running	Cardiorespiratory Endurance
Jump Rope	Cardiorespiratory Endurance, Muscular Fitness
Roller Blading	Cardiorespiratory Endurance
Martial Arts	Muscular Fitness, Flexibility
Spinning	Cardiorespiratory Endurance
Stability Ball Training	Muscular Fitness, Flexibility
Stair Climbing	Cardiorespiratory Endurance
Swimming	Cardiorespiratory Endurance
Walking	Cardiorespiratory Endurance
Water Aerobics	Cardiorespiratory Endurance, Muscular Fitness
Weight Training	Muscular Fitness
Yoga	Flexibility, Muscular Fitness
Zumba	Cardiorespiratory Endurance, Muscular Fitness, Flexibility

*Traditional sports (i.e., baseball, basketball, football, hockey, racquetball, soccer, softball, tennis, volleyball) were omitted because they address skill-related fitness more than health-related fitness on a recreational level. These activities can improve physical activity and to a lesser extent than health-related fitness, if modified properly.

3. *Who will you exercise with?*

The people you choose to exercise with or without can play an important role in your overall enjoyment of exercise. Some people like to exercise alone. They view exercise as "their own quality time," and they want to focus on themselves, how their body feels and how well they are doing. Some individuals like to work out with a partner or in small groups because it provides an opportunity to socialize with people of similar interests, make new friends or simply to catch up with old friends. This can provide a distraction from exercise which can make the workout time go by more quickly. It can provide a source of motivation, encourage-ment and support that many people need in order to give just a little more effort than might seem possible if they were exercising by themselves. Finally, for some people, exercising with a partner creates an opportunity to get together with someone they may not be able to see otherwise. (e.g., incompatible schedules, job responsibilities, live far away from each other, family obligations).

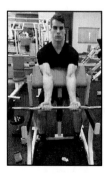 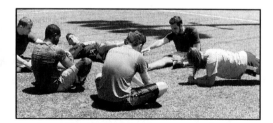 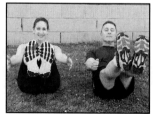

With whom will you exercise? Alone? In a group? Together?

Whatever environment you prefer to exercise in, it is important that you structure it into your workouts. If you like to work out alone, then find a place that is empty or a time when your exercise facility is not crowded. If you like to work out with a partner, then look for someone with the same schedule and interests as yourself. Contact family, friends, co-workers or neighbors that you would like to spend more time with and use exercising together as a means to accomplish this. Finally, if it is the class or group scene that you're looking for, then contact a nearby exercise facility, community center (e.g., local library, Y), or local college or university physical education or continuing education program to inquire about the courses offered in physical activity and exercise. For instance, many colleges and universities offer a wide variety of health-related fitness courses (e.g., aerobic dance, fitness for life, swim for fitness, weight training, yoga, cardio kickboxing, martial arts) specifically designed to address the health-related fitness needs and motives of their students. As their needs are identified and motives satisfied, students often recognize that they are not just taking the course(s) because they have to, but because they want to.

4. *Where do you plan to exercise?*

Whether it's at home, the local exercise facility, community center, college or university, or your workplace, you need to decide where you want to exercise. Therefore, you should weigh the strengths and limitations of each possible site to see what motivates you to want to exercise in that particular environment. For example, exercising at home may be convenient, but it may also be boring and difficult, especially if you spend all day at home and you are around young children or animals that require your constant attention. Exercising at a local gym can be rewarding if it is a well-run and well-equipped facility, but it may also be too costly for some people or unfulfilling for others if it is poorly managed and under-equipped. Table 5.2 provides a list of strengths and limitations for three popular exercise environments that can assist you in making the choices that work best for you.

Table 5.2
Strengths & Limitations of Popular Exercise Environments

	Strengths	Limitations
Exercising at home	Convenient Comfortable Surroundings Inexpensive Private	Can be boring Lack of Equipment Lack of Space Distractions
Exercising at a local gym	Wealth of equipment to choose ranging from cardio (i.e., bikes, treadmills, elypticals, arc trainers) to muscular fitness (i.e., free weights, machines, resistance bands) to flexibility (foam rollers, bands, mats) Spacious facilities Exercise professionals to assist you Day care facilities on premises	Membership can be costly Can get overcrowded Possible time limit on use of equipment Professionals may lack formal education in individualizing instruction to meet client's health-related fitness needs
Exercise in a college or university class	Expertise in instruction Opportunity to select from a wide range of classes Learn how to develop exercise programs that meet your needs Exercises are structured and scheduled for set days and times	Possibility of overcrowded classes Equipment may be outdated Facility may be old and run down Exercise time schedule is based on university schedule, not yours.

5. *When will you exercise? Time of day? Days of the week?*

Sometimes even when you intend to exercise, you may get distracted and suddenly run out of time by the end of the day and not get your workout in. Excuses like being too busy or not having enough time block your commitment to somehow get the workout in. The best way to ensure that you do indeed exercise is to create a plan that includes the time of day that you want to exercise, the amount of time that you exercise for, what your workout goal is and what exercise(s) you will do to reach your goals. It is important for you to view your exercise as a scheduled appointment, just as if it were a college class that you paid for, a doctor's appointment, sporting event or show that you had tickets for. You wouldn't think about canceling those appointments, unless you had an emergency, and that's exactly how you have to view your exercise: as a scheduled appointment. Write it down in your appointment book or day planner and treat your exercise time just as you would your other priorities, and stick to it because you're worth it!

6.   *How many days per week will you exercise?*

National sources (ACSM, CDC, U.S. Surgeon General's Report) suggest that in order to achieve health-related fitness benefits individuals should exercise between 3-5 days per week. However, if you are unfit or just getting back into exercising after a long layoff, you may not be committed or ready to start off exercising this much. The good news is that you do not have to. As you learned earlier in chapter 4, as long as you are doing a little more than what you were used to (principles of overload and progression), then you will improve and achieve positive results. Therefore, be proud of any number of day(s) that you have committed to start exercising, whether it be as few as one or as many as six because this represents an amazing starting point towards living a healthy lifestyle. Most important is the fact that you now have managed to find a way to fit exercise into your life without having to make significant changes. Think about it! Isn't it easier to start out exercising 1-2 or 2-3 days per week and add a day after a few weeks than it is to go from 0 to 3 days when first starting out?

So, if you are a beginner or someone who has not exercised in several months or more, you should start out slow (2-3 days per week at most). Remember that you cannot change your life around to fit exercise in. Instead, you must fit exercise into your life as it presently exists so that it works for you. Whether that is exercising 1 or 5 per week, be proud and acknowledge yourself for making the right decision. As time goes by, you will be the one to decide if and when you are ready to increase days per week or minutes per workout. As you become more physically active and start to see results, there's a good chance that you will want to find more time to exercise. Who wouldn't want to put more into something that they were getting a lot more out of!

7.   *What do you like to do that is fun and can be done during exercise?*

Many of you may know how to exercise properly. You may know how high your heart rate should be during cardiorespiratory exercise, how much weight to lift in order to shape your muscles and how long to hold a stretch for to improve your flexibility. However, as mentioned in chapter 1, knowledge of how to exercise properly does not seem to be enough of a motivating factor to keep people exercising continuously for the rest of their lives. The fact is if you do not enjoy your workouts, you are not going to stick with it. Therefore, it is paramount for you

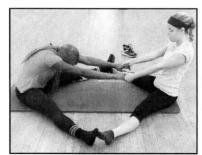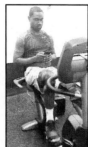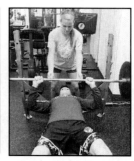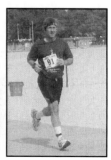

We stretch together. We play games. We lift together. We run!

to determine what it is that you enjoy and how you can make it part of your exercise program. So take a few minutes and jot down the things that you like to do. Then determine how you can incorporate these activities directly into your exercise program. Finally, take a look at Table 5.3 for a list of activities that you may not have jotted down that can be used to help you enjoy exercise.

So now that you have addressed seven important questions, it is time to really get started. Chapters 6-8 will help you to design your own exercise programs for cardiorespiratory endurance, muscular fitness, and flexibility. Each program will focus on your level of fitness (e.g., beginner-intermediate-advanced) as well as your level of commitment (e.g., low-moderate-high) to start exercising and live a healthy lifestyle. What more can you ask for? So let's get started!

Table 5.3
Activities to Help Make Exercising Fun

Please check the appropriate box to determine your level of interest in selecting these activities while you exercise.

	Not Interested	Somewhat Interested	Very Interested	
Listening to music				
Talking on your phone				
Texting, playing games, surfing the web, watching a movie or TV show on your phone				
Reading				
Playing hand-held video games				
Watching television				
Exercising with a partner				
Exercising outdoors—parks, beach, lakes				
Competition races				
Community Events, walkathon				
Other				

REVIEW QUESTIONS

1. Discuss the benefits of developing your own plan to exercise.

2. Explain why people want to start or continue exercising?

3. What are some of the things that individuals like to get out of exercise?

4. Explain why some people like to exercise by themselves and others like to exercise with a partner or in small groups?

5. What strategies can you incorporate to help individuals exercise by themselves? in pairs? small groups? exercise classes?

6. Name three different places people can go to exercise. What are the strengths and limitations of each place?

7. Explain the importance of planning the days of the week and times of the day can help someone to fit exercise into his/her life?

8. Why is having fun so important to exercising in the long-term (at least six months)?

9. What strategies can you implement to increase fun while exercising?

LAB ASSIGNMENT 5.1

1. Explain why you want to start exercising.

2. What would you like to get out of exercising in the next week, month, year and for the rest of your life?

3. Explain the benefits and limitations of exercising by yourself.

4. Explain the benefits and limitations of exercising with another person or in a class setting.

5. With whom to do plan to exercise with:

   by myself   with a partner   in a small group in an exercise class   not sure

6. Where do you plan to exercise?

   at home   local gym   college or university   local Y/community center   other

7. Using the Exercise Time Chart, list the days of the week, times of the day and amount of time you will allocate to exercising over the next few weeks (Appendix 5A to use the Time Chart).

8. List the activities that you enjoy doing and can be done while exercising.

9. Explain how you will incorporate the activities you listed above into your exercise program.

REFERENCES AND SUGGESTED READINGS

ACSM Guidelines (2006). www.acsm.org

ACSM fitness book (2003). pp 9 3rd edition. Champaign IL: Human Kinetics.

Blair, S. (1995). Exercise prescription for health. *Quest*, 47, 338-353

Blumenthal, J., Babyak, M., Moore, K., Craighead, W., Herman, S., Kharti, P., Waugh, R., Napolitano, M., Forman, L., Applebaum, M., Doraiswamy, M., & Krishman, R. (1999). Effects of exercise training on older patients with major depression. *Archives of Internal Medicine, 159,* 2349-2356.

Dishman, R.K., & Buckworth, J. (1996). Increasing physical activity: A quantitative synthesis. *Medicine and Science in Sport and Exercise, 28,* 706-719.

Dishman, R.D. (1988). *Exercise adherence: It's impact on public health.* Champaign, IL: Human Kinetics.

Dunn, A.L, Tirvedi, M.H., Kampert J.B, Clark, C.G. & Chambliss, H.(. (2005). Exercise treatment for depression. *American Journal of Preventative Medicine, 18,* 1, pp. 1-8.

Erling, J., & Oldridge, N.B. (1985). Effect of a spousal-support program on compliance with cardiac rehabilitation. *Medicine and Science in Sports and Exercise, 17,* 284.

Franklin, B.A. (1988). Program factors that influence exercise adherence; Practical adherence skills for the clinical staff. In R.K. Dishman (Ed.), *Exercise adherence: Its impact on public health* (pp. 237-258). Champaign, IL: Human Kinetics.

Landers, D.M., & Petruzzello, S.J. (1994). Physical activity, fitness, and anxiety. In C. Bouchard, R.J. Shepard, & T. Stevens (Eds.), *Physical activity, fitness, and health* (pp. 868-882). Champaign IL: Human Kinetics.

Long, B.C. (1984). Aerobic conditioning and stress inoculations: A comparison of stress management intervention. *Cognitive Therapy and Research, 8,* 517-542.

Long, B.C., & Haney, C.J. (1988). Coping strategies for working women: Aerobic exercise and relaxation interventions. *Behavior Therapy, 19,* 75-83.

Long, B.C., & Stavel, R.V. (1995). Effects of exercise training on anxiety: A meta-analysis. *Journal of Applied Sport Psychology, 7,*167-189.

Lox, C.L., Martin Ginis, K.A., & Petruzzello, S.J. (2006). *The Psychology of Exercise: Integrating Theory and Practice* pp. 393-394. Holcomb Hathaway Publishers.

Matteo, A. (2016). Exercise can protect against two major diseases. www.learningenglish.voanews.com/a/health-and-lifestyle-exercise-protexts-against-two-major-=diseases/3391399.html

Robbins, G., Powers, D., & Burgess, S. (2002*). A wellness way of life.* pp 50-110. McGraw-Hill.U.S. Surgeon General's Report. www.cdc.gov/needphp/sgr/adults.atm

Saxton, J.M. (2013). *Exercise and chronic disease: An evidenced-based approach.* New York: Routledge.

Weinberg, R.S. & Gould, D. (2003). *Foundations of sport and exercise psychology.* pp 414-415. Champaign, IL: Human Kinetics

Woodward, K. (2007). Exercise reduces chronic disease risks: Physical activity fights intra-abdominal fat that can fuel risk of cancer, heart disease, diabetes. *Hutch News*, July 1, 2007

www.mayoclinic.org/healthy-lifestyle/fitness/in-depth/exercise-and-chronic disease. June 20, 2015.

www.timesofindia.indiatimes.com/lifestyle/health-fitness/healthnews/.

www.webmd.comfitness-exercise/features/-do-you-have-sitting-disease? November 22, 2012

APPENDIX 5A
EXERCISE TIME CHART

	MON	TUES	WED	THURS	FRI	SAT	SUN
6AM – 7AM							
7AM – 8AM							
8AM – 9AM							
9AM – 10AM							
10AM – 11AM							
11AM -12 PM							
12PM – 1PM							
1PM – 2 PM							
2PM – 3PM							
3PM – 4PM							
4PM – 5PM							
5PM – 6PM							
6PM – 7PM							
8PM – 9PM							
9PM – 10 PM							
10PM – 11PM							
11PM – 12AM							
12 AM – 2AM							
2 AM – 4 AM							
4 AM – 6AM							

Chapter 6

Developing an Exercise Prescription
for Cardiorespiratory Endurance (CRE)

OBJECTIVES

After reading this chapter, you will be able to:

- Define cardiorespiratory endurance (CRE)
- Understand the benefits of CRE fitness
- Assess CRE
- Develop an exercise prescription for CRE that meets your needs
- Determine your level of commitment to CRE exercise
- Use SMAART goals to increase CRE performance and motivation
- Incorporate principles of health-related fitness into your CRE exercise prescription
- Evaluate the success of your CRE program
- Learn how to prevent injuries while engaging in CRE activities

Did you know that the normal resting heart rate (RHR) is said to be approximately 70-72 beats per minute (BPM)? With regular aerobic exercise this can drop 10 to 20 BPM or more. In fact, it is not uncommon for a resting heart rate (RHR) to be in the 60's, 50's or even 40's when you become aerobically fit. However, when you are aerobically unfit, your RHR can beat over 80 times per minute.

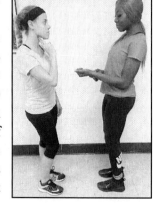

Imagine for a moment that when you were born, you were given a heart rate contract that stated your heart would beat two billion times and then stop forever. Having a RHR that beats 20 less times per minute translates to 1200 less beats per hour, 28,800 less beats per day, 201,600 less beats per week and over 10 million less beats per year. Moreover, how do you think you would feel if your RHR was 60 BPM compared to 80 BPM? Let's see. Imagine for a moment that you have improved your CRE and your RHR is indeed 60 BMP. (See Table 6.1 to see how many times your heart beats in one minute, one hour, one day, one week and one year).

Table 6.1
How many times does your heart beat?

RHR	1 Hour	1 Day	1 Week	1 Year
60	3600	86,400	604,800	31,536,000
70	4200	100,800	705,600	36,792,000
75	4500	108,000	756,000	39,420,000
80	4800	115,200	806,400	42,048,000
85	5100	122,400	856,800	44,676,000
90	5400	129,600	907,200	47,304,000

RHR indicates your resting heart rate or how many times your heart beats at rest

Wouldn't you feel better about yourself knowing that you chose to walk up a flight of stairs instead of having to take the elevator because you simply didn't have the energy to walk? Being aerobically fit will allow you to do just that and more. You will save millions of heart beats per year and not only will your heart beat less times per minute, but it will also give you more oxygen with each beat. More oxygen means more energy. Isn't it great to work so much less and get so much more out of it!

By now you should realize how important being aerobically fit is. Now it's time to develop the program that works best for you. This chapter will help you create a program that improves your CRE as well as identify exactly how committed you are towards becoming aerobically fit. Included are Exercise Prescriptions based on three levels of cardiorespiratory fitness as well as three levels of commitment. In addition, ACSM guidelines for aerobic fitness will be introduced and discussed in terms of both benefits as well as practicality. So have a heart and let's get ready to commit to becoming cardiovascularly fit.

WHAT IS CARDIORESPIRATORY ENDURANCE (CRE)?

CRE is defined as the ability of the circulatory and respiratory systems to supply oxygen and other fuels to the skeletal muscles during long periods of activity. In other words, CRE is a measurement of how well your heart, lungs and muscles work together to keep your body active over an extended period of time (Frey, 2016). CRE is an integral component of health-related fitness because so much of what we do requires the use of oxygen.

The Unfit Heart

Without a strong heart, a person may only be able to supply the oxygen necessary to perform minimal daily functions and thus be forced to reduce the amount of physical activity that can be done (e.g., walking up a flight of stairs, moving around continuously for more than a few minutes). An unfit heart has to work harder by pumping more often just to keep a person alive and thus, is subjected to more wear and tear than a well-conditioned heart. In situations that place strenuous demands on the heart such as running to class or catching the local bus or train to work, walking up several flights of stairs or carrying heavy packages to and from the car, the unfit heart may not be able to withstand the exertion. Consequently, the heart is forced to work harder by pumping more often, thus increasing one's level of fatigue as well as their susceptibility to heart disease.

The Fit Heart

The more fit a person's heart is, the more easily and efficiently it works. Simply put, this 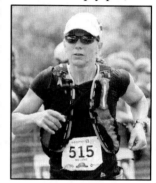 will provide you with more energy to be physically active without getting tired and here's why. When aerobically fit, the body is better able to consume, transport and use oxygen. With each heartbeat more blood is pumped throughout the body, blood volume increases, blood supply to the tissues improves, resting blood pressure decreases, resting heart rate slows down and the heart doesn't have to work as hard. Most important is the fact that as your CR fitness improves, you will reduce the risk of many lifestyle illnesses and diseases including heart disease, diabetes, colon cancer, stroke, hypertension, depression & anxiety.

BENEFITS OF CARDIORESPIRATORY ENDURANCE (CRE) TRAINING

By participating in Cardiorespiratory (CRE) activities, you will be rewarded with a wealth of physical and psychological benefits that include:

Physical Benefits

1. ***A stronger, more efficient heart***—Your heart will beat less times per minute and produce more blood to the working muscles. That is like having your car engine increasing in horsepower and giving you more miles to the gallon.
2. ***Decreased risk of lifestyle diseases***—As a result of your heart becoming stronger and more efficient, your risk or many diseases associated with inactivity and unhealthy lifestyle will decrease. These include heart disease, cancer, stroke, hypertension, and osteoporosis (just to name a few).
3. ***Increased VO2 Max***—The amount of oxygen your body is able to use will increase. You will be able to exercise longer and more vigorously without getting as tired.
4. ***Increased stroke volume***—Each time your heart beats, more blood is pumped. More blood means more energy.

5. *Improved physical appearance*—As you increase your CRE, your body will begin to use more stored fat as a source of energy and help you get rid of some of that excess, unwanted fat. This is one time in your life that you feel better about losing than gaining.

6. *Improved immune function*—As you improve your CRE, you also improve your body's resistance to illness and your susceptibility to common illness decreases (colds, flu, etc.).

7. *Increased job productivity*—Research has discovered that exercise will increase job productivity while decreasing worker absentiism. Consequently, many large businesses have either provided exercise memberships or built exercise facilities on site to be used by their employees.

8. *Better sleep*—As a result of exercise overload, your body will require more rest and this will help you fall asleep easier and improve the quality of your sleep, too.

9. *Increase in longevity*—Being physically active reduces risk factors for premature illness and death which results in living longer. In fact, research has indicated that leisure time physical activity is associated with longer life expectancy (National Institute of Health, Pate, et al., 1995; Blair, et al., 1998).

Psychological Benefits

1. *Enhances appearance and improved self-image*—When you exercise you will develop better muscular definition, reduce excess body fat and look better. These changes will make you feel good about yourself, as yesterday's difficult workout becomes tomorrow's easy workout. The challenges you set and conquer will improve your self-esteem and make you feel proud of who you are and what you have accomplished.

2. *Handle stress better*—By adapting to the positive stressors that exercise produces, your body becomes stronger and more resistant and better able to cope with some of the negative stressors associated with daily life (e.g., academics, job, money, relationships).

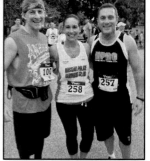

3. *Greater ability to relax*—After exercising, your body will begin to recuperate from your workout and your mind and body will feel relaxed, yet invigorated.

4. *Improved mental functioning*—You will learn how to concentrate on relevant aspects of your selected activity (e.g., heart rate, pace, breathing pattern, etc.). You will learn how to make effective choices within your workout such as knowing when to pick up or slow down the pace, when you should go a few extra minutes and when you have had enough. You will learn what to concentrate on and when it is ok to dissociate and listen to music or carry on a conversation with an exercise partner. This will carry over to other parts of your life as well and help you to be in control of your thoughts and think clearly and more productively.

5. ***Help in preventing and coping with depression and anxiety***—Research has demonstrated that exercise has had a positive effect on reducing anxiety, depression and ADHD while enhancing memory and boosting overall mood (Robinson, Segal & Smith, 2017; Otto & Smits, 2011, USDHHS, Morgan, 1997). In chapter 12, you will have an opportunity to explore your own stress levels and learn exactly how your stress changes on days that you exercise compared to days that you do not.

6. ***Enhanced quality of life***—One of the great things about exercise is that you begin to see your life more positively. The combination of both mental and physical achievements will help you to appreciate all that you have accomplished and all that you have to look forward to.

ASSESSING YOUR CRE

The purpose of assessing your CRE is to determine your actual level of CR fitness so that you can develop a program that will meet your needs and help you improve. Before participating in any of these assessments, you should practice them in order to familiarize yourself with their demands. Once you feel comfortable and confident that you can complete the test without overexerting yourself then you are ready to assess your CR fitness. There are several different assessments that you can perform in order to determine your CR fitness. Your selection of which assessment to use should be based on the following criteria:

1. ***Your current fitness level***—Each assessment has a different intensity or level of difficulty. The lower your CR fitness, the less intense the assessment should be.

2. ***Degree of enjoyment***—Selecting an assessment that you like will increase your level of motivation and commitment to do your very best. If you select an assessment and do not like it, you may not try very hard and thus get an inaccurate assessment of your current CR fitness level.

3. ***Facilities and equipment available***—Prior to beginning your CR fitness assessment, you have to decide where you are going to exercise and what equipment is available. Answering the following questions should help you to make the right decisions:

    a. Do you want to exercise at a public or private facility; in an individual or group setting?

    b. Is the equipment in satisfactory condition?

    c. How comfortable are you with using the equipment (e.g., track, treadmill, bicycle, pool, steps, elliptical, Stairmaster, etc.)?

FORMAL AND INFORMAL ASSESSMENTS

CR fitness assessments can be placed into two categories: (1) formal & (2) informal. *Formal Assessments* are more structured with a specific set of guidelines designed to create consistency in time, distance, pace, or rhythm. *Informal Assessments* are designed for individuals who possess a fitness level that is below the prescribed intensity, time or distance or are physically unable to withstand the overall demands of a formal assessment. This section provides a description of some of the more popular formal and informal CR fitness assessments.

Formal CRE Assessments

1.5-Mile Run: This test is used to determine your CR fitness by seeing how long it takes to run 1.5 miles. This test is recommended for individuals who have at least a moderate level of CRE and can jog or run 1.5 miles continuously without having to stop and walk.

Procedure for the 1.5-Mile Run

1. Start off by warming up either with a brisk walk or a slow job for a few minutes followed by a few dynamic stretches (see Chapter 8 for a list of dynamic stretches to consider).
2. Determine where you will run (standardized 440-yard track) or appropriately measured distance of 1.5 miles.
3. If possible, bring a friend to time you and keep track of your lap times as this can help to pace yourself. You can use the charts in Appendices 6A & 6B to record your lap times, overall time, heart rate and RPE. If you cannot bring a friend then bring a stopwatch and calculate the time it takes you to complete 1.5 miles.
4. Pace yourself by running consistently. Use your stopwatch to compare times on previous laps and adjust future laps accordingly (e.g., slow down if you are starting to feel tired or get out of breath; speed up if you feel comfortable and have lots of energy left). Do not sprint as this will cause your heart rate to go up too high and create an inaccurate assessment of your true intensity for most of the run.
5. After completing the 1.5-mile run, record you pulse for 10 seconds and multiply by 6. This will tell you your heart rate. Assess your pulse using carotid artery and radial pulse sites. Then walk slowly for one minute and check your pulse again for 10 seconds and multiply by 6. This will tell you your heart rate recovery (HRR). See Table 6.2 for a conversion of 10-second heart rate to one-minute heart rate.
6. Cool down and continue to walk or jog slowly for another 3-5 minutes and then stretch your muscles in order to reduce soreness.

When assessing your CRE using the 1.5-mile run, you can use either of these two charts. The first chart is used when running on a standardized ¼-mile track and the second chart is used when running on a 1/10 of a mile track. When using these charts for exercise classes simply divide your class into pairs and have one student record the individual and overall lap times while the other student is running. Once the run has been completed you can use the chart to record heart rate after run (HRAR) heart rate recovery lap (HRRL) and ratings of perceived exertion (RPE).

Table 6.2
Converting Your Heart Rate
to Beats Per Minute

10-Second Heart Rate	60-Second Heart Rate
15	90
16	96
17	102
18	108
19	114
20	120
21	126
22	132
23	138
24	144
25	150
26	156
27	162
28	168
29	174
30	180
31	186
32	192
33	198
34	204

1.5 Mile Run Assessment Form for Individuals and Groups
Using a ¼ of a Mile Track

Participant: Lilly   Date _____

	Lap 1	Lap 2	Lap 3	Lap 4	Lap 5	Lap 6	HRAR	HRRL	RPE
Overall Time	1:50	3.50	6.25	8.50	11.40	14.30	32=192	26=156	18
Lap Time X Min & Sec	1:50	2:00	2:35	2:25	115	2:50			

Using a 1/10 of a Mile Track

Participant: Jeremy   Date _____

Lap	1	2	3	4	5	6	7	8	9	10	11	12	13	14	15
Overall Time	46	1:36	2:24	3:12	4:00	4:46	5:30	6:12	6:54	7:38	8;20	9:04	9:46	10:3	11:1
Time X Seconds	46	50	48	48	48	46	44	42	42	44	42	44	42	44	40

Heart Rate after Run	Heart Rate Recovery Lap	RPE
30 = 180	18 = 108	12

Here is an example of how to record your 1.5 run using a standardized ¼ of a mile track or a 1/10 of a mile track commonly used in indoor, smaller exercise facilities. The top row represents each of the laps that you will complete. The middle row is where you record the time after you have completed each lap and the bottom row is used to calculate how many seconds each lap took you in order to determine how you paced yourself. Once you have completed the 1.5-mile run, check your heart rate for 10 seconds and record it in the HRAR (heart rate after run) box. Then go for a walk for one to two minutes and check your heart rate again and record it in the HRLL (heart rate recovery lap). Finally, use the RPE scale to determine how hard you perceived the difficulty this run was for you and record that in the box labeled RPE.

As you can see Lilly started out a little too fast in laps 1 and 2 causing her to have to slow down considerably in her remaining 4 laps. Her HRAR (32 = 192) indicated that she was running to maximum capacity and very tired at the end. Her HRRL dropped from 192 to 156, which is still pretty high after recovery. Finally, Lilly's RPE of 18 supports the fact that she thought she was very tired once she finished her run. Consequently, Jeremy paced himself extremely well throughout all 15 laps of his run. In fact, he ran his fastest overall lap at the end indicating that he had plenty of energy left to keep going. While his HRAR was high (30 =180), his HRRL dropped to 18 = 108 which means that he recuperated very quickly and his body was used to running at this pace. Finally, he rated his RPE at 12 which indicates that he thought his run was between light and somewhat hard.

Figure 6-1—1.5 Mile Run Assessment Form for Individuals and Groups

12-Minute Run: This test is recommended for individuals who enjoy running for time rather than distance. It is also recommended for exercise instructors who test moderate to large groups of people simultaneously and may be pressed for time. Rather than measuring the time it takes to complete a certain distance as done with the one-mile walk and 1.5 mile runs, the 12-minute run measures the distance completed in 12 minutes. Consequently, everyone finishes at the same time. (Use Figures 6.2 or 6.3 to measure distance covered in the 12-minute run).

Procedures for the 12-Minute Run

1. Start off by warming up either with a brisk walk or a slow jog for a few minutes followed by a few dynamic stretches (see Chapter 8 for a list of dynamic stretches to consider).

2. It is best to use a standardized track or distance and measure off different distances around the track (e.g., 20 yards, 40 yards). This way you can determine the exact distance covered in 12 minutes.

3. Pace yourself by running consistently. Use a stopwatch to remind yourself how many minutes you have been running and how many minutes you have left. This will help you to determine whether to keep the same pace, slow down and conserve energy if you are getting tired or pick up the pace if you have lots of energy left.

4. After completing the 12-Minute Run, check your pulse for 10 seconds and multiply by 6.

5. Then walk slowly for one minute and check your pulse again for 10 seconds and multiply by 6. Use Table 6.2 to convert your 10-second heart rate to a one-minute heart rate.

6. Continue to cool down by walking slowly for a few minutes and then select a few static stretches to stretch your muscles in order to reduce soreness (See Chapter 8 for a list of static stretches to choose from).

The benefits of the 12-Minute Run

(1) Many people can be tested within a short-period of time; (2) everyone is finished at the same time which is quite helpful for physical education teachers responsible for large numbers of students who are on a fixed time schedule. *The main limitation* is that some people may not be able to run 12 minutes continuously and thus have difficulty with the intensity of this assessment.

12-Minute Run Assessment Form: Pre-Test for 1/10 of a Mile Track

Lap	Lap 1	Lap 2	Lap 3	Lap 4	Lap 5	Lap 6	Lap 7	Lap 8	Lap 9	Lap 10	Lap 11	Lap 12	Lap 13	Lap 14	Lap 15	Lap 16	Lap 17	Lap 18	Lap 19	Lap 20
	¼ ½ ¾	¼ ½ ¾	¼ ½ ¾	¼ ½ ¾	¼ ½ ¾	¼ ½ ¾	¼ ½ ¾	¼ ½ ¾	¼ ½ ¾	¼ ½ ¾	¼ ½ ¾	¼ ½ ¾	¼ ½ ¾	¼ ½ ¾	¼ ½ ¾	¼ ½ ¾	¼ ½ ¾	¼ ½ ¾	¼ ½ ¾	¼ ½ ¾
Time																				
Pace																				

Circle the lap that has been completed each time the individual gets to the starting line. At the conclusion of the 12 minutes stop and record the distance that has been completed from the starting line.

Heart Rate after Run	Heart Rate Recovery Lap	RPE

12-Minute Run Assessment Form: Mid-Test for 1/10 of a Mile Track

Lap	Lap 1	Lap 2	Lap 3	Lap 4	Lap 5	Lap 6	Lap 7	Lap 8	Lap 9	Lap 10	Lap 11	Lap 12	Lap 13	Lap 14	Lap 15	Lap 16	Lap 17	Lap 18	Lap 19	Lap 20
	¼ ½ ¾	¼ ½ ¾	¼ ½ ¾	¼ ½ ¾	¼ ½ ¾	¼ ½ ¾	¼ ½ ¾	¼ ½ ¾	¼ ½ ¾	¼ ½ ¾	¼ ½ ¾	¼ ½ ¾	¼ ½ ¾	¼ ½ ¾	¼ ½ ¾	¼ ½ ¾	¼ ½ ¾	¼ ½ ¾	¼ ½ ¾	¼ ½ ¾
Lap time																				
Pace																				

Heart Rate after Run	Heart Rate Recovery Lap	RPE

12-Minute Run Assessment Form: Post-Test for 1/10 of a Mile Track

Lap	Lap 1	Lap 2	Lap 3	Lap 4	Lap 5	Lap 6	Lap 7	Lap 8	Lap 9	Lap 10	Lap 11	Lap 12	Lap 13	Lap 14	Lap 15	Lap 16	Lap 17	Lap 18	Lap 19	Lap 20
	¼ ½ ¾	¼ ½ ¾	¼ ½ ¾	¼ ½ ¾	¼ ½ ¾	¼ ½ ¾	¼ ½ ¾	¼ ½ ¾	¼ ½ ¾	¼ ½ ¾	¼ ½ ¾	¼ ½ ¾	¼ ½ ¾	¼ ½ ¾	¼ ½ ¾	¼ ½ ¾	¼ ½ ¾	¼ ½ ¾	¼ ½ ¾	¼ ½ ¾
Lap time																				
Pace																				

Heart Rate after Run	Heart Rate Recovery Lap	RPE

Figure 6.2—Assessing Your CRE Using the 12-Minute Run 1/10 of a Mile Track

12-Minute Run Assessment Form: Pre-Test for ¼ of a Mile Track

Distance	1	2	3	4	5	6	7	8
	¼ ½ ¾	¼ ½ ¾	¼ ½ ¾	¼ ½ ¾	¼ ½ ¾	¼ ½ ¾	¼ ½ ¾	¼ ½ ¾
Lap time								
Pace								

Circle the lap that has been completed each time the individual gets to the starting line. At the conclusion of the 12 minutes stop and record the distance that has been completed from the starting line.

Heart Rate after Run	Heart Rate Recovery Lap	RPE

12-Minute Run Assessment Form: Mid-Test for ¼ of a Mile Track

Distance	1	2	3	4	5	6	7	8
	¼ ½ ¾	¼ ½ ¾	¼ ½ ¾	¼ ½ ¾	¼ ½ ¾	¼ ½ ¾	¼ ½ ¾	¼ ½ ¾
Lap time								
Pace								

Heart Rate after Run	Heart Rate Recovery Lap	RPE

12-Minute Run Assessment Form: Post-Test for ¼ of a Mile Track

Distance	1	2	3	4	5	6	7	8
	¼ ½ ¾	¼ ½ ¾	¼ ½ ¾	¼ ½ ¾	¼ ½ ¾	¼ ½ ¾	¼ ½ ¾	¼ ½ ¾
Lap time								
Pace								

Heart Rate after Run	Heart Rate Recovery Lap	RPE

Figure 6.3—Assessing Your CRE Using the 12-Minute Run ¼ Mile Track

12-Minute Swim Test: This test is similar to the 12-minute run test in that the goal is to cover as much distance as you can in 12 minutes while swimming instead of running. This test is recommended only for those individuals who are skilled swimmers and plan on swimming as part of their CR exercise routine.

Procedures for the 12-Minute Swim

1. Enroll a friend or swim instructor to time you for 12 minutes.
2. Make sure there is a lifeguard on duty and that he/she knows you are being tested.
3. Warm up by swimming or treading water for a few minutes and then dynamically stretching both upper and lower body either in or out of the water.
4. Pace yourself throughout your swim and swim as many laps as you can.
5. After completing your swim, you can check your heart rate for 10 seconds in the same manner that you would for the 1.5 and 12-minute runs. However, it is important to note that your heart rate will be lower due to the water temperature in the pool. Therefore, it is recommended that you also use the RPE scale to determine your exercise intensity. (See section on CRE exercise prescription intensity and Figure 6.4).
6. Cool down by swimming slowly or treading water for a few minutes and then check your heart rate again.

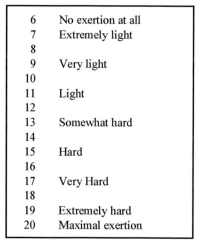

6	No exertion at all
7	Extremely light
8	
9	Very light
10	
11	Light
12	
13	Somewhat hard
14	
15	Hard
16	
17	Very Hard
18	
19	Extremely hard
20	Maximal exertion

Reference – Borg, G. (1998). Borg's perceived
exertion and pain scales.

Figure 6.4—Ratings of Perceived Exertion

The benefit of the 12-minute swim is that it is easier on the joints and the temperature in the pool is often regulated and more comfortable. ***The limitation*** is that not everyone is an efficient swimmer and while you may be cardiovascularly fit, you may not be an efficient swimmer and thus perform poorer than you would in other yore efficient.

The One-Mile Walk: This test is recommended for those individuals who have a low level of CR fitness and/or unable to run because of injuries or pre-existing conditions that prevent running or other more strenuous activities.

Proper Walking Technique—Proper walking includes keeping your upper body upright (do not lean forward or backward), extending opposite arms forward (e.g., as you step with your left foot, your right hand should be out in front of your body).

Procedures for the One-Mile Walk Test

1. Select the site where you will walk your one mile. You can use a standardized 440-yard track and walk four laps or if you do not have access to a track, simply measure out a distance of one mile at a location that is convenient to you (e.g., around your block; campus area; office; local park).
2. Bring a stopwatch and measure the time it takes you to walk one mile.
3. Walk as fast as you can.
4. Once you have finished walking, immediately check your pulse by counting the number of beats in 10 seconds.
5. Multiply your 10-second total by 6 to determine your heart rate in beats per minute. Then walk slowly for one minute and check your pulse rate again for 10 seconds and multiply by 6.

The benefits of the One-Mile Walk are: (1) it is easy to administer; (2) it requires only a low level of CRE and (3) it is virtually painless on the lower joints. ***The limitation*** is that sometimes individuals may not know how to walk properly and think they are going as fast as possible, yet still not get their HR up enough to determine if they working at a sufficient intensity.

Step Test: This test takes only three minutes to complete. All you need is a bench or gymnasium bleacher 16 ¼ inches high, a stopwatch and a metronome (to determine pace). This test is not recommended for anyone who suffers from joint, knee or leg problems, is significantly overweight, or has problems with balance, coordination or walking up and down stairs.

Procedures for the Step Test

1. Use a gymnasium bleacher or a staircase that measures 16 ¼ inches high.
2. Step up-up-down-down to the beat of 24 steps/minute for a man and 22 steps/minute for a woman.
3. Practice going up-up-down-down for a minute in order to get into the proper rhythm and pace.
4. Perform the test for three minutes.
5. After completing the test take your heart rate for 10 seconds.
6. Walk around for one minute and retake your heart rate.

The benefit of the step test is that it only takes three minutes to complete and it can be done with large numbers of people at one time in a variety of places (e.g., gymnasium, exercise facility, local park, at home). *The limitation* is that individuals may not be stepping to the correct rhythm (e.g., stepping more or less than the required number of steps) and have to adjust pace which may affect heart rate and cause an inaccurate assessment of the exercise intensity.

Informal Assessments

In case none of the CRE formal assessments listed above are right for you due to physical limitations (e.g., low CR fitness level, overcoming injuries, etc.) or psychological barriers (lack of motivation, social physique anxiety—not wanting to be around others while exercising, etc), you should consider an informal assessment and follow the guidelines listed below:

1. Select any rhythmic activity that you like (e.g., walking, bicycling, jogging, elliptical machine, Stairmaster, swimming, etc.)

2. Record the length of time that you exercised continuously and the total distance completed (if applicable). For walking or jogging, you can also use a pedometer and record the number of steps taken. For the Stairmaster, you can measure the number of floors climbed and for swimming you can count the number of laps swam.

3. Upon completion of your activity/exercise, you can check your heart rate to determine how hard you were working and use the RPE scale to evaluate perceived difficulty (See Figure 6.4).

4. You can use Table 6.3 to Informally Assess Your CRE and jot down your choice of activity, heart rate, post heart rate, RPE, minutes, distance, steps, laps, etc.

Table 6.3
Informally Assessing Your CRE

Date	Activity	Minutes	Distance	Laps	Floors	HRAA	HRR	RPE

Assessment. Select the aerobic activity that you would like to use to informally assess your CRE. Once you have completed your assessment, you can use the minutes' column to record the total number of minutes that you performed your activity before stopping. You can use the distance column to record the total distance that you achieved. You can use laps completed if you are assessing your CRE on a standardized surface (e.g., track, swimming pool with lap lanes) and plan to count how many laps you do. If you are using the Stairmaster, you can record the number of floors climbed. Once you have completed your CR assessment, immediately take your 10-second heart rate and record the total number of beats in the HRAA (Heart Rate After Activity) box. Then check your heart rate one minute later and record it in the HRR (Heart Rate Recovery) box. Finally, use the RPE box to record how hard you perceived your CR assessment to be.

Although Informal Assessments may not determine your true cardiorespiratory fitness level due to the limitations listed above, it is your starting point and something to be proud of for the following reasons:

- you now know where to begin your CR fitness program;
- you have moved from a sedentary to an active lifestyle;
- you are ready to begin improving and set your SMAART goals;
- your motivation to begin exercising should be high since you are not forcing yourself to do any more than you are physically or psychologically willing to do.

Regardless of which assessment(s) you choose (formal or informal), your results represent your starting point towards improving and enjoying exercise. You now have valuable numerical information that will assist you in evaluating your CR fitness level (e.g., ran 1.5 miles in 14:00; heart rate was 160 bpm after completing the 3:00 step test; walked for 10 minutes and then stopped; climbed 22 floors in 12 minutes on the Stairmaster). Most important, you can use your Stairway to Success to set SMAART goals to get you ready for action and improve your CRE. The important factor is not that you are less fit and unable to perform like you once did several years ago, but that you "got started" and for that you should be proud of yourself.

DEVELOPING YOUR EXERCISE PRESCRIPTION FOR CRE

Anyone who has taken prescribed medicine knows that on the bottle is information explaining what you are taking, the ingredients, how often and how long you should take it and what it is designed to do (e.g., fever reducer, cough suppressant, etc.) Well, like medicine, exercise has its own prescription commonly referred to as the FITT formula, which address the following four important questions about your exercise routine:

F—stands for frequency and addresses the question "How many days per week should I exercise?" It is generally recommended that in order to improve your CRE, you should do it at least 3 to 5 times per week. However, as you will learn later in this chapter that your commitment to CRE will ultimately determine just how many days it is appropriate for you to exercise whether it is one, two, three, four ....

I—stands for intensity and addresses the question, "How hard should my workout be?" There are two basic ways to measure intensity in your CRE program: (a) Heart Rate (HR) & (b) Ratings of Perceived Exertion (RPE).

(a) ***Heart Rate***—an objective measure of intensity that uses your heart rate to determine how hard you are working; the higher your heart rate, the harder you are physically working. Generally, you should work between 50%-85% of your heart rate reserve (HRR). (See below to determine how to get your HRR).

Let's use Sammy, a 20-year-old individual with a resting heart rate of 70 beats per minute (BPM), as an example of how to calculate proper intensity using HRR.

Predicted Max Heart Rate (pMHR) = 220 − age = 220 − 20 = 200

Resting Heart Rate (RHR) = 70

Heart Rate Reserve (HRR) = Max HR - RHR = 200 − 70 = 130

50%TI (Training Intensity) =	130 × .50 + RHR (70) = 135 beats per minute (BPM)
60%TI =	130 × .60 + RHR (70) = 148 BPM
65% TI =	130 × .65 + RHR (70) = 155 BPM
70% TI =	130 × .70 + RHR (70) = 161 BPM
75% TI =	130 × .75 + RHR (70) = 168 BPM
80% TI =	130 × .80 + RHR (70) = 174 BPM
85% TI =	130 × .85 + RHR (70) = 181 BPM

Using 50–85 percent of HRR, Sammy's proper cardiorespiratory (CR) intensity would be to exercise with a heart rate of 135 to 181 beats per minute. Individuals with low CR fitness levels should work between 50-70 percent and strive to conserve their energy so they can exercise for longer periods of time. As CR fitness improves, you will feel more comfortable working at a higher intensity (70%-85%) while still exercising for sufficient time periods (at least 30 minutes). While using your HRR is the most effective way to maximize working at the proper exercise intensity, it can be a complicated procedure for individuals with no formal background in exercise prescription. Therefore, a more simplified version of determining proper exercise intensity has been developed and implemented in both university and private exercise facilities. The formula looks like this:

1. Take your Max HR (220) and subtract your age.
2. Multiply by .50 to determine the low end of your training intensity and .85 to determine the high end of your training intensity.

For example, if you are 18 years old, then you would take 220-18 = 202. Then multiply 202 by .50 (low end) & .85 (high end). That would tell you to keep your heart rate between 101 and 172 beats per minute. This is also referred to as your target heart rate or area that you want your heart to be while exercising in order to achieve maximal benefits. See Table 6.4 to determine proper heart rate using the simplified formula.

Table 6.4
Calculating Your Target Heart Rate "Simply"

Age	10-Second Rate Count	Target Heart Rate Range in BPM
17-20	20-29	120-173
21-25	19-28	117-169
26-30	19-27	114-165
31-35	18-27	111-161
36-40	18-26	108-156
41-45	17-25	105-152
46-50	17-25	102-148
51-55	16-24	99-144
56-60	16-23	96-139
61-65	15-22	93-132
66-70	15-22	90-131
71-75	14-21	87-126
75+	14-20	85-119

b. ***Ratings of Perceived Exertion*** (RPE)—Developed by Borg in 1971, the RPE is a subjective measure of exercise intensity that asks you to determine how hard you perceive your workout to be. In theory, the higher your heart rate is, the harder you should perceive your workout to be. However, some people like to exercise at higher intensities and they perceive it to be quite comfortable. Others, however, are not used to the sudden demands that exercise places on their bodies and may perceive a workout to be quite hard even though their heart rate is well within or even below their target heart rate. Moreover, not everyone likes or remembers to check their heart rate during or even after their aerobic workout. Having the RPE allows you to evaluate just how hard you perceive you are working and thus determine if you should increase, decrease or maintain the same intensity. To get a complete understanding of the Borg scale, you can read Borg's Perceived Exertion and Pain Scales (1998). See Figure 6.4 to review the Borg Scale.

I recommend that you use both measures (HR & RPE) for the following reasons:

1. Checking your heart rate will provide you with the information you need to clearly see how hard your CR system is working.

2. The RPE scale allows you to be in touch with your thoughts and perceptions about how hard you are exercising without having to disrupt the flow of your workout. Simply ask yourself "How hard am I working?" Then determine if you need to make any mod-

ifications to your workout (i.e., slow down, speed up, change directions, switch equip-ment). For example, if you perceive your workout is very light then you can either keep the pace the same if you choose or pick it up a little. Conversely, if you perceive your workout is extremely hard, then you may want to slow it down a little to conserve your energy or change what you are doing (i.e., run to walk, ellyptical to bicycle, hills to flat surface).

Using both measures maximizes working at the right intensity, thus making your CR work-out challenging and productive rather than boring or painful.

T—stands for time and addresses the question, "How long should my workout be?"

Generally, it is recommended that you should exercise for 20-60 minutes. Of Frequency, Intensity and Time, Time is the most important component, especially for beginners or individuals with low level of CR fitness. By increasing minutes from one week to the next you are overloading your CR system and thus improving. In addition, increasing time is more prac-tical than either Frequency or Intensity for the following reasons:

1. if you feel pressed for time, you are not going to be able to find more days in the week to exercise;

2. if you are just getting started exercising, increasing intensity too much may cause you to overdo it and become excessively sore which will not only decrease the probability you can exercise productivity in the next day or two, but it will also decrease your motivation to want to;

3. the hardest part of beginning your workouts is usually getting to the exercise facility; once you are there, adding a few extra minutes to your workout not only increases your performance, but it will also make you feel good about yourself and increase your desire to do it again in the near future. So remember, it's **Time That Is On Your Side!**

T—stands for type and addresses the question, "What activities should I do? Any large muscle activity that is rhythmic in nature that you can do continuously for at least 15 minutes matches the criteria for the right exercise to improve your CRE. See Table 6.5 for a list of activities to choose from.

Table 6.5
CRE Activities to Choose From

Aerobics	Ice Skating	Roller Skating	Swimming
Aqua Aerobics	Jogging	Rowing	Stair Climbing (Stairmaster)
Bicycling	Jump Roping	Running	Tae Bo
Cardio Kickboxing	Kayaking	Skateboarding	Walking
Elyptical Machine	Pilates	Skiing	Yokibics
Hiking	Roller Blading	Spinning	Zumba

The most common way to develop a CR exercise prescription is to use the results from your CR fitness assessment and match your level of CR fitness to one of the three CR fitness prescriptions listed below. Choose whatever activities you like that will motivate you to want to exercise. There is no one exercise that you must do in order to improve your CR fitness. As long as you are working within your target heart rate for at least 15 minutes straight, you will be overloading your CRE and improving to a higher-level CR fitness. See Table 6.6 to select an exercise prescription based on your CRF level.

Table 6.6
Exercise Prescription Based on CR Level of Fitness

Low Level of CRF

	WEEK 1	WEEK 2	WEEK 3	WEEK 4	WEEK 5	WEEK 6
F	2-3	2-3	3	3-4	3-4	3-5
I-HRR RPE	50-60% 10-12	50-65% 10-14	60-75% 12-16	60-75% 12-16	60%-80% 12-18	60%-85% 12-18
T	15-16 min	16-18 min	18-20 min	20-22 min	22-25	25-30
T use Table 6.5						

Moderate Level of CRF

	WEEK 1	WEEK 2	WEEK 3	WEEK 4	WEEK 5	WEEK 6
F	3	3-4	4	4	4-5	4-5
I-HRR RPE	60%-75% 11-13	60%-75% 12-15	60%-80% 12-16	60%-80% 12-16	60%-85% 12-18	60%-85% 12-18
T	25-30 min	30-35 min	30-35 min	35-40 min	35-40	35-45
T use Table 6.5						

High Level of CRF

	WEEK 1	WEEK 2	WEEK 3	WEEK 4	WEEK 5	WEEK 6
F	4	4	4-5	4-5	5	5-6
I-HRR RPE	60%-85% 12-18	60%-85% 12-18	65%-85% 12-18	65%-85% 12-18	70%-85% 12-18	70%-85% 12-18
T	40-45 min	40-45 min	40-50 min	40-50 min	45-60 min	45-60 min
T use Table 6.5						

DETERMINING YOUR LEVEL OF COMMITMENT

Over the years, research from health and sport science organizations have suggested that you should exercise for 150 minutes per week or 30 minutes per day five times per week (AHA, 2016; ACSM, 2007). While this recommendation may work for some individuals, it may not work for others. The simple fact is that if you are not committed to exercise then you will not do it for very long! How else can you explain the fact that only 15-20% of our adult population exercises enough to achieve health-related fitness benefits? As long as you continue to perceive yourself to "have to," rather than "want to" exercise then it is unlikely that you will comply with this recommended prescription for the long haul "the rest of your life." You may give exercise a try for a short while, but after only a few months, you will find yourself in the category of exercise "dropout," along with the other 50-60% of the population. The bottom line is that you simply cannot change your life around to make exercise fit. You have to learn how to fit exercise into the way your life presently exists. This starts with identifying your level of commitment to exercise. In other words, what activities are you committed to? How many days per week and how many minutes per workout are you committed to? Your answers to these questions will help determine exactly what works for you.

Three Levels of Commitment

A low level of commitment is characterized by someone who's motives not to exercise exceed his/her motives to exercise. Generally, these individuals are either not exercising at all or doing so at a minimal level because they feel they "have to" not because they "want to" (e.g., doctor's recommendation, have to lose weight). Frequency of exercise is inconsistent at best and as time goes by the mere thought of exercise is often replaced with the barriers that stop one from actually getting started.

A moderate level of commitment is characterized by someone who either wants to start or is actually exercising, but is concerned he/she may not continue. Although there is a genuine concern to get started and be physically active, there is some doubt that compliance (short-term exercise participation) and ultimately adherence (long-term exercise participation) will occur. Attempts are made to exercise and sometimes achieved, however, consistency is lacking and exercise benefits are achieved sporadically.

A high level of commitment is characterized by someone who is able to fit exercise into his/her life. This individual looks forward to exercise, has positive thoughts about doing it, and feels great afterward. Uncertainty of where and when to exercise or of how to enjoy and be motivated to exercise have clearly been replaced with feelings of pride and accomplishment, confidence and self-desire to exercise.

So where are you on the commitment scale?

1	2	3	4	5	6	7	8	9
Low commitment			**Moderate Commitment**				**High Commitment**	

How many days per week and minutes per workout will you commit to exercise? Once you know exactly what you are committed to, you will miraculously find the time to exercise. You will feel good about what you are accomplishing and as time goes by, you will suddenly find more time to exercise because you "choose to" rather than because you "have to." Based upon your level of commitment, you should consider one of the three six-week cardio-respiratory fitness (CRF) programs listed in Table 6.7. Select the program that you have the highest commitment level to participate in. In other words, do what you want to do and what works for you, not what you think you have to do.

Table 6.7
CR Exercise Frequency Based on Level of Commitment

	Week 1	Week 2	Week 3	Week 4	Week 5	Week 6
Low	1-2	1-2	2	2	2-3	3
Moderate	2-3	2-3	3	3	3-4	4
High	4-5	4-5	4-5	4-6	4-6	4-6

USING SMAART GOALS TO INCREASE CR FITNESS AND MOTIVATION

In chapter 3, you were introduced to goal setting and learned the value of setting SMAART goals. Now it is time to incorporate SMAART goals into your CR fitness program so that you can increase your exercise performance as well as create and/or maintain a high level of exercise motivation. To illustrate how to use SMAART goals with your CR fitness program, let's use Arline as an example.

Presently, Arline is able to perform 15 minutes of CR activity, including jogging for 11 minutes and then biking for four minutes on level 1. Using the SMAART principle, Arline sets her goals. (See Figure 6.5.)

As you can see, Arline has a plan to improve her CRF by modestly increasing her workouts from 16 to 20 minutes over a three-week period. In addition, Arline has a backup plan to adjust her goal in the event that she either doesn't reach it or if it becomes too easy. Finally, Arline has selected several different activities (jogging and biking) to choose from to help her reach her CR fitness goals. By setting SMAART goals Arline has now increased her chances of improving her CR fitness and once she begins to see progress from weeks' 1 to 3, this will undoubtedly improve her motivation to continue, too.

In addition to setting SMAART goals, if you have CR fitness goals that you think may take longer than a few weeks to achieve, you can use Stairway to Success (STS) goals presented in Chapter 3. Here are two examples of how to use STS goals to improve your CRE.

Goals	Arline's SMAART Goals
SPECIFIC	Improve CRF
MEASURABLE	Be able to jog & bike continuously for 20 minutes.
ACTION-ORIENTED	Run and bike 2-3× per week at level 1 for 15-16 minutes in week 1; 16-18 minutes in week 2 and 18-20 minutes in week 3.
ADJUSTABLE	If the action is not achieved in week 1, Arline will either decrease 1-2 minutes or include walking into her actions. If the workouts become too easy, Arline will increase to level 2.
REALISTIC	Since Arline is currently up to 15 minutes of CR activity, increasing 1-2 minutes in the next week and 3-5 minutes over the next 3 weeks is certainly realistic.
TARGET DATE	Today is November 6 and Arline would like to reach her goal by November 27.

Figure 6.5—Using SMAART Goals to Increase CRF

First, Marc, who is a college student who used to run in high school, but has since taken a few years to concentrate on his studies. He decided it was time to improve his CR fitness once and for all so he enrolled in a course called Fitness for Life and ran 1.5 miles in 15:00 on 1/26. Using the STS, Marc has established both short-term and long-term goals along with target dates for reaching each of his goals. His long-term goal is to run 1.5 miles in 12:00 by 5/11, the last day of class. In order to get there, Marc will need to focus on his short-term goals and take one step at a time. His first short-term goal in one week (2/2) is to run 1.5 miles in 14:50. Once Marc reaches that goal, he will move up one step on his staircase where his next goal is to run 1.5 miles in 14:30 by 2/16. As you can see, each step up from Marc's baseline is specific, measurable, realistic and challenging. Moreover, as Marc progresses from one step to the next, he gets closer and closer to reaching his long-term goal of running 1.5 miles in 12:00 which will not only increase his CR fitness, but his confidence, motivation and commitment to keep working hard too. (See Figure 6.6 to view Marc's STS).

Now let's move on to Mae, a middle-aged family-oriented career woman who wants to increase her CRE by walking longer periods of time. Her ideal, long-term dream goal is to be able to walk continuously for 40 minutes within four months. Presently, she is able to walk for 10 minutes without stopping. Every two weeks Mae has set her short-term goal to increase walking by 2-3 minutes. Each time she reaches her short-term goal, Mae will move one step up her staircase to progress closer and closer to her long-term dream goal on the top of the stairs. Imagine what this will do to her confidence, motivation and commitment to be cardio-vascularly fit! See Figure 6.6 to review how Marc and Mae climbed the STS to reach their goals. Let's take full advantage and learn from Marc and Mae. Use the Stairway to improve your CRE, too.

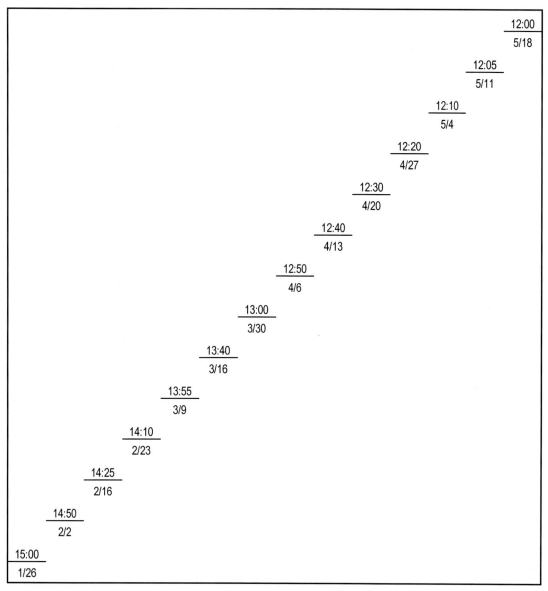

Stairway to Success... Marc ran 1.5 miles in 16:00. His goal is to be able to run 1.5 miles in 12:00. He knows this will not happen overnight and so he has set a long-term goal of being able to run 1.5 miles in 12:00 by 7/31. In the meantime, Marc has set several short-term goals that represents where he would like to be every two weeks. Each time Marc reaches his short-term goal, he will move up one step towards the next goal. If he does not reach his short-term goal, he can re-evaluate his actions and refer to Chapter 3 and BE SMAART.

Figure 6.6—Stairway to Success Based on 1.5-Mile Run

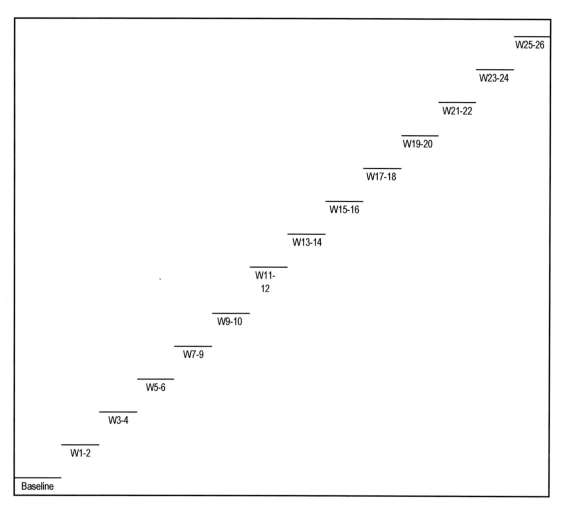

On the bottom of the stairs write down your present level of cardiovascular fitness in numerical terms (e.g., the number of continuous minutes you are exercising, distance covered, laps completed, etc. On the top of the stairs, write down what you would like to accomplish in 6 months. On the 2nd step to the bottom write down your first short-term goal and what you would like to accomplish within the next two weeks. When you reach your first short-term goal, proceed to the next step above and set your next short-term goal and so on until you reach your long-term goal. If at any time you are having difficulty reaching your short-term goals, return to Chapter 3 and review the section entitled "Exercise Barriers and Solutions.

Figure 6.6—My Stairway to Success

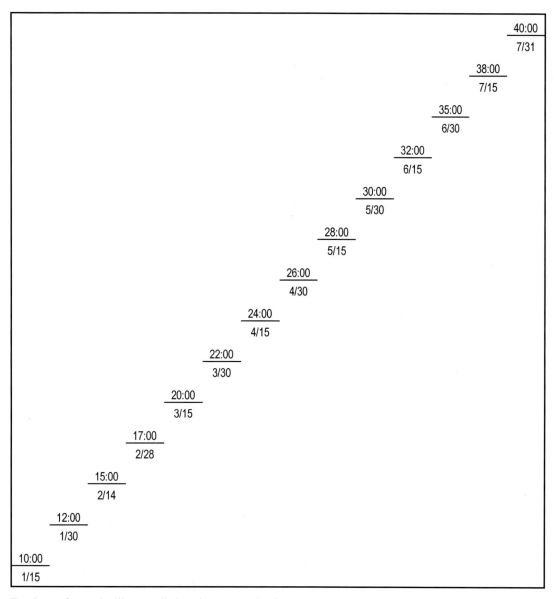

For those of you who like to walk, here is an example of how to use your stairway to success to set short-term and long-term goals to improve your CRE through walking. Mae is a middle-aged woman who performed an informal CRE assessment of walking for 10 minutes on 1/15. Her long-term goal is to be able to walk for 40 minutes. Using the stairway to success, Mae has set goals to improve a few minutes every two weeks. By July 15, Mae will be able to reach her goal of walking 40 minutes (and she'll do it walking faster and more comfortably, too)!

Figure 6.6—Stairway to Success Based on 10-Minute Walk

At the conclusion of this chapter, you will be able to set your own SMAART and Staircase goals which will help you to improve your CRF and increase your motivation to not only get fit, but stay fit, too. At this time, you are invited to review Chapter 3 and use the weekly goal sheets (in a SMAART way of course.). A copy of the weekly goal and the stairway to success goal sheets are included in Appendix 6A and Appendix 6B for you to use for your CRE program.

APPLYING THE PRINCIPLES OF FITNESS INTO YOUR CRF PROGRAM

Now that you have determined your level of CRF and commitment to begin working on your CRE, it is time to apply the principles of conditioning into your exercise program. This will help you design a program that will guarantee that you will improve your current level of CRE and enjoy the entire process (well, most of the time)!

Warm Up Principle—Whatever aerobic activity you choose for your CRF program, you will need to warm up by using that or a similar activity at a lower intensity. For example, if you plan to run, then warm up by walking briskly or jogging slowly for a few minutes. Once you feel your body has warmed up then you can begin to do a few dynamic stretches for a few minutes. This will prepare you to overload and improve your cardiorespiratory endurance system. (See Chapter 8 for a list of flexibility exercises to consider for your warm up).

Principle of Progression—When you review your exercise prescription for CRE, you should see systematic increases in any combination of frequency, intensity and time. Time should be increased first, followed by either intensity or frequency (whichever motivates you more) since it is a lot easier to add on a few more minutes once you have gotten started than it is to find an extra day to exercise or make yourself go harder than you may be used to. Once you achieve 30 minutes of aerobic activity, you can plan to increase intensity (e.g., running a few seconds faster per mile; going from level 1 to 2 on the stationary bicycle; walking up and down hills) provided you stay within your target heart rate or add an extra day to your weekly workout schedule.

Principle of Individuality—Your CRE exercise prescription should be based on your level of CRF and commitment. Therefore, you should be prescribing aerobic activities that you like to do rather than what someone else wants you to do. In addition, the length of time you exercise and the intensity that you work at should be based on your own CRF level and not someone else. So stick to the exercise prescription that's designed just for you.

Principle of Recuperation—Make sure that you do not overdo it and give yourself enough rest to recuperate from your exercise overload. If your CRF level is low then you should rest at least one and preferably two days in between workouts. If your CRF level is moderate than you should rest every other day or every third day and if your CRF level is high, then you give yourself at least one, preferably two or even three of days rest if your workouts exceed 60 minutes. Most important, you should always listen to your body. It is always better to take an extra day's rest and feel ready for your next workout than to overwork yourself by exercising too many days in a row resulting in feeling sluggish, tired and sore. See Figure 6.7 to see how you can incorporate the POR into your CRE program based on your present level of fitness and commitment to exercise 2-5 days per week.

Principle of Fun—You can make exercise fun by incorporating activities that you like to do directly into your workout. So, if you like to listen to music then plan to use your CD, MP3, IPOD or radio while exercising. If you like to exercise with a partner than invite someone you know to exercise with you, join a gym or take an exercise class that appeals to you and look to meet someone in class whose interests and workout schedules match yours. If you like to exercise alone then find a quiet time in the gym or another place that is unoccupied or spacious to exercise like parks or trails. Once you blend what is fun for you into your exercise routine, you will look forward to and enjoy working out more.

Principle of Reversibility—Another way of stating the principle of reversibility is "use it or lose it." To avoid this principle you must stick to your exercise routine. Based on your level of commitment, you have decided how many days per week you will exercise. To keep you on task, you should write down your exercise schedule at the beginning of every week. Include day, time, length, activity, and facility into your day planner. Make a copy of it and place it in areas that you frequent such as your car, office desk, locker, book bag and cell phone and stick to it. This way you won't have to worry about reversing what you have gained. You can use Figure 6.7 to help you.

CRE	Day 1	Day 2	Day 3	Day 4	Day 5	Day 6	Day 7
Low CRE 2× @ WK	EXERCISE	REST	REST	REST	EXERCISE	REST	REST
Low CRE 3× @ WK	EXERCISE	REST	EXERCISE	REST	EXERCISE	REST	REST
Low CRE 3× @ WK	EXERCISE	REST	REST	EXERCISE	REST	EXERCISE	REST
Mod CRE 3× @ WK	EXERCISE	REST	EXERCISE	REST	REST	EXERCISE	REST
Mod CRE 4× @ WK	EXERCISE	EXERCISE	REST	REST	EXERCISE	EXERCISE	REST
MOD CRE 4× @ WK	EXERCISE	REST	EXERCISE	EXERCISE	REST	EXERCISE	REST
High CRE 4× @ WK	EXERCISE	REST	EXERCISE	EXERCISE	REST	EXERCISE	REST
High CRE 5× @ WK	EXERCISE	EXERCISE	REST	EXERCISE	EXERCISE	REST	EXERCISE
High CRE 5× @ WK	EXERCISE	EXERCISE	EXERCISE	REST	EXERCISE	EXERCISE	REST

Figure 6.7—Incorporating the Principle of Recuperation into Your CRE Program

EVALUATING THE SUCCESS OF YOUR CRE PROGRAM

After your first week has been completed, it is now time to evaluate the success of your program. Did you reach your goals and exercise the number of times per week and minutes you committed to? Do you think you have more energy to exercise longer in this upcoming week? Are the workouts getting a little easier? If you answered "YES" to all of these questions then you are ready to set new goals and move on to week 2. If you answered "NO" to any of these questions, it is time to identify what stopped you. Did you not reach your goals because the goals were too hard? If so, you should probably consider modifying your goals and make them a little more realistic to your present CRF level and commitment. Perhaps you need to reduce the frequency by a day or the time by a few minutes. If you didn't reach your goal, but improved, you may just be a workout or two away so keep the same goal for next week and write down a strategy for how you will reach your goal and stick to it. Perhaps you did not reach your goal because you were lazy or maybe you just didn't feel like you had the energy or desire to exercise? For whatever the reason, be aware that something "stopped you." Now determine what your action plan is for next week. Incorporate specific strategies that will help you to stay on task and overcome what stopped you from reaching your goal(s) last week. For example, write down your SMAART goal(s), the days and time(s) you plan to exercise, what exercises you will do, how long you will exercise for, where you plan to exercise and how you plan to make your workouts fun and something you look forward to doing. Remember, striving to reach your goal will only help you to enjoy the exercise more. Most important, it will remind you that you are committed to getting fit and staying fit for life (what a catchy name for an exercise class).

Hopefully by now you realize how much control you have over your own progress. You discovered how cardiovascularly fit you were, how committed you were to improving and what you were actually going to do in your workouts. Then you set a SMAART goal and evaluated your success. You came up with strategies to motivate yourself and stay on task and this should have enhanced your desire to continue exercising in upcoming weeks. If at any time you get stopped over the next few weeks and thereafter, all you need to do is re-examine your exercise prescription along with your perceptions of what stopped you. Then incorporate the strategies that make it more fun for you to continue and increase your commitment level. Once you make the commitment to have fun and improve, you will. Do you see how simple it is!

Regardless of what exercises you choose to do to improve your CRE, it is important to chart your results and monitor your progress. This will help you to determine if you are improving and what you can do to maximize your progress (e.g., add minutes, add days per week, increase speed or level). Please review the Appendices at the end of this chapter for Cardiovascular Endurance Workout Cards and Goal Sheets that can assist you in monitoring your workouts.

HOW TO PREVENT INJURIES WHILE ENGAGING IN CRE ACTIVITIES

The best way to deal with injuries is not to get them so follow these basic guidelines towards an injury free exercise routine.

1. ***Consult Your Physician***—Before embarking on your CRE exercise program it is recommended that you consult your physician and discuss your desire to begin exercising especially if you are over 40 or you have been diagnosed with certain preexisting conditions such as arthritis, asthma, tendonitis, heart condition, diabetes or epilepsy.

2. ***Warm up first***—Before beginning your CR exercise, you should warm up your muscles in the same or similar way you plan to overload them just at a lower intensity. So, if you plan to go for a run, then you should warm up by walking and jogging lightly for a few minutes. Then, proceed to stretch your muscles and then you will be ready to run.

3. ***Start out slowly***—Sometimes we want to get fit quick and overdo it by working out too intensely or too long. We may push ourselves beyond our normal capacity resulting in excessive soreness and possible injury. So start out slowly and listen to your body. If you are feeling excessive tension or you are getting out a breath then stop. These are signs that you may be doing too much, too soon and increasing your chances of injury.

4. ***Select the right shoes***—Select a shoe that is designed for the exercise you plan to do. Try the shoe on in a store that specializes in the activities that you do. Then walk or jog with it on to make sure that it feels comfortable. Inform the shoe specialist about your activities (e.g., walking, jogging, running, aerobic dance, bicycling, stair climbing, cross training), your planned exercise program (e.g., days per week, # of miles walking or running per week, etc.), desired exercise facility (e.g., at home indoors, local gym, outdoor park), and surface being exercised on (e.g., treadmill, grass, track, street, hardwood floor). Examine your feet to see if you step straight or curved inward or outward. You want to make sure that the shoe provides ample support and comfort in the working areas (e.g., heel, arch, ball of foot, toe).

5. ***Cool down***—After you complete your workout, your body may be tired and your muscles may feel a little tight. Therefore, you should cool down by walking slowly for a few minutes and then stretch using static or passive static stretches to alleviate any excessive tension created from your exercise overload. (See Chapter 8 for a list of static and passive static stretches that you can do after a workout).

6. ***Exercising in the Heat and Cold***—Exercising in hot weather can cause cramping, dehydration, heat exhaustion and heat stroke. To avoid this, you should make sure you are hydrated by drinking 10 to 20 ounces of water or a lightly salted liquid (e.g., Gatorade) about 15-30 minutes before exercising and every 15 minutes while exercising. In addition, on days that you are planning to exercise, you should increase your daily water/fluid consumption prior to exercising to make sure that you are appropriately hydrated. You should wear a hat or bandana to cover your head from the sun and your

clothes should be light and comfortable. In hot weather, avoid wearing sweat suits or long-sleeved shirts as this will only increase body temperature. In cold weather, it is important to protect yourself from getting hypothermia or frostbite. Therefore, you should wear layers of clothing and protect exposed areas by keeping them covered. Wear gloves or mittens to cover your hands and thick athletic socks to keep your feet warm. Wear a hat to cover your head and ears and in extreme cold and windy conditions you should consider a scarf or ski mask to protect your face.

7. ***Learn proper form***—Sometimes injury can be caused by improper form/technique (e.g., length of your stride, how your feet hit the ground, the way you balance yourself). Therefore, before beginning your exercise program, become familiar with the proper form. If necessary, practice a few times and examine your form to see if it is correct. If you are having trouble then you should consider consulting with a qualified exercise professional as well as reading books that explain how to do the activities you have chosen properly.

This chapter has introduced cardiorespiratory endurance and explains the importance of being aerobically fit. A variety of CRE assessments, both formal and informal, based on one's level of CRF (low-moderate-high) are presented. In addition, exercise prescriptions are included and integrated based on CRF as well as level of commitment. Principles of fitness are reintroduced to help you improve your present level of CRF. Finally, strategies to prevent injuries are introduced to help you exercise safely.

REVIEW QUESTIONS

1. Define cardiorespiratory endurance.
2. Explain the differences between a fit vs. an unfit heart.
3. List at least eight physical and psychological benefits of being CR fit.
4. What is the purpose of assessing your CR fitness?
5. List three ways you can formally assess your CRE and explain the strengths and limitations of each.
6. What is an informal assessment and explain when it is beneficial to use this methodology to assess CR fitness?
7. Define the four components of an exercise prescription and include an example of each.
8. Discuss two ways you can measure the exercise intensity for CRE activities.
9. What strategies do you have planned to prevent the principle of reversibility from occurring?

10. Explain how you have been overloading your CRE from weeks 1 to 4.

11. Discuss how you would determine if your CR fitness program was successful?

12. Describe how you can incorporate the principles of progression, specificity, individuality, warm up, recuperation, reversibility, and fun into a CRF program.

13. What strategies can you incorporate to reduce and prevent the chances of injuries from CR exercise?

LAB ASSIGNMENT 6.1

Questions 1-9 should be answered prior to beginning your CR fitness program.

1. How committed are you to improving your CR fitness over the next 4 weeks? If you have a low level of commitment, what strategies will you incorporate to increase your level of commitment?

2. What are your SMAART goals for improving your CRE over the next 4 weeks?
   A. _____
   B. _____
   C. _____

3. Using the Stairway to Success, convert your SMAART goals into stairway goals over the next four weeks.

                                                             _____

                                   _____

                     _____

       _____

4. Develop an exercise prescription to improve your CR fitness over the next four weeks.

	Week 1	Week 2	Week 3	Week 4
F				
I				
T				
T				

5. Explain how you will be progressing in CR fitness from weeks 1 to 4?

6. Describe how you plan to incorporate the principle of recuperation into your CR fitness program?

7. What do you plan to do to satisfy the warm up principle?

8. What strategies are you considering to incorporate the principle of fun?

9. What strategies do you plan to prevent the principle of reversibility?

Questions 10-14 should be answered at the conclusion of each week.

10. Explain how you have been overloading your CR endurance system from Weeks 1-2-3-4?

11. How has your recuperation time changed from weeks' 1-4?

12. How successful were you in preventing the principle of reversibility? Be specific!

13. How much have your improved from weeks' 1-4?

14. If you did not have fun, first explain why and then discuss what you plan to do to make your CR workouts more fun for next week (e.g., music, working out with a partner, setting SMAART goals, etc.).

REFERENCES

American College of Sports Medicine.com (2005).

Blair, S.N., Kohl III, W., Paffenbarger, Jr., R.S., Clark, D.G., Cooper, K.H., & Gibbons, L.W. (1998). Physical fitness and all-cause mortality: A prospective study of healthy men and women. *Journal of the American Medical Association, 262*, 2395-2401.

Borg G. (1998). Borg's perceived exertion and pain scales. Champaign, IL, Human Kinetics.

Burton, W.N., McCalister, K.T., Chen, C.Y & Edington, D.W. (2005). The association of health status, worksite fitness center participation, and two measures of productivity. *Jorunal of Occupational and Environmental Medicine. 47*, 4, 343-351.

Fahey, T.D., Insel, P.M., & Roth, W.T. (2005). Applying the FITT Equation pp 68 in Fit and well: Core concepts and labs in physical fitness and wellness. 6th edition, McGraw Hill. Griest, J.H., Klein, M.H., Eischens, R.R., & Faris, J.T. (1978). Running out of depression. *Physician and Sportsmedicine, 6*, 49-56.

Frey, M. (2016). www.verywell.com/what-is-cardiorespiratory-endurance-34...

Lox, C.L., Martin Ginis, K.A., Petruzzello, S.J. (2006). Health-related quality of life and exercise, pp, 389-415, in C.L. Lox, K.A. Martin Ginis, & S.J. Petruzello, *The Psychology of exercise: Integrating theory and practice,* (pp. 389-415) 2nd edition, Holcomb Hathaway Publishers

Morgan, W.P. (1997). Physical activity and mental health. Washington, DC: Taylor & Francis. Morgan, W.P., & Goldston, S.E. (1987). Exercise and mental health. Washington, DC: Hemisphere.

Otto, M. & Smits, J.A.(2011). *Exercise for mood and anxiety, proven strategies for overcoming depression and enhancing well-being.* Oxford University Press.

Pate, R.R., Pratt, M., Blain, S.N., Haskell, W.L., Macera, C.A., Bouchard, C., Buckner, D., Ettinger, W., Heath, G. W., King, A.C., Kriska, A., Leon, A.S., Marcus, B.H., Morris, J., Paffenbarger, R.S., Jr., Patrick, P., Pollock, M.L., Rippe, J.M., Sallis, J., & Wilmore, J.H. (1995). Physical activity and public health. *Journal of the American Medical Association, 273,* 402-407.

Pollack, M.L., Rippe, J.M., Sallis, J., & Wilmore, J.H. (1995). Physical activity and public health. *Journal of the American Medical Association, 273,* 402-407.

Robinson, L., Segal, J., & Smith J. (2017). The mental health benefits of exercise: The exercise prescription for depression, anxiety, stress and more. www.helpguide.org/articles/exercise-fitness/emotional-benefits-of-exercise.html

Ryan, A.J. (1983). Exercise is medicine. Physician and Sportsmedicine, 11, 10. United States Department of Health and Human Services, 1996. Physical activity and health: A report of the Surgeon General. Report DHHS publication no. (PH5) 017-023-00196-5. Atlanta: U.S. Department of Health and Human Services, Centers for Disease Control and Prevention, National Center for Chronic Disease Prevention and Health Promotion.

Sharifzadeh, M. (2013). Does fitness and exercise increase productivity? Assessing fitness and productivity relationship. *American Journal of Management, 13,* 1, 32-52.

United States Department of Health and Human Services, 1996. Physical activity and health: A report of the Surgeon General. Report DHHS publication no. (PH5) 017-023-00196-5, Atlanta, U.S. Department of Health and Human Services, Center for Disease Control and Prevention, National Center for Chronic Disease Prevention and Health Promotion.

www.cancer.gov/new-events-press-release/2012.

APPENDIX 6A
WEEKLY GOAL SHEET FOR CRE

Name _____ Date: _____

Select 1-2 goals that will help you improve your CRE. Write down your goal(s) in the "Goal(s) Selected" column next to the category of goal that you have selected. Using the 7 Day Chart down below, record each day's workout next to the appropriate activity and under the actual day. After the week is up, add up your total workout performances and put them in the "Performance Results" column. If you achieved you weekly goal, mark an "A" across from your goal category in the "Achieved" column. If you did not reach your goal, mark an "NA" across from you goal category and under the "Not Achieved" column.

Category of Goals to Select From	Goal(s) Selected	Performance Results	Achieved = A	Not Achieved = NA
CRE Goals				
Frequency of Weekly Workouts				
Time in Minutes Exercised for Week				
Activity Selected				
Run / Walk				
Bicycle				
Elyptical				
Rowing				
Stairmaster				
Other				

	Day 1	Day 2	Day 3	Day 4	Day 5	Day 6	Day 7
CRE							
Run/Walk							
Bicycle							
Elyptical							
Rowing							
Stairmaster							
Other							

Name _____ Date: _____

APPENDIX 6B
STAIRWAY TO CRE SUCCESS

6-MONTH CRE STAIRWAY TO SUCCESS

Name _____ Date: _____

APPENDIX 6C
CARDIOVASCULAR ENDURANCE WORKOUT CARD

Date	Activity	Time	Distance	Level	HRAR	HRRL	Total Minutes	Total Distance
GOAL								

Chapter 7

Developing an Exercise Prescription for Muscular Fitness

OBJECTIVES

After this chapter, you will be able to:

- Define muscular fitness and distinguish between muscular strength & muscular endurance
- Understand the benefits of being muscularly fit
- Assess your muscular fitness safely
- Develop an exercise prescription for muscular fitness
- Determine your level of commitment to being muscularly fit
- Spice up your muscular fitness program
- Incorporate principles of fitness into your muscular fitness program
- Evaluate the success of your muscular fitness program
- Learn how to minimize and prevent injuries while engaging in muscular fitness activities
- Have fun while working on your muscular fitness

Over the past thirty years, the popularity of weight training has grown tremendously with more men and women participating in weight training programs in both public and private exercise facilities than ever before.

At one time, however, weight training was viewed as a masculine activity, designed to help people "bulk up" or increase their muscular size. This decreased interest for many people, specifically women who were simply motivated to shape their bodies by firming and defining their muscles, yet not increase their muscular size. Consequently, there were less women enrolling in weight training classes and participating in the weight rooms of local exercise facilities. While this common misconception still exists today, more and more people have become educated about the benefits of muscular fitness, particularly, weight training. Specifically, they have learned that the hormonal differences between men and women do not allow women to gain muscular size in the same way that men do. Men have more testosterone which is a growth producing hormone and one of the main factors in producing increases

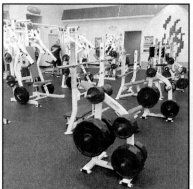 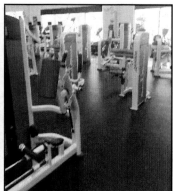

Free Weights   *Weight Training Machines*

in muscular size. So, not only will women not bulk up, those who choose to participate in weight training will notice better shape in their muscles (Hesson, 2007). Just remember, weight training is equally beneficial for men and women. In this chapter, you will learn how to assess your muscular strength and endurance and design a muscular fitness (MF) program that clearly meets your needs (e.g., body shape, tone and define muscles, improve strength and build muscle and/or increase muscular size). You will become an educated consumer and learn how to weight train safely and productively so that you can do what is best for you! Ready! Set! Lift your fingers to the next page and let's get started.

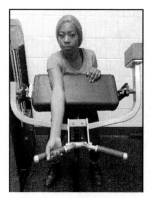 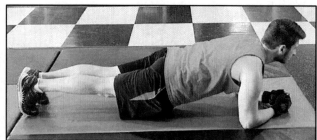

One Arm Preachers   *Planks*

WHAT IS MUSCULAR FITNESS?

Muscular Fitness consists of two components of health-related fitness: (1) muscular strength and (2) muscular endurance. ***Muscular strength*** is the ability of the muscles to generate maximum force. For example, you are working on your muscular strength when you are lifting heavy weights that can only be done for a few reps or if you are carrying heavy objects that you can only hold for a short period of time before your muscle(s) fatigue. ***Muscular endurance*** is the ability of a muscle to produce submaximal force repeatedly over time by contracting the muscles or holding a contraction for a long period of time. An example of muscular endurance is performing many repetitions of an exercise (e.g., 20 crunches) or holding a package for several minutes. While muscular strength and endurance are interrelated, training for each is somewhat different. Specifically, if you want to develop muscular strength, then you should lift heavier weights for less reps (e.g., 2-8 reps per set or 70%-90% of your 1-rep max) and if you want to develop muscular endurance, then you should lift lighter weights for more repetitions (12-20 reps per set or 50% -60% of your 1-rep max). Finally, if you want to develop both muscular strength and endurance then you should lift a moderate amount of weight that you can do for 8-12 repetitions or 60%-70% of your one-rep max for each set.

BENEFITS OF MUSCULAR FITNESS TRAINING (MFT)

There are many benefits to MFT. The key is to find the one(s) that attract(s) you most towards getting started and improving your MF. Listed below are 11 different benefits that can be achieved from MFT.

1. ***Reduced rate of injury***—As your muscles get stronger, they are more resistant to fatigue and will not break down as easily. This will decrease your susceptibility to getting injured.

2. ***Reduced rate of low back problems***—One of the main causes of back problems is having weak back and abdominal muscles. MFT will help to strengthen these areas and reduce and possibly even prevent back problems.

3. ***Reduced risk of Osteoporosis***—Improving strength with increase bone density and make you less prone to bone fractures and weak bones.

4. ***Weight control***— One of the main reasons why people are interested in MFT is to change the way their body looks. For those of you who want to lose body fat, working on MF will help you increase your metabolism and burn off "fat weight" while you develop, shape, and strengthen your muscles. For those of you who want to gain weight, it is important to note that muscle weighs more than fat (although it takes up a lot less space). By working on increasing your muscular strength, you will increase your muscle mass and gain "muscle weight." In both scenarios, you are striving to maintain your proper body weight through MFT.

5. ***Improved athletic performance***—Many sport teams employ strength and conditioning coaches to help their athletes build muscular strength and endurance, speed and power which aid in improving athletic performance across a wide variety of sports.

6. ***Improved recreational performance***—All recreational activities require some degree of muscular fitness. When you have poor levels of either muscular strength, endurance or both, it limits your ability to successfully perform in many activities that involve the following movements: (1) walking; (2) jogging; (3) running; (4) sprinting; (5) jumping; (6) throwing; (7) kicking; Increasing your muscular fitness can improve your per-

formance in these areas and quite possibly increase your enjoyment to participate and be more physically active, too.

7. ***Better quality of life***—As a result of being muscularly fit, you will be able to accomplish more on a daily basis without getting tired (e.g., lifting heavy objects; carrying your books around all day; walking up and down stairs; Having more energy means more productivity which will make you feel better and improve the quality of your life.

8. ***Increase self-esteem & self-confidence***—Your confidence will increase as you see improvements in your MF workouts (i.e., performing more reps, sets, exercises, increasing the amount of weight you lift). Yesterday's hard workout becomes today's easier workout. You will challenge yourself to conquer new and exciting goals (e.g., getting to the next weight, adding a few more reps, learning a new exercise) as your early hesitation about muscular fitness training has now been replaced with a strong belief that you can accomplish whatever you set your mind and body towards.

9. ***Looking better***—Working on your MF will develop, shape and define your muscles, which will make you look and feel better about yourself.

10. ***Manage stress and anxiety better***——Making the commitment to build up your MF and challenging yourself to improve will help to take your mind off of daily stressors. When you begin to see and feel the results, it will decrease the anxiety that often confronts you when you are not taking good care of yourself. In chapter 12, you will learn more about identifying your stressors and using exercises as a way to cope with and eventually get rid of unwanted stress in your life.

11. ***Improve health and slow down the aging process***—As you improve your MF, your health will improve, too. Your muscles will become stronger and the natural aging process will slow down which can prevent certain illnesses from occurring. What a great feeling to get older and feel younger!

ASSESSING YOUR MUSCULAR FITNESS

Although muscular strength and endurance are related, the ways they are measured and trained for are different. This section provides information about how to assess your muscular strength and endurance.

Assessing Muscular Strength

The most common way to assess your muscular strength is with a 1-rep max test. This involves lifting the heaviest amount of weight you can for one repetition (rep) and only one rep. For example, let's say you want to find out how strong your legs are so you go over to the Leg Press and lift 200 lbs. If you can do more than one rep, then you would raise the weight until you could no longer lift one complete rep. The heaviest weight that you can successfully lift for one rep represents your "max" and your true muscular strength for that exercise/muscle group.

Procedure for the One-Rep Max Test

1. Familiarize yourself with the equipment (proper sitting positions, lying down or standing positions, appropriate range of motion, use of bars, handles or cables).
2. Select 1-2 exercises that work the major muscle groups of the body (See Table 7.1 for a list of exercises to max on).

Table 7.1

Exercises to Max On

Chest	Back	Shoulders
Free Weight Bench Press	Lat Pull Down	Rear Deltoid
Isolateral Bench Press or Chess Press	Low Row	Shoulder Press
Seated Fly Machine	T Bar/Incline Row	
Legs	**Triceps**	**Biceps**
Leg Press	Tricep Pull Down	Barbell Curl
Leg Curl	Tricep Extension	Preacher Curl
Leg Extension		

3. Learn proper form by practicing a few times with a low or minimal amount of weight. If performing the max test is part of a class requirement (e.g., weight training, physical conditioning, fitness for life) then one class should be devoted to practicing and the next class to max testing. (See Table 7.2 for a list and explanation of common mistakes and corrections of popular resistance training exercises and view pictures of these exercises.
4. Have a spotter with you to make sure you are performing each exercise safely and correctly.
5. Warm up first by lifting a light amount of weight for 8-12 reps.
6. Proceed to raising the weight and lifting for one repetition.
7. If successful, continue to lift the heaviest amount of weight that you can for only one repetition.
8. Record your results on your Muscular Fitness Assessment Form located in Appendix 7A).

Muscular endurance can be assessed by performing the maximum number of repetitions of a submaximal resistance or by the length of time a person can hold a contraction (e.g., flexed arm hang) (Hoeger & Hoeger, 2005). For example, if you maxed 100 lbs. on the bench press, how many reps of 50 lbs. (50% of your max) can you perform? How many push-ups can you do continuously without stopping or how long can you hang on a chin up bar? Some of the more popular exercises to assess your muscular endurance include: push-ups, sit ups and curl ups. (Use Appendix 7A to record your results on your Muscular Fitness Assessment Form).

SAFE AND UNSAFE WAYS TO LIFT WEIGHTS

Although lifting weights has been around for many years across a variety of settings (e.g., school gyms, military, sports, exercise facilities, local Y), proper form and technique have not always been emphasized. Consequently, many individuals have developed bad habits and use incorrect form resulting in a higher risk of injuries and decrease in productivity. Table 7.2 includes a list of popular resistance training exercises along with their common mistake(s) and correction(s). Figure 7.1 includes pictures of these exercises demonstrating both incorrect and correct form.

Table 7.2
Common Mistakes and Corrections of Popular Resistance Training Exercises

Exercise	Common Mistake	Correction
Free Weight Bench Press	Arching the back—creates stress on the lower and central parts of the back;	Place feet flat on the floor and keep back flat on the bench as you expand your chest;
Isolateral Bench Press	Lifting head up and/or tilting head forward creates stress on the neck, upper body and spinal column;	Keep your head flat on the bench so you can look straight up toward the ceiling with no tension on your neck;
	Lifting bar unevenly occurs when one side of the body is significantly stronger than the other. This can cause possible injury to the upper body.	Lift bar evenly by concentrating on the weaker side which will slow down the stronger/dominant side.
Seated Flys	Tilting head forward—creates stress in the neck, shoulders and upper back;	Keep head and back straight by resting up against the back cushion;
Lat-Pulldown	Arching back/leaning backwards—creates stress on the lower back;	Keep back straight throughout the lift;
	Bringing handles behind the neck—causes stress on the neck, upper back and spinal column.	Avoid using machines that place handles in the back of the neck and instead use machines that place handles in the front of the chest or use cables which are situated in the front of the shoulders.

Seated Row	Arching back on the exertion phase—causes stress on the lower back;	Lean forward on the resting phase and keep back straight up on the exertion phase and pull the handles toward your abdominal section keeping your shoulders back.
Shoulder Press	Leaning and tilting head forward—creates stress in the neck and upper back;	Keep hands in an upright position over your shoulders with your head and back aligned straight and resting on the back rest;
Leg Press	Moving too fast and locking knees on the exertion phase—causes excessive strain on the knees;	Proceed a little slower than usual on the exertion phase and extend your legs to a point where the knees remain slightly bent and never straightened;
Leg Extension	Moving too fast and locking knees—causes excessive strain on the knees;	Proceed slowly on the exertion phase and extend your legs to a point where knees remain slightly bent and never straightened;
Behind the Neck Squats	Knees Over Toes, leaning slightly forward – causes stress on the knees and back;	Sit back first with heels on the floor and knees behind toes;
Tricep Pulldown	Raising bar above your chest causes your elbows to move away from the sides of your body—allows your upper body to help you lift the weight, thus reducing the workload for the triceps;	Keep elbows next to your sides and bring the bar up slowly on the resting phase to chest height or slightly below;
Tricep Extension	Locking elbows-causes excessive strain on the elbows;	Proceed slowly on the exertion phase to the point where your arms are almost fully extended keeping elbows slightly bent;
Lying Tricep Extension	Extending bar away from back of the head – causes stress on the shoulders and lower back; Bending Wrists – creates strain on the wrist and assists in the lifting of the exercise;	Allow bar to move to the forehead or slightly behind the back of the head; Keep wrists locked and forward on the resting phase with palms facing upwards towards the ceiling;
Bicep Curls	Arching backwards on the exertion phase in order to complete the full range of motion which can cause excessive stress on the lower back;	Keep back straight throughout the lift and avoid leaning forward or backward; consider sitting on a utility bench or a swiss ball and focus on sitting upright and keeping your body weight centered;

Sit Up	Interlocking hands behind the neck causes stress on the neck and spinal column	Place fingers behind ears or cross arms in front of body with no space between elbows and body;
	Lifting buttocks off the ground – causes stress in lower back	Keep your buttocks on the ground at all times to stabilize the lower back; you can also keep your feet slightly off the ground to stabilize the lower back;
Crunches	Knees are over chest—this reduces the range of motion and significantly decreases the amount of tension in the abdominal muscles creating "less results."	Keep your knees over your hips and point your elbows toward the top of your knees with the ultimate goal to touch your knees with your elbows over your hips. This will create a greater range of motion and more tension on the upper abdominal section which creates "better results."
Push Ups	Raising buttocks too high prevents full range of motion and decreases tension thus producing less results;	Keep your shoulders, back, buttocks and legs in a straight line so chest and abdominal section can move comfortably down towards the ground.

Figure 7.1—Correct and Incorrect Ways to Perform Resistance Training Exercises

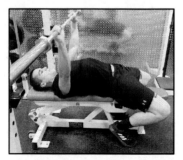

Bench Press Incorrect Form
Arching Back

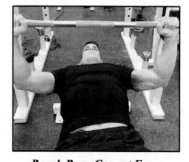

Bench Press Correct Form

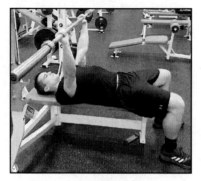

Bench Press Correct Form
Side Angle

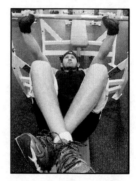

Bench Press Correct Form
Feet Up and Ankles Crossed

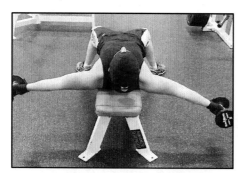

Dumbbell Flys Incorrect Form
Elbows Locked and Arms Below Shoulder
Height

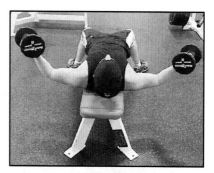

Dumbbell Flys
Correct Form

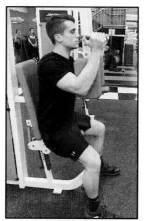

Seated Fly—Incorrect Form.
Leaning Forward

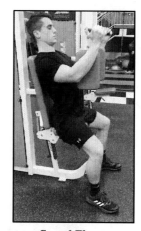

Seated Fly—
Correct Form

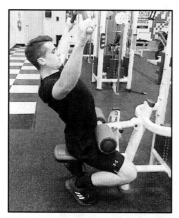

Lat Pulldown Incorrect Form.
Arching Back

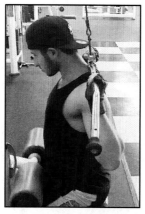

Lat Pulldown Incorrect
Form. Bar behind Neck
Side View

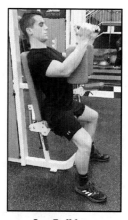

Lat Pulldown
Correct Form

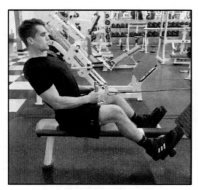
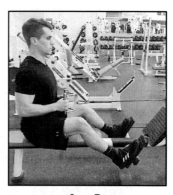

Low Row Incorrect Form
Arching Back

Low Row
Correct Form

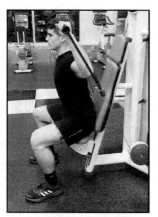
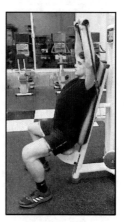

Shoulder Press Incorrect Form.
Leaning Forward

Shoulder Press
Correct Form

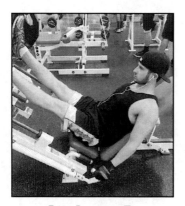
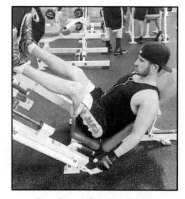

Press Incorrect Form
Knees Locked

Leg Press Correct Form

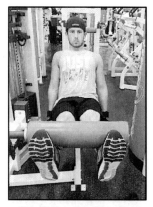 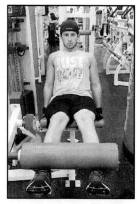

Leg Extension Incorrect Form. Knees Locked.	***Leg Extension Correct Form. Knees Slightly Bent***

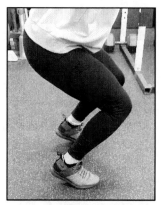 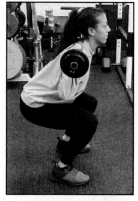

Behind-the-Neck Squats Incorrect Form. Weight on Toes. Knees over Toes.	***Behind-the-Neck Squats Correct Form. Sitting Back. Knees behind Toes.***

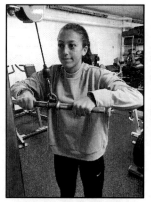 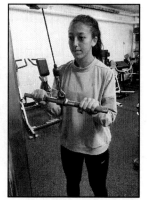

Tricep Pulldown Incorrect Form Elbows away from Body	***Tricep Pulldown Correct Form***

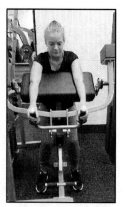 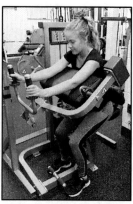

Tricep Extension Incorrect   *Tricep Extension Correct*
Form. Elbows Locked   *Form. Elbows bent.*

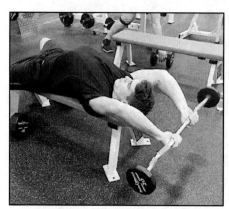 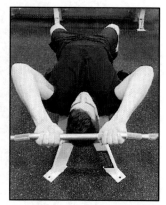

Lying Tricep Extension Incorrect Form.   *Lying Tricep Extension*
Bar Too Far Away from Head   *Correct Form*

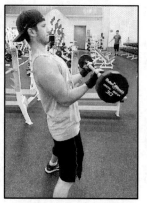 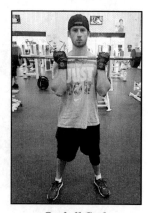

Barbell Curls Incorrect   *Barbell Curls*
Form. Arching Back   *Correct Form*

DEVELOPING AN EXERCISE PRESCRIPTION FOR MUSCULAR FITNESS (MF)

The four components of an exercise prescription for MF are identical to the ones introduced in Chapter 6 for CRE (F-I-T-T). However, the way you measure each component for MF is slightly different than for CRE.

Frequency—There are two ways to determine frequency of a MF program: (1) days per week you will work on MF and (2) days per week you will work on a specific muscle group. Generally, if you are doing a split routine then it is recommended that you work on each of the major muscle groups 1X per week. However, if you are doing a total body workout, then you should be working on each muscle group a minimum of 2X per week and preferably 3X-5X per week depending on your level of MF.

Intensity—Since MFT does not focus on overloading the heart, checking your HR will not define how hard you are working on your MF. Instead, intensity for MF is measured in one of two ways: (1) percent max or (2) range of reps being used. For example, if you wanted to work on your muscular strength and you maxed 100 lbs. on the seated fly machine, you would start with at least 70% of your max or 70 or more lbs. which would produce a range of 2-8 reps in a set.

Intensity can also be determined by the number of desired reps to be achieved. For example, if you want to body shape and tone your muscles, you would be striving to achieve 12-15 reps per set. Once you have achieved 15 reps in a given set, then you should raise the weight on the next set or next workout. If you cannot achieve 12 reps, the the weight is too heavy and you should lower the weight on the next set. See Table 7.3 for a description of proper intensity using both percent max and range of reps for muscular fitness training.

Table 7.3
Determining Proper Intensity for Muscular Fitness Training Using Percent Max and Desired Range of Reps

Type of Training	% Max	Desired Range of Reps	Recommendations
Muscular Strength	70% or greater	2-8	Increase weight once 8 reps are achieved in a set
Muscular Strength and Endurance	60%–70%	8-12	Increase weight once 12 reps are achieved in a set and decrease weight on next set if 8 reps cannot be achieved
Muscular Endurance "Body Toning"	50%–60%	12-15	Increase weight once 15 reps are achieved in a set and decrease weight if 12 reps cannot be achieved

Time—Typically, you would measure time by how long your workout lasts in terms of minutes or hours. However, with MF, minutes would not be appropriate measures of time since the majority of time spent during MFT is sitting down or resting in between sets. Moreover, expressing that you worked on MF for an hour doesn't explain what you have accomplished. Therefore, you should measure time by answering 5 basic questions:

1. What body parts will you work on today?
2. How many exercises will you do for each body part?
3. How many sets will you do for each exercise?
4. What is your range of reps for each exercise that you plan to do (e.g., 2-8, 8-12, 12-15)?
5. How much rest time will you take in between sets?

For example, let's say Josh wants to work on his legs and shoulders, today. He selected 3 exercises for each body part and he performed 2 sets of each exercise. Since he wants to work on his strength, he will be striving to lift 2-8 reps per set and take 90 seconds off in between sets to recuperate. His workout is complete when he finishes the last rep of his last set from his last exercise.

Type— addresses all of the exercises you will consider doing for each of the major muscle groups. Generally, exercises facilities will have three different types of resistance training equipment to choose from: (1) free weights; (2) plate loaded equipment and (3) selectorized equipment. Free weights come in the form of barbells and dumbbells. Plate loaded equipment include machines that are plate loaded with free weights and selectorized equipment are machines that have a stacked amount of weight where a pin is inserted into the slot of the desired amount of weight to be lifted.

Of course, the place you choose to work on your MF can play a significant role in the exercises you select (e.g., equipment available, crowdedness of facility). However, there is no one specific exercise that you have to do in order to improve a specific body part(s) and therefore it is a good idea to have a list of different exercises to choose from in the event that someone is using the equipment that you intended to use (i.e., bench press to dumbbell press; seated fly machine to dumbbell flys; barbell curls to dumbbell curls). See Table 7.4 for a list of muscular fitness exercises to choose from by body part and Figure 7.2 for pictures of these exercises.

Table 7.4
Muscular Fitness Exercises to Choose From

CHEST	BACK	SHOULDERS
Dumbbell Bench Press	Barbell Row	Barbell Upright Row
Universal Bench Press	One-arm Dumbbell Row	Dumbbell Upright Row
Decline Bench Press	Incline Dumbbell Row	Front Raises
Incline Bench Press	Lat Pulldown (See Exercise 3)	Lateral Raises
Decline Dumbbell Press	Low Row (See Exercise 4)	Bent Over Lateral Raises
Bent Arm Dumbbell Flys	High Row (See Exercise 5)	Shoulder Shrugs
Bent Arm Decline Flys	Hack Squat (See Exercise 6)	Dumbbell Press
Incline Dumbbell Flys		Shoulder Press (See Exercise 6)
Dumbbell Chest Press		Rear Deltoid (See Exercise 7)
Bench Press (See Fig 7.1 Exercise 1)		
Seated Fly (See Exercise 2)		

TRICEPS	BICEPS	LEGS
One Arm Tricep Extension	Barbell Curl	Dumbbell Lunges
Two Arm Tricep Extension	Hammer Curl	Wall Sit
Dip Machine	Seated Curl	Abductor
Bench Dips	Concentrations	Adductor
Lying Tricep Extension	Incline Dumbbell Curl	Leg Press (See Exercise 8)
Tricep Press	Alternating Dumbbell Curl	Leg Curl (See Exercise 9)
Lying Tricep Dumbbell Extension	Preacher Curl	Leg Extension (See Exercise 10)
Kickbacks	(See Exercise 14)	Hack Squat (See Exercise 11)
Tricep Pulldown (See Exercise 12)		
Tricep Extension (See Exercise 13)		

ABDOMINALS

Seeing Through Your Legs
Shoulders to the Sky
12-18's
Crossovers
Bicycles
SETK (Same Elbow to Knee)
Opposite Leg Raise
Sit Up
Touch My Toes Above
Reach My Toes
Climb the Rope
Crunches
Crossover Crunches
Standing Twists
Seated Twists
Squeeze Me

Figure 7.2—Pictures of Muscular Fitness Exercises to Choose From by Body Part

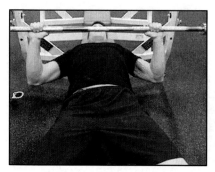

Bench Press Resting Phase

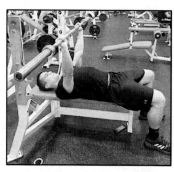

Bench Press Exertion Phase

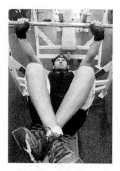

Bench Press Form. Feet up and ankles crossed for low back support

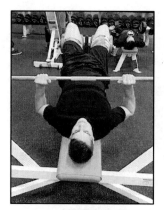

Decline Bench Press Resting Phase

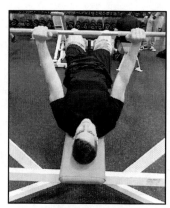

Decline Bench Press Exertion Phase

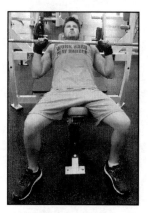

Incline Bench Press Resting Phase

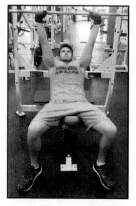

Incline Bench Press Exertion Phase

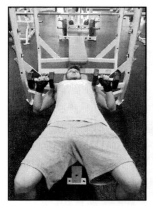

*Dumbbell Press
Resting Phase*

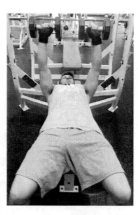

*Dumbbell Press
Exertion Phase*

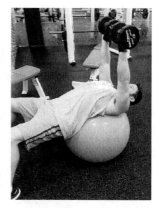

*Dumbbell Press on Ball.
Side Angle for additional
back support*

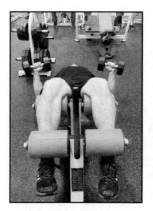

*Decline Dumbbell Press
Resting Phase*

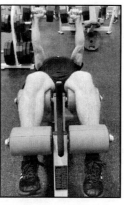

*Decline Dumbbell Press
Exertion Phase*

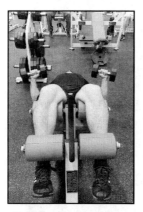

*Decline Dumbbell Press
Opposite View Resting
Phase*

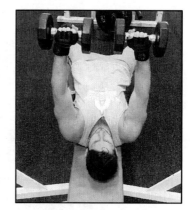

*Decline Dumbbell Press
Opposite View Exertion Phase*

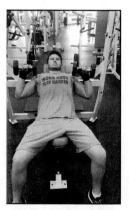 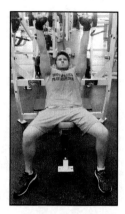

*Incline Dumbbell Press
Resting Phase*

*Incline Dumbbell
Press Exertion Phase*

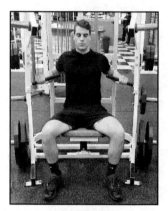 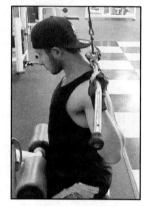

*Iso Lateral Press
Resting Phase*

*Iso Lateral Press
Exertion Phase*

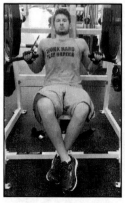 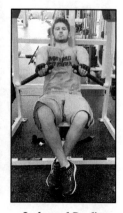

*Isolateral Decline Press
Resting Phase*

*Isolateral Decline
Press Exertion Phase*

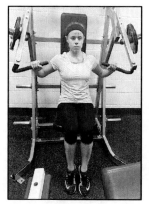 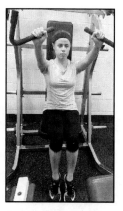

Isolateral Incline Press   *Isolateral Incline Press*
Resting Phase   *Exertion Phase*

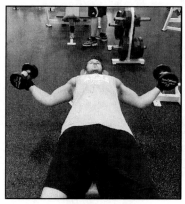 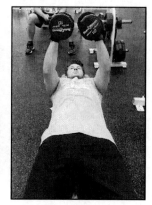

Dumbbell Flys   *Dumbbell Flys*
Resting Phase   *Exertion Phase*

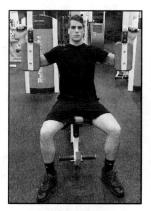 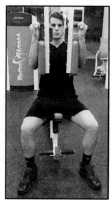

Seated Flys   *Seated Flys*
Resting Phase   *Exertion Phase*

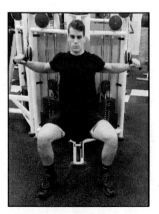
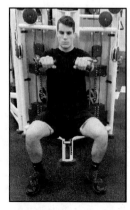

Chest Press Cables
Resting Phase

Chest Press Cables
Exertion Phase

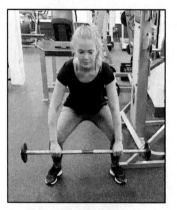
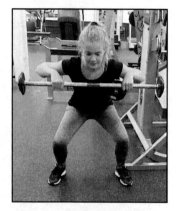

Barbell Row
Resting Phase

Barbell Row
Exertion Phase

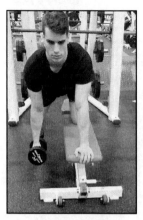
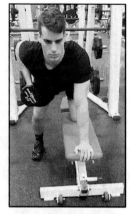

Bent Over One Arm
Dumbbell Row
Resting Phase

Bent Over One Arm
Dumbbell Row
Exertion Phase

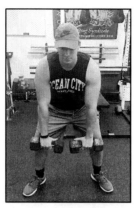 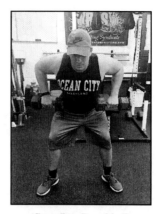

Standing Dumbbell Row Resting Phase   *Standing Dumbbell Row Exertion Phase*

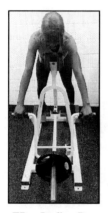 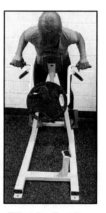 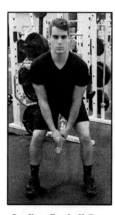 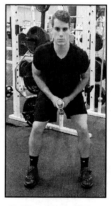

TBar Incline Row Resting Phase   *TBar Incline Row Exertion Phase*   *Incline Barbell Row Resting Phase*   *Incline Barbell Row Exertion Phase*

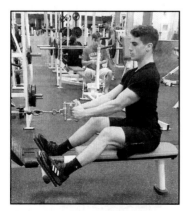 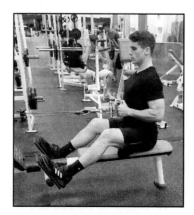

Low Row with Cables Resting Phase   *Low Row with Cables Exertion Phase*

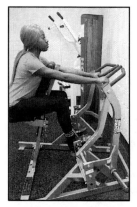
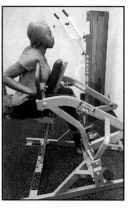
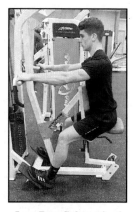
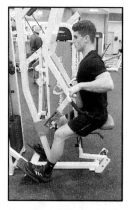

Low Row Plate Loaded Resting Phase   *Low Row Plate Loaded Exertion Phase*   *Low Row Selectorized Resting Phase*   *Low Row Selectorized Exertion Phase*

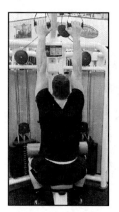
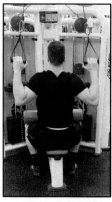
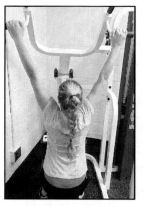
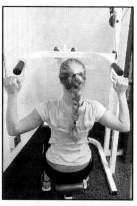

Lat Pulldown with Cables Resting Phase   *Lat Pulldown with Cables Exertion Phase*   *Lat Pulldown Selectorized Resting Phase*   *Lat Pulldown Selectorized Exertion Phased*

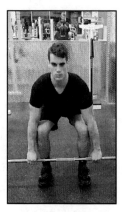
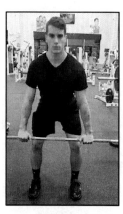

Deadlift Resting Phase   *Deadlift Exertion Phase*

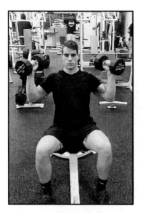
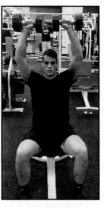
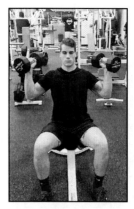
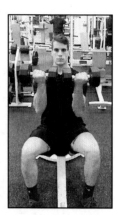

*Arnold Press
Extend Out*

*Arnold Press
Extend Up*

*Arnold Press
Bring Down*

*Arnold Press
Rotate In*

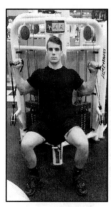
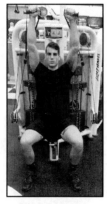
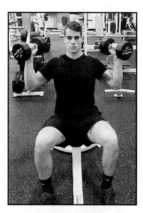
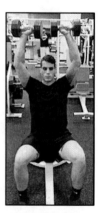

*Shoulder Press
with Cables
Resting Phase*

*Shoulder Press
with Cables
Exertion Phase*

*Shoulder Press
with Dumbbells
Resting Phase*

*Shoulder Press
with Dumbbells
Exertion Phase*

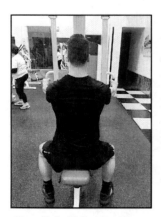
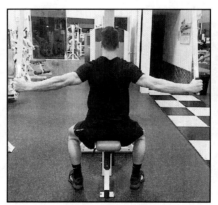
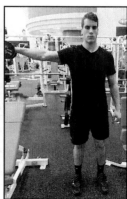

Rear Deltoid Resting Phase　　　*Rear Deltoid Exertion Phase*　　　*Lateral Raise*

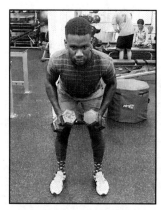

Standing Bent-over Lateral Raise
Resting Phase

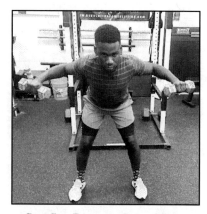

Standing Bent-over Lateral Raise
Exertion Phase

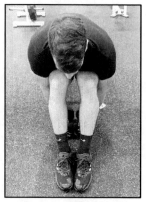

Seated Bent-Over Lateral
Raise Resting Phase

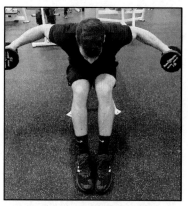

Seated Bent-Over Lateral Raise
Exertion Phase

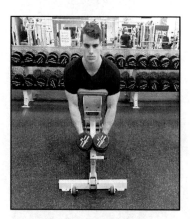

Incline Lateral Raise
Resting Phase

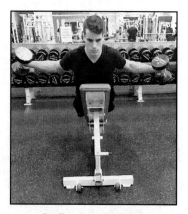

Incline Lateral Raise
Exertion Phase

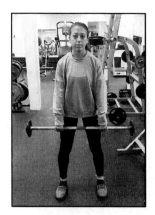 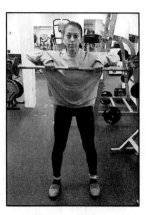 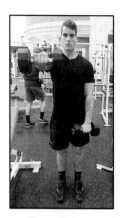

**Upright Row
Resting Phase**

**Upright Row
Exertion Phase**

Front Raise

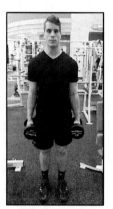 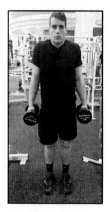

**Shoulder Shrugs
Resting Phase**

Shoulder Shrugs

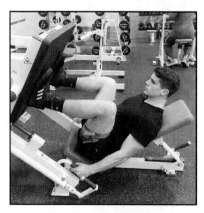 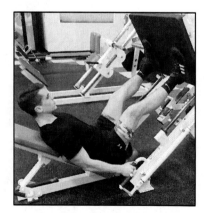

Leg Press Resting Phase

Leg Press Exertion Phase

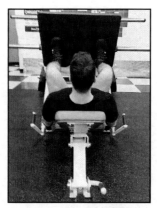 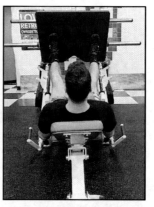

Leg Press Resting Phase   *Leg Press Exertion Phase*
Over the Top Angle   *Over the Top Angle*

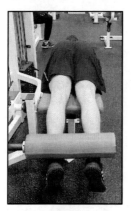 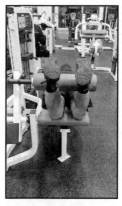

Leg Curl   *Leg Curl*
Resting Phase   *Exertion Phase*

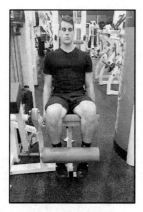 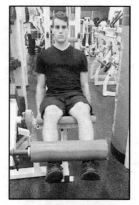

Leg Extension   *Leg Extension*
Resting Phase   *Exertion Phase*

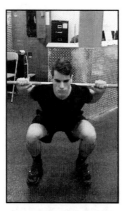 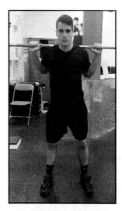

Behind the Neck Squat
Resting Phase

Behind the Neck Squat
Exertion Phase

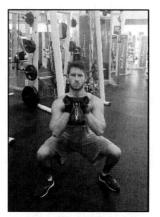 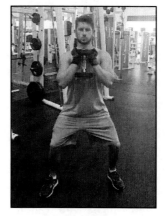

Front Squat
Resting Phase

Front Squat
Exertion Phase

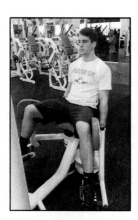 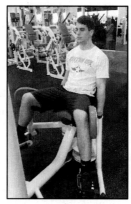 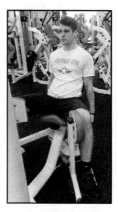 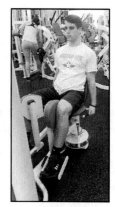

Abductor
Resting Phase

Abductor
Exertion Phase

Abductor
Resting Phase

Abductor
Exertion Phase

How Many Days Should I Work on Muscular Fitness?

Ideally, it is recommended that you work on MF two to five times per week. Of course, a lot depends on your level of MF. For example, if you are a beginner then it is probably best to start out with 1-2 days per week so you can you can get your body used to the demands of MFT. This will allow your mind to feel comfortable finding the days and time that fits best for you to start training. Now, if you want to progress to an intermediate level of MF then you should increase to 3X-4X times per week and if you are advanced then you should be training at least 4X per week. This will give you an opportunity to sufficiently overload each of the major muscle groups while also providing enough days in the week to rest and recuperate so you can be ready for next week's workouts. However, for those individuals who are only willing to commit one day per week towards working on MF, acknowledge yourself for getting started. While you may not see significant improvements in MF from only one day per week of training, you will certainly see some modest gains from where you started and you will be able to perform more reps, sets and exercises from one week to the next. Most important, you should notice how much better you feel particularly after you have completed your workout. Hopefully, this will motivate you to consider adding more day(s) per week in the future to achieve even greater gains in your MF and body composition. Moreover, once you find that second, third or possibly a fourth day, you will notice that the benefits far outweigh the limitations.

What Do I Want to Accomplish?

Muscular strength (MS) programs are designed for those individuals whose primary goals are to get stronger and increase their muscular size. Muscular endurance (ME) programs are designed for those individuals who want to shape and define their muscles without increasing muscular size. The combination programs (MSME) are designed for those individuals who want a little bit of everything (increases in MS and ME, body shape, tone, define muscles).

What type of MF workout do I want to do?

Once you have determined the frequency and intensity of your MF program, the next step is to choose the type of workout that you want to participate in. Generally, there are two different types of MF workouts: (1) Split Routine (SR) and (2) Total Body Workout (TBWO). A split routine is when you select different body parts to work on alternate days of the week. For example, working on Chest, Triceps and Shoulders on one day and Back, Biceps and Legs on another. A Total Body Work Out (TBWO) involves addressing all 6 major muscle groups (Chest, Back, Shoulders, Legs, Triceps & Biceps) in each days' workout. In the SR workout, you will be performing a series of different exercises for each muscle group/body part selected, however, in the TBWO you will only perform one exercise for each muscle group/body part and then change the exercises for each additional day that you plan to work on your MF. For both types of workouts, you can determine the number of sets per exercise based on your level of fitness and your range of reps based on your physical goals (MS, ME, MS & ME). Tables 7.5-7.8 are split routine workouts that display four different muscular fitness workouts based on the number of days per week that you commit to working on your MF. In addition, each workout includes three different programs based on your level of MF (e.g., beginner, intermediate, advanced). Table 7.9 includes a list of exercises for those of you interested in executing a TBWO from one to five days per week. Trust me, give this one a try.

Training for Muscular Fitness One Day Per Week

If you are planning to work on your MF one day per week then you should address all six of your major muscle groups in a TBWO. You can determine how many sets to do for each exercise based on your current level of MF. Please see Table 7.9 for a list of exercises to be used in a TBWO.

Training for Muscular Fitness Two Days Per Week

By adding a second day to your MFT, you will obviously accomplish more than working out one day per week. Rather than working all six major muscle groups in one day (chest, back, shoulders, legs, triceps, biceps), you can break down your workouts and focus on three different muscle groups for each workout. This is more common known as a **"Split Routine"** and there are two different ways to determine how to split up your muscle groups for each days' workouts. The first is the agonist-antagonist method which explains that whenever you contract a muscle "agonist" there is an opposing muscle group that must relax "antagonist." Therefore, when choosing an exercise that works a joint in one direction, you should also slect another exercise that works the joint in the opposite direction. For example, after working your Chest, you should work your Back. After working the Biceps, you should work the Triceps.

The second way to choose what exercises to work on is to pair a large muscle group with a related small muscle group. For example, when you are working your Chest, you are also working your Triceps and when you are working your Back, you are also working your Biceps. Therefore, it makes sense to group Chest with Triceps and Back with Biceps during a workout.

Remember, when you work your Triceps and Biceps, you do not have to perform as many sets of total work as you did with your larger muscle groups because the Triceps and Biceps are smaller and they will fatigue sooner and thus do not need as much work to overload them. For those of you interested in working the large muscle group with the related small (Chest-Tricep; Back-Bicep), please always remember that you work the large muscle group first. By working the large muscle group first, you are also working the related small muscle group, too. However, if you work the smaller muscle group first, it will fatigue sooner and not be able to be used efficiently. This will result in you not overloading the larger muscle group properly (chest, back and shoulders) and overworking the smaller muscle group (biceps and triceps). This end result is you will wind up lifting less weight than you should for the larger muscle group exercises and needing more time to recuperate the smaller muscle groups. Here are a few examples of workouts for you to consider using at two-day format of training.

Day 1	Day 2
Chest-Back-Shoulders	Triceps-Biceps-Legs
Chest-Back-Legs	Shoulders-Triceps-Biceps
Chest-Triceps-Shoulders	Back-Biceps-Legs
Chest Triceps-Legs	Shoulders-Back-Biceps

Training for Muscular Fitness Three Days Per Week

Adding a third day to your MFT will allow you to concentrate on two body parts per workout instead of three. This can help you create a greater overload for each body part by doing more exercises, sets and of course overall reps. Remember, a greater overload means greater results. Here are a few examples of workouts for each of the three days: Day 1 Chest-Back; Day 2 Shoulders-Legs; Day 3 Triceps-Biceps; Day 1 Chest-Triceps; Day 2 Back-Biceps; Day 3 Shoulder-Legs.

Day 1	Day 2	Day 3
Chest-Back	Shoulders-Legs	Triceps-Biceps
Chest-Triceps	Back-Biceps	Shoulders-Legs

Training Four Muscular Fitness Four Days Per Week

If you choose to work on your MF four days per week, you will begin to work one or two body parts per workout. One advantage of training more times per week is if you are pressed for time on a given day, your workouts can be completed in a shorter time span because you are working less body parts. Moreover, you may be able to accomplish more work on a given body part while also giving each muscle group a significant amount of time to recuperate. Here are a few examples of workouts for each of the four days:

Day 1	Day 2	Day 3	Day 4
Chest	Back	Legs-Shoulders	Triceps-Biceps
Chest-Back	Legs	Shoulders	Triceps-Biceps
Chest-Triceps	Legs	Shoulders	Triceps-Biceps
Back-Biceps	Legs	Chest-Triceps	Shoulders

Training for Muscular Fitness Five Days Per Week

If you choose to work on your MF five days per week, you will be performing a one-body part workout on four of those days and a two-body part workout on one day. There are multiple ways you can organize your workouts and here are a few examples. Just remember to give your smaller muscle groups enough time to recuperate in between workouts.

Day 1	Day 2	Day 3	Day 4	Day 5
Chest	Back	Legs	Shoulders	Triceps-Biceps
Back	Chest	Shoulders	Legs	Biceps-Triceps

Table 7.5
Training for Muscular Fitness Two Days Per Week Using Split Routine

	Week 1	Week 2	Week 3	Week 4
F	2	2	2	2
I - MS	70%-90% of 1-rep max or 2-8 reps per set	70%-90% of 1-rep max or 2-8 reps per set	70%-90% of 1-rep max or 2-8 reps per set	70%-90% of 1-rep max or 2-8 reps per set
I – MS & ME	60%-70% of 1-rep max or 8-12 reps per set	60%-70% of 1-rep max or 8-12 reps per set	60%-70% of 1-rep max or 8-12 reps per set	60%-70% of 1-rep max or 8-12 reps per set
I – ME	50%-60% of 1-rep max or 12-15 reps per set	50%-60% of 1-rep max or 12-15 reps per set	50%-60% of 1-rep max or 12-15 reps per set	50%-60% of 1-rep max or 12-15 reps per set
T	**Beginners** 2-3 exercises per body part; 2 sets per exercise	**Beginners** 3 exercises per body part; 2 sets per exercise	**Beginners** 3 exercises per body part; 2-3 sets per exercise	**Beginners** 3 exercises per body part; 2-3 sets per exercise
	Intermediate 3 exercises per body part; 3 sets per exercise	**Intermediate** 3-4 exercises per body part; 3 sets per exercise	**Intermediate** 3-4 exercises per body part; 3 sets per exercise	**Intermediate** 4 exercises per body part; 3 sets per exercise
	Advanced 4-6 exercises per body part; 4-6 sets per exercise Day 1 Chest-Triceps-Shoulders Day 2 Back-Biceps-Legs	**Advanced** 4-6 exercises per body part; 4-6 sets per exercise Day 1 Chest-Triceps-Shoulders Day 2 Back-Biceps-Legs	**Advanced** 5-6 exercises per body part; 4-6 sets per exercise Day 1 Chest-Back-Shoulder Day 2 Legs-Triceps-Biceps-	**Advanced** 5-6 exercises per body part; 4-6 sets per exercise Day 1 Chest-Back-Shoulders Day 2 Legs-Triceps-Biceps

Table 7.6
Training for Muscular Fitness Three Days Per Week Using a Split Routine

	Week 1	Week 2	Week 3	Week 4
F	3	3	3	3
I - MS	70%-90% of 1-rep max or 2-8 reps per set	70%-90% of 1-rep max or 2-8 reps per set	70%-90% of 1-rep max or 2-8 reps per set	70%-90% of 1-rep max or 2-8 reps per set
I – MS & ME	60%-70% of 1-rep max or 8-12 reps per set	60%-70% of 1-rep max or 8-12 reps per set	60%-70% of 1-rep max or 8-12 reps per set	60%-70% of 1-rep max or 8-12 reps per set
I - ME	50%-60% of 1-rep max or 12-15 reps per set	50%-60% of 1-rep max or 12-15 reps per set	50%-60% of 1-rep max or 12-15 reps per set	50%-60% of 1-rep max or 12-15 reps per set
T	**Beginners** 2-3 exercises per body part; 2 sets per exercise	**Beginners** 3 exercises per body part; 2 sets per exercise	**Beginners** 3 exercises per body part; 2-3 sets per exercise	**Beginners** 3 exercises per body part; 2-3 sets per exercise
	Intermediate 3 exercises per body part; 3 sets per exercise	**Intermediate** 3 exercises per body part; 3 sets per exercise	**Intermediate** 3-4 exercises per body part; 3 sets per exercise	**Intermediate** 4 exercises per body part; 3 sets per exercise
	Advanced 4-6 exercises per body part; 4-6 sets per exercise Day 1 Chest-Triceps Day 2 Back-Biceps Day 3 Shoulders-Legs	**Advanced** 4-6 exercises per body part; 4-6 sets per exercise Day 1 Chest-Triceps Day 2 Back-Biceps Day 3 Shoulders-Legs	**Advanced** 5-6 exercises per body part; 4-6 sets per exercise Day 1 Chest-Back Day 2 Shoulders-Legs Day 3 Triceps-Biceps	**Advanced** 5-6 exercises per body part; 4-6 sets per exercise Day 1 Chest-Back Day 2 Shoulders-Legs Day 3 Triceps-Biceps

Table 7.7

Split Routine Training for Muscular Fitness Four Days Per Week Using Split Routine

	Week 1	Week 2	Week 3	Week 4
F	4	4	4	4
I - MS	70%-90% of 1-rep max or 2-8 reps per set	70%-90% of 1-rep max or 2-8 reps per set	70%-90% of 1-rep max or 2-8 reps per set	70%-90% of 1-rep max or 2-8 reps per set
I – MS & ME	60%-70% of 1-rep max or 8-12 reps per set	60%-70% of 1-rep max or 8-12 reps per set	60%-70% of 1-rep max or 8-12 reps per set	60%-70% of 1-rep max or 8-12 reps per set
I - ME	50%-60% of 1-rep max or 12-15 reps per set	50%-60% of 1-rep max or 12-15 reps per set	50%-60% of 1-rep max or 12-15 reps per set	50%-60% of 1-rep max or 12-15 reps per set
T	**Beginners** 2-3 exercises per body part; 2 sets per exercise	**Beginners** 3 exercises per body part; 2 sets per exercise	**Beginners** 3 exercises per body part; 2-3 sets per exercise	**Beginners** 3 exercises per body part; 2-3 sets per exercise
	Intermediate 3 exercises per body part; 3 sets per exercise	**Intermediate** 3 exercises per body part; 3 sets per exercise	**Intermediate** 3-4 exercises per body part; 3 sets per exercise	**Intermediate** 4 exercises per body part; 3 sets per exercise
	Advanced 4-6 exercises per body part; 4-6 sets per exercise Day 1 Chest-Triceps Day 2 Shoulders Day 3 Legs Day 4 Back-Biceps	**Advanced** 4-6 exercises per body part; 4-6 sets per exercise Day 1 Chest-Triceps Day 2 Back-Biceps Day 3 Legs Day 4 Shoulders	**Advanced** 5-6 exercises per body part; 4-6 sets per exercise Day 1 Chest Day 2 Back Day 3 Shoulders-Legs Day 4 Triceps-Biceps	**Advanced** 5-6 exercises per body part; 4-6 sets per exercise Day 1 Chest-Back Day 2 Legs Day 3 Shoulders Day 4 Triceps-Biceps

Table 7.8
Training for Muscular Fitness Five Days Per Week Using A Split Routine

	Week 1	Week 2	Week 3	Week 4
F	**5**	**5**	**5**	**5**
I - MS	70%-90% of 1-rep max or 2-8 reps per set	70%-90% of 1-rep max or 2-8 reps per set	70%-90% of 1-rep max or 2-8 reps per set	70%-90% of 1-rep max or 2-8 reps per set
I – MS & ME	60%-70% of 1-rep max or 8-12 reps per set	60%-70% of 1-rep max or 8-12 reps per set	60%-70% of 1-rep max or 8-12 reps per set	60%-70% of 1-rep max or 8-12 reps per set
I - ME	50%-60% of 1-rep max or 12-15 reps per set	50%-60% of 1-rep max or 12-15 reps per set	50%-60% of 1-rep max or 12-15 reps per set	50%-60% of 1-rep max or 12-15 reps per set
T	**Beginners** 2-3 exercises per body part; 2 sets per exercise	**Beginners** 3 exercises per body part; 2 sets per exercise	**Beginners** 3 exercises per body part; 2-3 sets per exercise	**Beginners** 3 exercises per body part; 2-3 sets per exercise
	Intermediate 3 exercises per body part; 3 sets per exercise	**Intermediate** 3 exercises per body part; 3 sets per exercise	**Intermediate** 3-4 exercises per body part; 3 sets per exercise	**Intermediate** 4 exercises per body part; 3 sets per exercise
	Advanced 4-6 exercises per body part; 4-6 sets per exercise	**Advanced** 4-6 exercises per body part; 4-6 sets per exercise	**Advanced** 5-6 exercises per body part; 4-6 sets per exercise	**Advanced** 5-6 exercises per body part; 4-6 sets per exercise
	Day 1 Chest	Day 1 Chest	Day 1 Back	Day 1 Back
	Day 2 Back	Day 2 Back	Day 2 Chest	Day 2 Chest
	Day 3 Legs	Day 3 Legs	Day 3 Legs	Day 3 Legs
	Day 4 Shoulders	Day 4 Shoulders	Day 4 Shoulders	Day 4 Shoulders
	Day 5 Triceps-Biceps	Day 5 Triceps-Biceps	Day 5 Biceps-Triceps	Day Triceps-Biceps

Total Body Workouts

As mentioned earlier, there are two different ways of training for MF, a Split Routine (SR) and a Total Body Workout (TBWO). All of the workouts presented above from two to five days were for the SR and while the SR appears to be the more popular way of training, the TBWO is beginning to gain more attention for the following reasons: (1) the workout takes less time; (2) the workouts are more intense yet the recuperation time is less; (3) all the major muscle groups are addressed in each workout so the individual doesn't have to worry if they missed a day then they missed body part(s) for the week like in a SR. So, for those of you interested in a TBWO, here's how it works:

1. In each workout, you will address the following 6 major muscles in any of the following ways:

   Chest-Back-Legs-Shoulders-Triceps-Biceps
   Chest-Back-Shoulders-Legs-Triceps-Biceps
   Back-Chest-Legs-Shoulders-Biceps Triceps
   Back-Chest-Shoulders-Legs-Biceps-Triceps

2. Body parts will be addressed in a superset fashion (See #3 on Spicing Up Your MF Program). That means you will perform one set of an exercise one (chest or back) followed immediately by one set of the other body part and then rest (and repeat 2-4X based on your level of MF and how many sets you plan to do for each exercise.

3. Once you have completed working on your Chest and Back, you then proceed to the Legs and Shoulders and again work them in superset fashion. That means Leg Exercise followed by Shoulder Exercise or vice-versa and then rest (and repeat 2-6X based on you level of MF).

4. After finishing working on your Legs and Shoulders, proceed to working on your Triceps and Biceps, again in super set fashion.

By working on two different muscle groups simultaneously, your overall rest time in between sets is decreased and thus the intensity of your workouts is increased. In contrast, when incorporating a SR, I have noticed both in the classes I teach as well as the gym that I work out in that all too often individuals become fixated on their cell phones, texting, playing games or watching videos/T.V. while resting in between sets. This "dramatically" increases the overall time it takes to complete a workout. So why not give the TBWO a try! See Table 7.9 for a list of exercises to perform in a TBWO from one to five days per week

Table 7.9
Total Body Work Out (TBYO)

Body Part	Day 1	Day 2	Day 3	Day 4	Day 5
Chest	Decline Bench Press or Decline Dumbbell Press	Flat Bench Press or Dumbbell Press	Incline BP	Seated Flys	Chest Press, Push Ups or Bench Push Ups
Back	Barbell Row or Two Hand Dumbbell Row	Lat Pull Down Cables	Incline Row	Dead Lift	Lat Pull Down Selectorized
Legs	Behind the Neck Squats or Front Squats	Leg Press & Calf Raises	Leg Curls &Leg Extensions	Farmer's Carry	Wall Sit or Abductor & Adductor
Shoulders	Arnold Press	Front Raise	Incline Lateral Raise	Shoulder Shrugs	Upight Row or Bent Over Lateral Raise
Triceps	Lying Tricep Extension	Tricep Pulldowns	Tricep Dips on Bench	Tricep Pushdowns	Tricep Extension or Tricep Pressdown
Biceps	One Arm Preacher Curls	Hammer Curls	Incline Curls	Barbell Curls or Two Arm Preacher Curls	Concentration or Reverse Curls
Abdominal Exercises	Pick 2-4 exercises from Table 7.4	Pick 2-4 exercises from Table 7.4	Pick 2-4 exercises from Table 7.4	Pick 2-4 exercises from Table 7.4	Pick 2-4 exercises from Table 7.4

Beginning Levels of MF should perform 2 sets per exercise
Intermediate Levels of MF should perform 3 sets per exercises
Advanced Levels of MF should perform 4-5 sets per exercise

Determining Your Level of Commitment to Muscular Fitness Training

As you learned in the previous chapter, your level of commitment, more than your actual fitness level, will determine how much, how often, and how hard you will exercise. For some reason, one of the hardest parts of an exercise program seems to be scheduling the actual days(s) and times(s) to do the workout and then getting to the exercise facility to get started. Therefore, it is imperative that you determine how many days per week you will commit to MFT. In addition, you should also identify what your MF goals are. Do you want to work on muscular strength and increase your muscular size? Do you want to work on your muscular endurance and develop, shape and define your muscles or do you want to work on both areas of muscular fitness and increase muscular strength and endurance in order to enhance muscular size and shape? In the previous section, you were introduced to three different MF programs designed to improve muscular strength, muscular endurance, or a combination of the two. Each program is also based on the number of days per week that you are committed toward working on your MF.

So where are you on the commitment scale?

1	2	3	4	5	6	7	8	9

Low commitment   **Moderate Commitment**   **High Commitment**

How many days per week will you commit to working on MF?

1	2	3	4	5

Based upon your level of commitment, you should consider one of the four-week MF programs introduced above and presented in Tables 7.5 – 7.9. Simply select the program that you have the highest level of commitment to follow over the next four weeks. Most important, enjoy yourself and have fun body shaping and strengthening your muscles.

SPICING UP YOUR PROGRAM

After a few weeks of training your muscles, doing the same exercises in the same order with the same number of sets and reps, your body as well as your mind begins to get used to the "same old routine" and your early performance gains will slowly diminish, not to mention you getting bored with your workouts. Physically, you are not challenging your body as much because your muscles have grown accustomed to the same workout. Mentally, you may become bored doing the same routine over and over again and you might lose motivation and stop challenging yourself to get that extra rep or set in or raise the weight or add a new exercise. To get the spice back into your workout, you should consider incorporating one or more of the following workout strategies: (1) pyramids; (2) reverse pyramids; (3) supersets; (4) circuit training; (5) total body workout:

1. *Pyramids*—occur when you increase the weight from the first set to the last which creates a greater intensity on each rep resulting in achieving fewer reps per set. Although this tends to be a popular method of weight training, pyramids are recommended to be used as a means to spice up your workouts rather than as your usual way of training since performing pyramids on every set of every exercise makes it difficult to overload properly. For example, if you are working on a smaller muscle group like biceps, it is unrealistic to raise the weight on each set simply because the intensity would become too great. Let's say your goal is to shape, define and strengthen your muscles and you are up to 50 lbs. on the barbell curl striving to achieve between 8-12 reps per set. Last week you did 10, 9 and 8 reps, respectively. This week, you started with 50 lbs. and you did 11 reps on the first set. Adopting a pyramid method of training, you raised the weight on the next set to 55 lbs. and achieved 7 reps. You are already below the minimum number of reps you should achieve and now you plan to raise the

weight to 60 lbs. on set 3. How many reps do you think you would achieve by raising the weight almost 10%? The end result is you will achieve significantly less reps using the pyramid method and while you will definitely improve your strength, you will not be addressing your goals to shape and define your muscles.

It is important to note that sometimes a pyramid may be used incorrectly. This occurs when you purposely keep the weight too low on the earlier sets just so you can raise the weight on the later sets. Doing so will only create exercise overload on the later sets, thus reducing the amount of overall progress you are achieving. Let's take a more in-depth look. Logically, you are the strongest in the beginning of your workout and if you want to improve your MF, then you must overload your muscles properly throughout all phases of your workout (e.g., at the beginning, middle and end). That means lifting as much weight as you possibly can for the desired amount of reps that you are striving to achieve (e.g., 2-8, 8-12, 12-15) on all sets. It may be tempting to stop after achieving a certain number of reps in a given set even though you can continue to do a few more reps just so you can raise the weight in the later sets. The fact remains, if you can do more reps and you choose not to then you are minimizing your overload and thus reducing your performance gains. Therefore, keep going until you cannot do any more reps and then raise the weight on the next set.

Pyramids are an excellent way to spice up your workout from time to time by changing the intensity so that your body does not get used to lifting the same amount of weight on every set. However, using pyramids should not become your regular workout routine simply because you do not need to raise the weight from set to set just to increase overload and decrease reps. If you are overloading properly then the reps will decrease from one set to the next with the same weight, simply because your muscles are getting weaker after each set and thus not able to do as much in the latter sets then in the earlier sets. Table 7.10 demonstrates how to incorporate a pyramid correctly and incorrectly.

Table 7.10
Correct and Incorrect Ways of Pyramid Training

Body Part = Chest	Correct Pyramid	Incorrect Pyramid
Exercise = Bench Press	100 lbs 10-12×	100 lbs 12×
	105 lbs 8-9×	120 lbs 10×
	110 lbs 5-6×	140 lbs 6×
	115 lbs 2-4×	160 lbs 4×
	120 lbs 1-2×	180 lbs 2×

As you can see in the correct pyramid, each time the weight was slightly increased the number of reps decreased, naturally. In other words, the workload from set to set increased in difficulty resulting in performing a few less reps per set. However, in the incorrect pyramid, the weight is substantially increased from 100 lbs. in the first set to 180 lbs. in the 5th set, yet the reps have only decreased, slightly. This indicates that the individual could have lifted substantially more weight in the early sets and by not doing so the overload was minimalized until the later sets, thus reducing the overall benefits of this method of training.

2. ***Reverse Pyramids***—are when you start with the heaviest weight that you can lift for 1-2 reps and then you decrease the weight each set from the first set to the last resulting in achieving more reps per set. Again, just like pyramids, this way of training is recommended to be used as a means to spice up your workouts rather than as your usual way of training. (See Table 7.11 for a proper way of performing a Reverse Pyramid).

Table 7.11
Spicing Up Your MF Workout Using a Reverse Pyramid

Body Part = Chest	Reverse Pyramid
Exercise = Bench Press	120 lbs. 1-2×
	110 lbs. 3-5×
	100 lbs. 6-8×
	90 lbs. 8-10×
	80 lbs. 10-12×

3. ***Supersets***—involves two exercises that work opposing muscle groups performed consecutively without resting in between. For example, let's say you are working your chest and back and you plan to do two exercises for each body part. Instead of doing all of your chest exercises first and then all of your back exercises next, a superset would involve performing your first set of your first chest exercise followed immediately with your first set of your first back exercise and then a rest period before beginning your second set of chest and back exercises. By decreasing your overall rest time, you are increasing the intensity of your workout creating a greater overload which will result in improving your muscular fitness at a more accelerated rate. However, it is important to note that fatigue will set in more quickly with supersets which may result in the need to decrease weight and/or reps or increase rest time in the latter part of your workout. (See Table 7.12 for an example of how-to superset in a SR workout.

Table 7.12
Spicing Up Your Workout with Supersets

Chest Exercise 1
Decline Dumbbell Press
Back Exercise 1
Barbell Row
Repeat for 3 Sets
Chest Exercise 2
Bench Press
Back Exercise 2
Lat Pulldown
Repeat for 3 Sets
Chest Exercise 3
Incline Dumbbell Press
Back Exercise 3
T Bar or Incline Row
Repeat for 3 Sets
Chest Exercise 4
Seated Flys
Back Exercise 4
Low Row
Repeat for 3 Sets

4. ***Circuit Training***—combines muscular fitness exercises with aerobic exercises in the same workout using a format like this: (1) select 8-12 resistance training exercises that incorporate all of the major muscle groups; (2) use approximately 40 to 50 percent of your max or select a weight that you can perform for 20-30 reps; (3) superset two related, but different resistance training exercises followed by an aerobic exercise for 1:00 to 2:00 that will elevate your heart rate into your training zone (e.g., jogging in place, stationary bicycle, stairmaster, shadow boxing, dancing, jump rope, jumping jacks, lunges, farmer's carry, hill climbing). The shorter the period you do your aerobic exercises for, the higher your intensity should be. For example, if you normally run a mile in 10 minutes and you put the treadmill on 6.0 for two minutes then raise it to 6.5 if you plan to go for one minute. Repeat cycle 2-6 times based on your level of health-related fitness.

Circuit training is an excellent way to address multiple components of both health and skill related fitness (e.g., muscular fitness, cardiovascular endurance, speed, power, coordination, agility) and a creative way to train especially when you might be pressed for time and not able to work all the areas of fitness that you normally would do for longer time periods. However, it is important to note that circuits are not a replacement for working on CRE and MF separately simply because when you have more time, you will accomplish more in terms of exercises, sets and reps for MF and distance, steps and time for CRE. See Table 7.13 for a list of exercises that you can perform in a circuit training workout and **Appendix 7**…. to create your own circuit training workout.

Table 7.13
Spicing Up Your Muscular Fitness Workout
Using Circuit Training

Begin by warming up with an aerobic exercise for 2-5 minutes	Desired # of Reps	Minutes & Reps Completed
Dumbbell Press	20-30	
Barbell Row	20-30	
Rhythmic Exercise	1-2 minutes	
Shoulder Press	20-30	
Leg Press	20-30	
Rhythmic Exercise	1-2 minutes	
Tricep Pulldowns	20-30	
Pump 'N' Walk	20-30	
Push Ups	1 minute or 20-40 reps	
Rhythmic Exercise	1-2 minutes	
Sit Ups	1 minute or 20-40 reps	
Rhythmic Exercise	1-2 minutes	
Farmer's Carry	1 minute	

If you are at the beginning level of fitness, then I recommend that you do one complete cycle which should take between 12-14 minutes to complete.

If you are at the intermediate level of fitness, then I recommended that you do 2-3 cycles which should take between 30-45 minutes to complete.

If you are at the advanced level of fitness, then I recommended you should complete 4-5 cycles which should take between 45-60 minutes to complete.

Feel free to add or change exercises if you are doing more than one complete cycle. Simply refer to Figure 7.2 for a list of additional exercises by body part to choose from.

Incorporating the POC into your MF Program

To make sure your muscular fitness program is going to produce your desired results, you need to be certain that you are incorporating each of the 8 principles of fitness into your workouts. Here are strategies for you to accomplish that.

Warm Up Principle—An effective way to physically warm up before beginning to work on your MF is to select the exercise that you plan on starting with and perform a set of either a light or no weight for about 12-15 reps. This will activate your muscles and let your body know exactly what you will be working on before you actually get started overloading. Another way to physically warm up is to do a few minutes of an aerobic activity (e.g., walking, jogging, stationary bicycle). This will increase your body temperature which will make it easier to overload your muscles while lifting.

While warming up physically is very important, it is equally important to warm up mentally because no matter how ready your body is to exercise, if your mind is not then you are going to have a difficult time enjoying your workout and challenging yourself to improve your MF. You can warm up your mind and prepare it for working out in any or all of the following ways: (1) listening to music that makes puts you in a positive mood state and makes you feel energized and happy; (2) having a conversation with your exercise partner(s) to clear your mind and prepare it for your workout; (3) using positive slogans that make you feel confident (e.g., "I'm going to have a great workout. I feel great. This is awesome. I am so ready.") (4) writing down your SMAART goals and paying specific attention to what you plan to do and how you plan to get it done; (5) using a journal to write down your thoughts about what is going through your mind, what barriers may arise that can stop you from having a productive workout and what strategies you plan to utilize to overcome these barriers so you can have an awesome workout. This will help to erase any negative thoughts that often sit with you before you begin to exercise (e.g., I'm tired. I don't want to do this).

Principle of Progression (POP)—The simplest way to incorporate the POP is to first use your workout card and add up what you accomplished in your workouts. In other words, how many exercises, sets and reps did you do last week? Then look to systematically increase what you did last week by starting with reps first, then sets and then exercises. You should be able to do at least one more rep in every exercise that you did last week, right? Once you have achieved the desired amount of reps in a given set (8, 12 or 15) then it's time to raise the weight. For those of you who are beginners, you can add a set from one to two and two to three every few weeks. In addition, once your body gets used to the same exercises you may want to consider adding a new exercise to your workouts. By challenging yourself to add reps, sets and/or exercises you will create a strong sense of accomplishment and keep yourself on the road to improving your muscular fitness each and every workout.

Principle of Individuality—Determine the number of days you will work on your MF along with the exercises, weight, sets and reps based on your own MF needs and not anyone else(s). The easiest way to accomplish this is to use the information from your MF assessment form along with your present schedule to determine your level of MF and how many days you are willing to commit to working on your MF. Select the exercises that are appealing to you rather than only doing exercises that you see other people doing.

Principle of Recuperation—Since working on MF is somewhat more intense on the muscles than CRE training, you should make sure to provide adequate rest (at least 72 hours) after your muscles have been overloaded before you plan to work them out again. Generally, working on each major muscle group once per week (for a Split Routine) will give you sufficient rest time to recuperate from your workout overload and get you back stronger in the next week. When working the large muscle group with the related small muscle group (e.g., chest with triceps; back with biceps), you are giving each body part six days of rest before being worked on again. When using the agonist-antagonist method (e.g., chest with back, triceps with biceps), you should work the larger muscle groups earlier in the week and give yourself at least 72 hours before working on the related small muscle groups. For example, if you plan on working out three times this week, you can start off working chest with back on day 1, shoulders with legs on day 2 and triceps with biceps on day 3. The only exception is when you are doing a total body workout. Then you will be working the same muscle groups multiple times per week, yet performing significantly less sets and exercises per body part each workout day. Therefore, you should consider taking 3-4 days of rest in between each days' workout for beginners, 2-3 days of rest for intermediates and at least 1 day, preferably 2 days of rest for advanced lifters per week.

Principle of Fun—You can make your MF program fun in the identical way you are making your CRE program fun. Identify what you like that you can incorporate into your MF program (e.g., listening to music, working out with an exercise partner, joining a gym, selecting exercises that you enjoy, choosing a time that works for you, setting and striving to reach SMAART goals, using positive slogans to make you fun good – i.e., I got this! I'm awesome! Keep going! Nobody better than me!)

Principle of Reversibility——In order to avoid losing what you have gained from overloading, you must work each of your major muscle groups every week. If you are accustomed to working on your MF at least three times per week and your schedule suddenly changes and you only have one or two days per week to exercise, you can modify your workout in the following manner to maintain or possibly even increase your MF: (1) switch from a split routine to a total body workout; This will allow you to address all of the major muscle groups in one workout; (2) add more sets or exercises to your workout; So, even though your frequency has decreased and you are missing days, you can compensate for that by doing more work on the days you exercise. (3) change the intensity; If your body is used to working on strength then change it to working on endurance or vice versa; This will shock your body and create an entirely different overload; (4) incorporate supersets, pyramids, reverse pyramids or circuits; Again, this is just another way to change the overload your body has grown accustomed to resulting in creating different challenges for yourself. By incorporating any of the above-mentioned strategies, you will be able to maintain and quite possibly improve your MF until you get back to your usual schedule.

Using SMAART Goals to Increase Muscular Fitness Motivation and Performance

To use SMAART goals to increase your MF, start with your baseline level of MF. Simply take the results of what you maxed on or use the amount of weight that you can presently lift for the exercises that you plan to use in your workouts and set any of the following goals: (1) increase max; (2) increase amount of weight being used during workouts; (3) increase exercises being performed each week; (4) increase sets and reps being performed each week or (5) increase the number of days working on MF. Of course, you will need to name your exercise(s) and numerically include what you are up to. For example, let's say you maxed 150 lbs. on the leg press in week 1. You can set a goal to increase your max to 200 lbs. by week 5. Perhaps you are lifting 6 sets per body part. Maybe you want to set a goal to achieve 7 sets by next week. Whatever motivates you the most to challenge yourself to improve your MF is the SMAART goal for you. Table 7.14 includes an example of Howie, a man who wants to improve his MF and get stronger. He starts off by maxing 130 lbs on the bench press and he sets a measurable goal to be able to max 150 lbs. He creates an action plan to lift weights 3X per week over the next 4 weeks and increase his total number of sets per workout by two each week during the 4-week period. If he does not improve each week, he will change his program around by either increasing his frequency to a fourth day or adding 1-2 sets of chest exercises to his workouts.

Now let's see if Howie's goal fits the SMAART principle. His goal is specific because he states that he wants to improve him MF and get stronger. It is measurable because he sets a numerical goal to max 150 lbs. on the bench press. He has an action plan of working out 3X per week over the next 4 weeks and increase his number of sets per workout by two each

Table 7.14
SMAART Goal #1

	Howie's SMAART Goals	My SMAART Goals
S	Improve Muscular Fitness & Get Stronger	
M	Max 150 lbs on the Bench Press	
A	Lift weights 3× per week and increase 2 sets per week over the next four weeks	
A	Work out a fourth day in a week to add 1-2 sets of chest exercises per week.	
R	Increasing Max on the Bench Press from 130 lbs to 150 is a challenging goal and certainly within reach if the plan of action is followed.	
T	Howie's target date to max 150 lbs. on the bench press is 4 weeks from the day he first started working on his MF.	

week. His goal is adjustable because he has created strategies to employ in the event that he is not improving from week to week. His goal is realistic because he started with a max of 130 pounds and he is giving himself 4 weeks to increase 20 lbs. Finally, he has a target date of 4 weeks after the day he first started lifting. Consequently, Howie's goal is very SMAART. Now let's see if your goals are SMAART. Use Table 7.14 to set your own SMAART goal for MF this week. In addition, you can use Appendices' 7D and 7E to set weekly goals for muscular fitness as well as SMAART goals for individual and weekly workouts.

SETTING STAIRWAY TO SUCCESS GOALS TO IMPROVE YOUR MF

In addition to setting SMAART goals, if you have MF goals that you think may take longer than a few weeks to achieve, you can use the Stairway to Success to set both short and long-term goals. Let's use Leslie as an example of how to use the Stairway to Success. On September 8, Leslie did 25 sit-ups on the 3:00 sit-up test and she would like to achieve 80 by December 6.

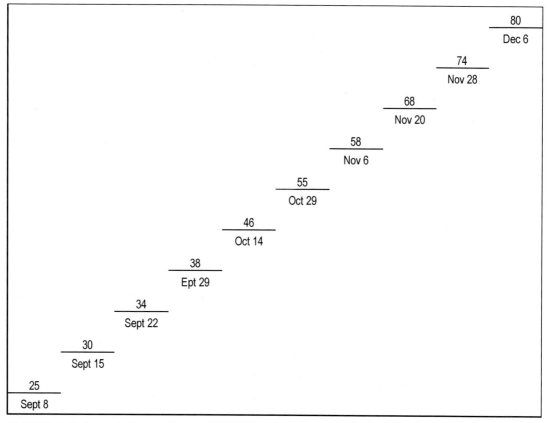

10-20 Week Stairway to Success.

Figure 7.3—Leslie's Stairway to Success

Using the Stairway to Success, Leslie wrote down her baseline of 25 sit-ups along with the date she accomplished that on the bottom step. Then she set her long-term goal of 80 sit-ups on the top set along with her target date of December 6. Then she set her first short-term goal of 30 sit-ups by September 15. Each time Leslie reached her short-term goal she climbed one step up the stairway to her next short-term goal until she was able to reach the top of the stairs and complete 80 sit-ups in 3:00. See Figure 7.3 to review Leslie's Stairway to Success as well as Appendix 7F to set your own stairway to success goals.

EVALUATING THE SUCCESS OF YOUR MUSCULAR FITNESS PROGRAM

Have you followed your exercise prescription for MF? Are you as committed to improving your MF as you thought you would be? Have you identified and overcome any barriers that may have stopped you from reaching your SMAART goals for MF?

Have you seen improvements from Weeks' 1 to 4 in any of the following: (1) amount of weight lifted; (2) number of reps and sets achieved; (3) amount of exercises being performed or (4) frequency of weekly workouts? Do you feel better after your workout? Has your recuperation time decreased? Does soreness or discomfort subside quicker? Do you look forward to working on your MF? Has your body improved in muscular size? definition? tone? firmness? Did you reach your SMAART goals? Your answers to each of these questions is a perfect way to evaluate the success of your MF program.

If you answered "NO" to any of these questions, then you should re-evaluate your workouts and determine if you need to do any of the following: (1) change your workouts around by adding more or different exercises; (2) increase the weight you are working out with to challenge yourself more; (3) add sets to your workouts; You must determine what is stopping you and then develop a plan of action to overcome these barriers and get back on track.

Preventing Injuries

There are several strategies that you can incorporate to reduce and possibly prevent injuries and they include:

Warming up—Prior to overloading your muscles you should warm up both physically and mentally by doing any and all of the following: (1) choose an aerobic exercise (bike, Stairmaster, treadmill, elliptical) to use for 3-5 minutes and identify what's in your mind; (2) allow your thoughts to enter and exit without evaluation; (3) then plan your workout—what you are going to do; the order you plan to do it; how you will reach your SMAART goals; (4) go to your first exercise and perform 12-15 reps with no weight or a light weight; (5) repeat #4 each time you begin working on a new body part;

Learning proper form of exercises—Before selecting an exercise, make sure you know how to do it properly. If you are taking an exercise class, the instructor should demonstrate how to perform each exercise properly. If you belong to a gym and you are unfamiliar with the exercise equipment, ask the manager or exercise staff to demonstrate how to do any of the exercises that you are interested in learning. Take the textbook with you and model the pictures labeled "correct form." Finally, using either "no" or "very light" weight, practice these exercises a few times and concentrate on using the correct form, proper starting position, incorporating the right range of motion and going slowly.

Spotting—Use a partner to assist you in your workout; The spotter's primary responsibility is to maximize safety! That means knowing the correct form of the exercise being performed, the ability of the individual lifting, (e.g., how many reps he/she is planning on doing), proper breathing techniques and the correct positioning of the exercise(s) being performed (e.g., range of motion, incline, decline, lying on back, lying on stomach, sitting, standing, balancing). Remember that the spotter is not there to help the individual lift the weight. He/she is there only to make sure the individual is lifting the weight safely.

Breathing Properly—You should exhale on the exertion phase (lifting the weight) and inhale on the resting phase (when the weight returns to its starting position). Generally, the exertion phase should take 1-2 seconds while the resting phase should take 3-4 seconds. That means that each rep should take approximately 4-6 seconds to complete.

Know your exercise—Some popular exercises can cause injuries if done improperly and they include: (1) arching your back on the Flat Bench Press or standing Barbell Curl; (2) locking your knees on a Leg Press or Leg Extension or (3) extending the bar behind your neck on the Lat Pulldown. Therefore, know your exercises and how to execute proper form before planning to use them in your MF program.

In this chapter, you have learned the benefits of participating in a muscular fitness program. You have been introduced to two different methods of assessing your MF as well as a variety of different MF programs to choose from. You should be able to find at least one program that you are at least moderately and hopefully highly committed to using so that you can enjoy working on improving your MF. Please proceed onto to the review questions and lab assignments for Chapter 7 so you can test your knowledge and continue to develop your expertise.

REVIEW QUESTIONS

1. Describe a common myth associated with women who participate in weight training and explain how you would disprove this myth.

2. Define the two components of muscular fitness?

3. List five or more benefits of being muscularly fit. Which of these benefits increases your motivation to start or continue working on your muscular fitness?

4. Explain how you could accurately assess someone's muscular strength.

5. Explain how you could accurately assess someone's muscular endurance.

6. How would you measure the four components of an exercise prescription for muscular fitness?

7. Explain the difference in intensity for someone who wants to "body shape" or tone and define his/her muscles and someone who wants to increase their muscular size.

8. List the five questions that determine time for a muscular fitness prescription.

9. List 3-5 muscular fitness exercises that are commonly performed incorrectly and explain how you would correct each.

10. Compare and contrast the differences between a split routine and a total body workout? Which method of training do you like best and why.

11. Describe two strategies that you can use to spice up your muscular fitness program.

12. Explain the correct and incorrect ways of using a pyramid to work on muscular fitness.

13. Discuss how you plan to use goal setting (SMAART Goals and Stairway to Success Goals) to improve your muscular fitness and create a high level of motivation to continue over the next 6 months?

14. What can you do to prevent injuries while working on your muscular fitness?

LAB ASSIGNMENT 7.1

Questions 1-9 should be answered prior to beginning your MF fitness program.

1. How committed are you to improving your MF fitness over the next six weeks?

<table>
<tr><td>1</td><td>2</td><td>3</td><td>4</td><td>5</td><td>6</td><td>7</td><td>8</td><td>9</td></tr>
</table>

　　Not　　　　　　　　　　　　　　　　　　　　Extremely
Committed　　　　　　　　　　　　　　　　　Committed

If you have a low level of commitment, what strategies will you incorporate to increase your level of commitment?

2. Using the box below, what are your SMAART goal(s) for improving your MF over the next 6 weeks. You can use Appendix 7C to create your action plan for reaching your SMAART goals?

S	
M	
A	
A	
R	
T	

3. Create 1-2 Stairway to Success Goals for MJ over the next six weeks.

**Long-term
goal. Date:
6 weeks from
when you start**

Baseline

Long-term
goal. Date:
6 weeks from
_____ when you start

_____

_____

_____

Baseline

4. Develop an exercise prescription to improve your MF fitness over the next six weeks.

	Week 1	Week 2	Week 3	Week 4	Week 5	Week 6
F						
I						
T						
T						

5. Explain how you plan to adhere to the 8 principles of conditioning over the next 6 weeks.

Questions 6-10 should be answered at the conclusion of the 6 weeks

6. How has your overload changed from weeks' 1 to 6?

7. How has your recuperation time changed from weeks 1-6?

8. What strategies did you use to prevent the principle of reversibility from occurring?

9. How much you have improved from weeks' 1-6? You can use the chart in Appendix 7B to numerically jot down your workouts over the 6 weeks to determine your overall improvement?

10. Did you have fun while working on your MF? If so, explain the strategies that you have incorporated to have fun? If you did not have fun, explain what you plan to do over the next few weeks to make your MF workouts more fun (e.g., music, exercise with a partner, etc.).

LAB ASSIGNMENT 7.2

1. Discuss how you feel about the improvements that you have made over the last 6 weeks?

2. Circle the answer that best represents your motivation to continue working on MF.

   decreased   remained the same   increased

3. If your motivation to work on your MF has decreased or remained the same, explain why and then list your strategies to increase your motivation to improve your MF over the next 6 weeks.

4. What goals will you strive to achieve over the next 6 weeks. Use Appendix 7C to set your weekly MF goals.

REFERENCES AND RECOMMENDED READINGS

American College of Sports Medicine (2002). Position Stand: Progression Models in Resistance Training for Healthy Adults. Medicine and Science in Sport and Exercise, 34(2), 364-380.

Brzycki, M. (1999). "Free weights and machines." *Fitness Management, 15*, 36-37 40.

Hakkinen, K. (2004). Changes in muscle hypertrophy in women with periodized resistance training. *Medicine and Science in Sports and Exercise, 36, 4*, 697-708.

Hesson, J. (2007). Weight training for life, 8th addition. Wadsworth/Thomson Learning.

Hoeger, W. WK., Hopkins, D.R., Barette, S.L., & Hale, D.F. (1990). Relationship between repetitions and selected percentages of one repetition maximum: A comparison between untrained and trained males and females. *Journal of Applied Sport Science Research, 4*, 47-51.

Kraemer, W.J., & Ratamess, N.A. (2004). Fundamentals of resistance training: Progression and exercise prescriptions. *Medicine and Science in Sports and Exercise, 36, 4*, 674-689.

Powers, S.K., & Howley, E.T. (2004). Exercise physiology: Theory and application to fitness and performance. 5th edition. McGraw-Hill.

Rhea, M.R., Alvar, B.A., Ball, S.D., & Burkett, L.N. (2002). Three sets of weight training superior to 1 set with equal intensity for eliciting strength. *Journal of Strength Conditioning Research, 16*, 525-529.

Smith, D., & Bruce-Low, S. (2004). Strength training methods and the work of Arthur Jones. *Journal of Exercise Physiology, 7, 6,* 52-62.

www.acsm-msse.org.

APPENDIX 7A
MUSCULAR FITNESS ASSESSMENT FORM

Name _____   Pre Test Date _____   Post Test Date _____

Body Part	Exercise	Pre Test		Post Test	
		Max *Sub Max*		*Max* *Sub Max*	
Chest	Free Weight Bench Press				
	Isolateral Bench Press				
	Chest Press				
	Seated Fly Machine				
Back	Lat Pull Down				
	Low Row				
	T Bar/Incline Row				
Shoulders	Rear Deltoid				
	Shoulder Press				
	Lateral Raise				
Legs	Leg Press				
	Leg Curl				
	Leg Extension				
Triceps	Tricep Pulldown				
	Tricep Extension				
Biceps	Barbell Curl				
	Preacher Curl				
Upper Body	Push Ups				
	Pull Ups				
	Flexed Arm Hang				
Abdominals	3:00 Sit Ups or Curl Ups				

Circle whether you chose a max or a sub max test. For max tests—record the highest amount of weight lifted for one repetition.

For sub max tests—record the amount of weight lifted and the total number of repetitions achieved.

For Flexed Arm Hang—record the total number of seconds held on the chin up bar.

APPENDIX 7B
HOW MUCH HAVE YOU IMPROVED OVER THE LAST SIX WEEKS?

	WEEK 1	WEEK 2	WEEK 3	WEEK 4	WEEK 5	WEEK 6
# OF DAYS EXERCISED						
# OF BODY PARTS ADDRESSED						
# OF EXERCISES SELECTED						
# OF SETS ACHIEVED						
# OF REPS ACHIEVED						
# OF TIMES YOU INCREASED WEIGHT						

APPENDIX 7C
DEVELOPING YOUR ACTION PLAN
FOR IMPROVING YOUR MUSCULAR FITNESS

	Week 1	Week 2	Week 3	Week 4	Week 5	Week 6
The actions I will take over the next 6 weeks to improve my muscular fitness and reach my SMAART goals are						
Action 1						
Action 2						
Action 3						
Action 4						

APPENDIX 7D
WEEKLY GOAL SHEET FOR MUSCULAR FITNESS

Muscular Fitness Goals to Choose	Goal(s) Chosen	Performance Results	Achieved = A	Not Achieved = NA
Frequency of Weekly Muscular Fitness Workouts				
# of Exercises Completed for the Workout/Week				
# of Sets Completed for the Workout/Week				
# of Reps Completed for the Workout/Week				
Exercises Increasing in Weight for the Workout/Week				

Muscular Fitness	Day 1	Day 2	Day 3	Day 4	Day 5	Day 6	Day 7
Exercises Completed							
Sets Completed							
Reps Completed							
# of Exercises Increasing in Weight							

APPENDIX 7E
MY SMAART GOALS FOR MF

SMAART Goal #1

S	
M	
A	
A	
R	
T	

SMAART Goal #2

S	
M	
A	
A	
R	
T	

APPENDIX # 7F
MY STAIRWAY TO SUCCESS GOALS FOR MF

10-20 Week Stairway to Success.

Stairway to Exercise Success

10-20 Week Stairway to Success.

Chapter 8

Developing Your Exercise Prescription for Flexibility

Objectives

After this chapter, you will be able to:
- Understand the benefits and importance of being flexible
- Formally and informally assess your flexibility
- Develop an exercise prescription to improve your flexibility
- Determine your level of commitment to being more flexible
- Set S-M-A-A-R-T goals to improve and enjoy your flexibility workouts
- Learn how to minimize and prevent injuries while engaging in flexibility exercises
- Spice up your flexibility workouts so you look forward to stretching

Did you know that flexibility is one of the most important components of health-related fitness? In fact, it is the one component of health-related fitness that is directly connected to both cardiovascular endurance (CVE) and muscular fitness (MF) performance. For example, if you feel tight and inflexible when working on your CVE then your performance may suffer due to the discomfort you are experiencing. Factors like tight hamstrings, quads, glutes and calves may make it too uncomfortable to exercise in a consistent, comfortable manner and thus reduce the overall quality of your workout and force you to exercise for less time at a lower intensity and possibly less days per week.

When you work on your MF, it is quite common to be sore the next day or two after your workout. By neglecting to work on flexibility during or after your MF workouts, you can increase the intensity as well as the duration of your soreness. This can create excessive amounts of discomfort while exercising and again reduce the overall quality of your workout, resulting in lifting less weight, reps, sets, exercises and less days per week than you had originally committed to. Now, if you work on your flexibility and develop a good range of motion then your CRE & MF workouts will flow more smoothly which can enhance your performance, decrease the severity and longevity of soreness and minimize the risk of injuries.

Today, much research has been conducted on the importance and benefits of being flexible as well as the proper methods of how to stretch properly (Millar, 2016, Therien, 2015, Alter, 2004, Liemohn, 2003). Nevertheless, flexibility continues to be the least worked on component of health-related fitness. Factors such as boredom, not seeing tangible results, not stretching properly, lack of motivation, misinterpreting tension for pain have all been recognized as barriers that stop individuals from improving their flexibility. By the end of this chapter, you will be motivated to "stretch out your schedule" and fit flexibility into your workout routine.

WHAT IS MUSCULAR FLEXIBILITY?

Flexibility is defined as the ability of a joint to move through its full range of motion. Being flexible means feeling "loose" and being able to move your body around freely and comfortably without pain. However, being flexible in one part of the body does not mean that you are equally as flexible in another. For example, you can be very loose in your upper body and have full range of motion in your arms, shoulders and chest and have a limited range of motion in your legs and have difficulty touching your toes.

As you get older, your flexibility naturally decreases which increases your chances of aches, pains, and injuries. The only solution is to be "flexible" and make the commitment to find the time to work on increasing your range of motion.

Benefits of Flexibility

There are many benefits to being more flexible and they include:
1. increased ability to move around freely
2. reduced injury frequency and severity
3. increased motor performance
4. increased joint mobility
5. improve athletic performance
6. improved posture
7. decreased muscle soreness
8. fewer aches and pains
9. fewer low back problems
10. reduction of stress

Assessing Your Flexibility

As you learned in Chapter 6, there are both formal and informal ways to assess health-related fitness. While both cardiorespiratory endurance and muscular strength may be assessed in a variety of ways (e.g., 1.5-mile run, step test, 12-minute swim, max testing, sub max test), flexibility assessments are limited due to a lack of joint specific equipment. Presently, there are only a handful of formal assessments, none of which measure flexibility in all parts of the body.

Therefore, in order to determine one's true level of flexibility, a combination of formal and informal assessments should be considered in order to gain more accurate information on how flexible you are in all areas of the body rather than in one or two places.

Formal and Informal Assessments

The two most common formal assessments for flexibility are the sit and reach (see Figure 8.1) and the trunk rotation tests (see Figure 8.2).

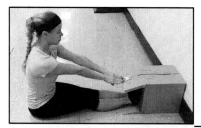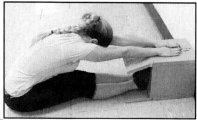

Figure 8.1 Sit and Reach Test

Procedures for Sit and Reach Test

1. Warm up first by moving around continuously for a few minutes (e.g., walking briskly, light jogging, stationary bicycle).
2. Take your shoes off and sit on the floor.
3. Extend your legs forward so that your heels are up against the sit & reach box.
4. Keep your knees locked.
5. Place one hand on top of the other and move the lever as far forward as possible. Repeat twice for a total of three trials.
6. Record your highest number in either inches or centimeters to the nearest half.

Procedures for Performing Trunk Rotation Test

1. Tape two yardsticks to the wall at shoulder height, one right side up and the other upside down. The numbers should read 1-36 right side up on the left side and 1-36 upside down on the right side.
2. Stand with your left shoulder arm's distance from the wall. Toes should be facing straight ahead, perpendicular to the wall and even with the 15-inch mark of the left yardstick.
3. Drop the left arm and raise the right arm to the side.
4. Without moving your feet, rotate your trunk to the right as far as possible as you reach along the yardstick.

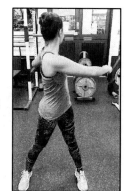

Figure 8.2. Trunk Rotation

5. Hold for 3-4 seconds and do not move your feet or bend the trunk. You can bend your knees slightly.

6. Have a partner record the distance reached to the nearest half-inch. Repeat two times and record your highest score.

7. Change directions with your right shoulder arm's distance from the wall. This time you will rotate to the left and use the second yardstick (the one that is upside down).

While these assessments provide valuable information about how flexible you are in these specific areas, they do not tell you how flexible you are throughout the rest of your body. So in order to design an individualized flexibility program, you will need to conduct a series of informal assessments using a variety of commonly used flexibility exercises. You want to select at least one flexibility exercise for each major joint or body part that is used in sport, exercise and daily life and measure the following three criteria; (1) your tension point or furthest area you can hold a stretch; (2) how long you can hold each stretch for and (3) how comfortable you feel while holding each stretch. Table 8.1 includes the format for informally assessing your flexibility. Column 1 includes a list of popular stretches that individuals use when they want to improve their flexibility. Column 2 identifies the areas of the body being stretched. Column 3 is used to measure the furthest spot a stretch was held for. Column 4 is used to measure the length of time the stretch was held for. Column 5 is used to measure the level of comfort felt during each stretch and column 6 is used to reveal the enjoyment experienced while engaging in each stretch.

By using a combination of standardized (formal) assessments with traditional flexibility exercises and measuring your tension point along with the amount of time you held each stretch, you will learn exactly how flexible you are throughout your body; with this knowledge, you can design a flexibility program that is just right for you. You can use Appendix 8A to informally assess your own level of flexibility.

Table 8.1
Informally Assessing Your Flexibility

Flexibility Exercises	Area(s) Being Addressed	Tension Point Achieved	Length of Time Held	Level of Comfort Experienced	Level of Enjoyment Experienced

To determine your level of comfort and enjoyment while performing each stretch during your informal flexibility assessment, please answer the following questions.

How comfortable did you feel during this exercise?

1	2	3	4	5	6	7	8	9

extremely
uncomfortable

extremely
comfortable

How much did you enjoy this exercise?

This exercise was comfortable

1	2	3	4	5	6	7	8	9

not at all

very much

TYPES OF STRETCHING TECHNIQUES

There are a variety of stretching techniques that you can use to improve your flexibility. Each one has their strengths as well as their limitations so read on and see which ones(s) work best for you.

Static Stretch (SS)—This type of stretch occurs when you stretch a muscle or joint to where you feel tension and hold it for a prescribed length of time, usually 10 to 30 seconds. The *benefits* of static stretching are: (1) that it is easy to do; (2) it is the safest of all flexibility techniques; (3) you can do it by yourself and (4) you will certainly improve your flexibility. The *limitation* is that you may not be able to reach your true tension point by yourself due to certain physical limitations. For example, when performing a seated toe touch, you will only be able to reach to a certain point by yourself. However, with some assistance from a partner, you will be able to stretch further and reach your true tension point. See Figure 8.3 to familiarize yourself with static stretching.

Figure 8.3.
Static Stretch

Passive Static (PS)— Passive static stretching usually involves the use of a partner to help you stretch and achieve your full range of motion. The partner serves as an external force to assist you in the desired direction of the stretch. For example, let's say you want to stretch your hamstrings and lower back and you are performing a sitting toe touch stretch. By yourself, you can reach your ankles, but not any further. Now your partner kneels behind you and places some force in the lower and center parts of your back which allows you to stretch further and touch your toes. Or, how about this one. You are laying down on a mat and you move your leg as far to you as possible which gets to the front of your shoulders. Now your partner assists you by holding the heel of your foot and slowly begins to move your leg towards you and now your foot is several inches past your shoulders. Amazing!

In addition to using a partner, you can also perform passive static stretches by using certain objects like a towel or a resistance band to assist you in creating an enhanced range of motion. Let's use the lying hamstring stretch as an example. Simply lay flat on your back and raise one leg in the air and place a towel around your ankle, holding the edges of the towel on each side. Slowly begin to move the towel towards your face until you cannot go any further. By holding the towel in this position you will be able to move your leg a further distance than without it which will allow you to stretch towards your true tension point, thus creating a greater range of motion. The benefit of passive static stretching is that it will enable you to reach your true tension point and stretch further than a static stretch. Moreover, having a partner with you may also increase your motivation to stretch. The main limitation of passive static stretching is lack of communication. When working with a partner, the following information must be discussed: (1) the exercise(s) being performed; (2) how long the stretch is to be held for; (3) the desired tension point and (4) when the individual has had enough and needs to stop; The partner must know the proper form of all exercises being performed as well as the ability of the individual stretching. It is also important for the partner to listen to the individual and not force him/her to overstretch by going past the proper tension point or holding longer than can be comfortably withstood. Failure to do so can result in injury. (See Figure 8.4 to familiarize yourself with passive static stretching).

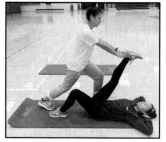 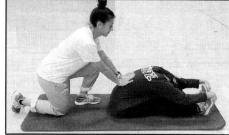

Figure 8.4. Passive Static Stretch

Proprioceptive Neuromuscular Facilitation (PNF)—PNF stretching is a more advanced form of flexibility training that was originally developed as a type of rehabilitation to help individuals who were injured to regain flexibility, mobility and muscular strength. PNF stretching involves the use of a partner to assist you in the stretching process. It is based on a contract-relax sequence where your partner creates some force by pushing you slowly in the direction of your desired stretch. You then apply force in the opposite direction against your partner, thus inhibiting or delaying the movement. The amount of resistance applied by your partner should be relevant to one's individual level of muscular fitness and flexibility. Ideally, your partner should hold you in a position for 5-10 seconds, thus creating an isometric contraction with force exerted without any movement. Then, if possible, your partner should increase the resistance slightly by holding you at a greater angle. You repeat the isometric contraction for another 5-10 seconds and then relax. The process can be performed anywhere from 2-5 times for as little as 5 seconds or as long as 30 seconds depending on your level of muscular fitness and flexibility. The *benefits* of PNF stretching are: (1) it creates a better range of motion than static stretching because of the use of a partner to help you stretch and (2) it will improve muscular fitness due to the isometric contraction being performed for prescribed lengths of time (5-30 seconds). The *limitations* are: (1) PNF stretching has been known to cause muscle stiffness and soreness; (2) PNF stretching takes more time to complete than static stretching and (3) PNF stretching requires a knowledgeable partner who knows how to perform the exercises correctly and understands your present level of flexibility and how much resistance is necessary to exert in order to improve flexibility safely and productively. (See Figure 8.5 to familiarize yourself with PNF stretching).

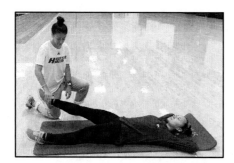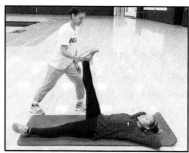

Figure 8.5 PNF Stretch

Ballistic Stretch—"Ballistic" refers to a bouncing motion and when you perform a ballistic stretch you are bouncing up and down, forward and back on in and out, repeatedly. The *benefit* of of a ballistic stretch is that by bouncing you are elongating your muscles at a faster rate and that can improve your flexibility provided you bounce slowly, gently and in a controlled motion. The *limitation* is that ballistic stretching can be dangerous if bouncing is done in a rapid, thrusting, jerky motion. This can cause overstretching which can lead to soreness and possible injury due to the tearing of soft tissue. A simple way to view ballistic stretching is to imagine your muscles being like a frozen rubber band. You take the rubber band out of the freezer and look to stretch it back and forth very quickly. The end result would be a broken rubber band because it needed to be warmed up first. Out of all of the different flexibility techniques, ballistic stretching is the least recommended due to the high risk of stretching improperly and causing injury.

Dynamic Stretch—involves the combination of moving around while elongating the muscles. For example, when doing lunges you are walking and elongating your stride, thus you are warming up your muscles while simultaneously stretching them out. Consequently, dynamic stretching is the one flexi-bility technique that should be done to warm up before exer-cising. (See Figure 8.6 to familiarize yourself with dynamic stretching).

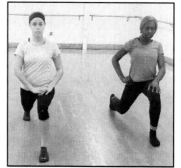

Figure 8.6. Dynamic Stretch

COMMON PROBLEMS AND SOLUTIONS ASSOCIATED WITH STRETCHING

For many years, flexibility was equated with warming up. Whether at the start of physical education class, the beginning of sports' practice or getting ready for your morning workout, it has often been common practice to start out with a few static stretches and then begin your sport or exercise activity. Although flexibility and warming up are related, they are not the same thing. Warming up means getting your body ready for action, usually through large muscle activity (e.g., brisk walk, light jog, stationary bicycle) for a few minutes prior to the start of your workout. It also means working the same muscle groups that you plan to overload at a slower or lighter intensity motion (e.g., performing 8-12 reps with a light weight before increasing to a weight that will create overload), while stretching involves moving your joints through their full range of motion. To put it "coldly" stretching before warming up is like taking that frozen rubber band out of the freezer and trying to elongate it. "Ouch!" When you first start to exercise, your muscles are cold and tight and really cannot be stretched effectively without being warmed up first. In other words, take your frozen rubber band and put it in some warm water so the ice melts and then stretch it out. "Ah, the amazing advances of modern science. Now, doesn't that feel better!" Below are some common problems that occur when stretching, along with ways of preventing them.

Going too fast—Sometimes we stretching is viewed as a prelude to another activity where you rush through a few stretches by quickly moving to a point of light to moderate tension and holding it briefly just so you can move on to your desired activity (e.g., jogging, lifting weights, playing sports). The problem is that you aren't giving yourself enough time to hold the stretch long enough or far enough to truly improve your flexibility. *Solution*: Go slow. Stretch to a point where you feel tension and hold it for at least 10 seconds. Then stretch just a little bit further. The slower you go and the longer you can hold a stretch, the further you will be able to stretch and the better you will feel.

Not reaching tension point—It is tempting to stretch until you feel a little bit of tension and then stop. While doing so will improve your flexibility somewhat (provided you hold the stretch for at least 10 seconds), if you are not stretching to your true tension point then you will not be stretching as effectively as you can. To give you a clear example of what this is like imagine if you were lifting 40 percent of your and stopping after 10 reps or jogging with your heart at 30% MHR. *Solution:* Stretch as far as you can and hold for at least 10 seconds. Every 5 seconds stretch a little further.

No pain no gain—Some people believe that in order to see results they must feel pain. That is simply not true. There is a fine line between tension and pain. Feeling tension while stretching indicates that you are overloading the intended area which means that you are improving your flexibility. Feeling pain while stretching often means overstretching or not using the proper form which can result in injury. *Solution:* Learn where your tension point is and challenge yourself to reach it and not go past it. You should be experiencing a moderate amount of tension while stretching, and the longer you hold the stretch, the less tension you should feel. If you are experiencing pain, then shorten the distance that you are stretching. Remember that is is vital to always avoid full flexion and extension of the knees and neck

Holding your breath—Sometimes people hold their breath while stretching. This makes it difficult to stretch for prolonged periods of time or concentrate on stretching to the true tension point. *Solution*: Inhale before you start to feel tension and then slowly exhale once you begin to hold at your tension point. As you exhale, imagine the tension being evaporated from the part of your body that you are stretching. You can also count to yourself while inhaling and exhaling. This will help you to stretch longer and make sure you are breathing properly and not holding your breath.

Not seeing results—The physical changes in one's body is not as apparent with flexibility as it is with CRE and MF. Moreover, there is less equipment available for flexibility than for CRE and MF workouts and less material (e.g., workout cards, progress sheets) to record your flexibility workouts and determine your numerical progress. Consequently, it is easy to forget what may have been accomplished in a flexibility workout and thus your level of motivation may decrease. *Solution*: Record your results. Write down the exercises that you do, the length of time that you hold each stretch, your present tension point for each exercise that do and your SMAART goals for flexibility. (See Appendix 8C to record your workouts on your Flexibility Workout Card).

Boredom—Holding a stretch for a certain length of time can become quite boring especially for those people who enjoy high intensity, non-stop workouts that require consistent movement (e.g., interval training, supersets, spin classes, boot camp). *Solution*: Find something you like to do while stretching. For example, listen to your favorite types of music, play games on your phone, text your family or friends, watch a movie on your phone on in an exercise facility that has cardio theatre, read a book or stretch with a friend/partner and engage in a friendly conversation. This will help you to associate stretching with what you like to do and thus increase your motivation to improve your flexibility. In Chapter 11, you will be introduced to cognitive strategies that teach you how and what to think during various modes of exercise (e.g., flexibility, CRE, MF).

DEVELOPING AN EXERCISE PRESCRIPTION FOR IMPROVING YOUR FLEXIBILITY

By now you should realize that working on flexibility is a very important part of your health-related fitness. Now it is time to develop your own exercise prescription for flexibility so that you can get started working in this area and feel good about what you are accomplishing. While the same four components of an exercise prescription are used (F-I-T-T), the way each is measured is slightly different for flexibility than CRE or MF.

Frequency—How many days will you commit to flexibility? While it is commonly recommended by fitness experts that you should work on flexibility at least 3-5 days per week, this may or may not be realistic for you especially if you are not presently active or if your motivation to work on flexibility is low. Therefore, you should decide how many days you will commit to working on flexibility and remember that stretching does not have to take as long as CRE or MFT to see and feel good results.

Intensity—the intensity of your flexibility program is defined and measured by your tension point. Your tension point is the furthest area that you can hold a stretch for a prescribed amount of time which is usually 10 to 30 seconds. For example, if the furthest spot you can reach to on the modified hurdler's stretch is your shins, then your tension point is your shins for that stretch.

Time—Time can be defined and measured in three ways: (1) the number of exercises that you plan to do; (2) the number of sets that you plan to do and (3) the length of time that you plan to hold a stretch for. For example, Lila has selected 6 stretches to do and she plans on doing two sets of each and holding each stretch for 15-20 seconds. Therefore, Lila will be stretching for a total of 3-4 minutes.

Type—Type is also defined and measured in two ways: (1) the flexibility technique that you are using (e.g., static, passive static, PNF) and (2) the name of the stretches you select (e.g., butterfly, pigeon, towel stretch).

Table 8.2
Flexibility Exercise Prescription Form

	Week 1	Week 2	Week 3	Week 4
F	1-2-3-4-5-6-7	1-2-3-4-5-6-7	1-2-3-4-5-6-7	1-2-3-4-5-6-7
I–	Include the names of the flexibility exercises that you plan to do and your present tension points for each.	Include the names of the flexibility exercises that you plan to do and your desired tension points for each.	Include the names of the flexibility exercises that you plan to do and your desired tension points for each.	Include the names of the flexibility exercises that you plan to do and your desired tension points for each.
T– list the number of stretches you will do each week & how long you plan to hold each stretch for;				
T– list the flexibility technique(s) that you will use (SS, PS, PNF).				

For "F" – circle the number of days that you plan to work on improving your flexibility.
For T – SS = Static Stretch; PS = Passive Static Stretch; PNF = Proprioceptive Neuromuscular Facilitation Stretch.

Of the four components of your exercise prescription, the one that is the most related to your level of commitment is "Frequency." Once you have decided how many days per week you will commit to working on flexibility, the Intensity, Time, and Type should be easy for you to follow. Starting with "Type," select different stretches that work all of your major muscle groups and/or the areas of your body that you are least flexible. Then choose which flexibility "Techniques" work best for you (e.g., Static, Passive Static, PNF). Next is "Time" where you should choose how long you would like to hold each stretch for and how many sets you plan to do for each exercise. Finally, "Intensity" where you can discover exactly where your tension points are for each of the exercises that you have selected. Each time you stretch you can start at your present tension point and strive to reach a new, desired tension point. This will help you to visualize and quantify your flexibility workouts and make it more tangible to recognize your results. See Table 8.2 to familiarize yourself with the format for creating your own exercise prescription for flexibility.

Below is an example that demonstrates how to create an exercise prescription for flexibility over a 4-week period. Lincoln is a college freshman who worked on his flexibility two times in Week 1. He performed 4 stretches listed on his Flexibility Workout Card (See Appendix 8C) and he held each stretch for 10 seconds. As a result of his performance in Week 1, Lincoln designed the following exercise prescription for himself in Weeks' 2-4. (See Table 8.3 to view Lincoln's Flexibility Exercise Prescription).

Table 8.3
Lincoln's Flexibility Exercise Prescription

	WEEK 1	WEEK 2	WEEK 3	WEEK 4
F	1-**2**-3-**4**-5-6-7	1-**2**-3-**4**-5-6-7	1-**2**-3-**4**-5-6-7	1-**2**-3-**4**-5-6-7
I	Butterfly Knees 2 inches off ground Seated Toe Touch Fingertips to shins Kneeling Lunge Hips Forward & Knees Behind Toes Standing Quad Stretch Heel to Buttocks	Butterfly Knees 1.5 inches off ground Seated Toe Touch Fingertips to ankles Kneeling Lunge Hips Forward & Knees Behind Toes Standing Quad Stretch Heel to Buttocks Fingers to the Sky	Butterfly Knees 1 inch off ground Seated Toe Touch Palms to Ankles Kneeling Lunge Hips Forward & Knees Behind Toes Standing Quad Stretch Heel to Buttocks Fingers to the Sky	Butterfly Knees 0.5 inches off ground Seated Toe Touch Fingertips to Toes Kneeling Lunge Hips forward & Knees Behind toes Standing Quad Stretch Heel to Buttocks Fingers to the Sky Back Extension on Swiss Ball Fingertips Toward Ground
T	4 stretches held for 10 seconds each	4-5 stretches held for 12 seconds each	5 stretches held for 15 seconds each	6 stretches held for 20 seconds each
T	SS	SS	SS	SS

SS—static stretch; PS—passive static stretch; PNF—proprioceptive neuromuscular facilitation stretch

As you can see, Lincoln has increased the length of time he stretched, holding each stretch for :10 in Week 1 and increasing to :12, :15 and :20 in Weeks' 2, 3 and 4, respectively. In addition, Lincoln has identified where he would like his tension points to be in each of the flexibility exercises that he plans to do over the 4 weeks. Since he now strives to stretch further and longer each week, Lincoln will definitely see a significant improvement in his flexibility over time. Now it's your turn. By now, you should have a clear understanding of how to develop and implement your Flexibility Exercise Prescription and record your results. If Lincoln can do it, then so can you!

Below is a procedure for you to follow that will help you design and implement your flexibility exercise prescription over a four-week period.

1. Using your Flexibility Exercise Prescription Form (Appendix 8B) circle the number of days that you are committing to work on flexibility in Week 1.

2. Skip down to the first "T" and choose how many different stretches you will do, the number of sets you will do for each stretch and how long you plan to hold each stretch.

3. Now go to the last "T" and select the flexibility technique(s) that motivate you the most to improve your flexibility. Now list the names of each stretch that you plan to do.

4. Finally, move back up to "I" and include your present tension points for each of the stretching exercises that you listed.

Once you have completed your flexibility exercise prescription, it is now time to stretch. Please follow these guidelines to ensure that you are stretching safely, properly, and productively (and of course having lots of fun, too).

1. Warm up before stretching—physically this means to start moving around and get the blood flowing and your body temperature up. You can go for a walk, get on the exercise bike or even jog for a few minutes; mentally this means that you are thinking positively and ready to begin stretching. Using words or phrases that encourage you to stretch can ensure that you are mentally ready (i.e., relax, awesome, feels great). You want to look forward to stretching because you know it will make you feel better.

2. Breathe properly—inhale for 4 seconds before you begin to stretch and then slowly exhale once you begin to hold your stretch;

3. Stretch slowly and gently—as you begin to stretch you should concentrate on where you feel tension and slowly keep moving towards your tension point;

4. Stretch to your tension point—stretch as far as you can and once you cannot stretch any further then you have reached your tension point;

Once you have finished, you can record your results on your flexibility workout card located in Appendix 8C. Then you can use your results from week 1 (e.g., number of days you worked on flexibility, number of stretches completed, seconds held for each stretch, tension points achieved for each exercise) to design your Flexibility Exercise Prescription for weeks 2, 3, & 4. (See Appendix 8B for your Flexibility Exercise Prescription Form). You see, once you have completed week 1, you can use those results to improve your flexibility by adding more stretches in the upcoming weeks, striving to hold each stretch a few seconds longer and reaching new tension points.

DETERMINING YOUR LEVEL OF COMMITMENT TO BEING MORE FLEXIBLE

No matter how much information there is to explain the importance of flexibility, no many how many assessments (formal or informal) there are to measure your level of flexibility, no matter how many charts you can use to monitor your progress, the bottom line is this. The only way you are going to work on improving your flexibility is to be committed to it. So let's find out just exactly how committed you are. How committed are you to improving your flexibility?

How many days per week are you committed to work on your flexibility?

1   2   3   4   5   6   7   8   9

How many minutes per workout will you commit towards working on your flexibility?

1-2 3-4 5-6 7-8 9-10 11-12 13-15 16-19 20-25 26 or more

The most important factor in developing and eventually maintaining a high level of commitment is to find the time that fits for you. Instead of changing around your lifestyle to find the time to work on flexibility, simply write down the available time(s) that you have right now. You are better off having a high level of commitment to work on flexibility two times per week than a low level of commitment to work on flexibility five times per week. As each week progresses and you begin to experience the many benefits associated with being more flexible, you should inevitably find some more time to continue improving. Think about it! Why wouldn't you want to find the time to do something that will benefit your health and make you feel good? (See Table 8D to determine your time commitment to flexibility).

Spicing Up Your Flexibility Program

In order to make your flexibility program fun, enjoyable and something you look forward to doing, there are a few strategies for you to consider while stretching.

1. First, determine the environment/location where you would like to stretch.

    A. *At home (inside)*—This may be the perfect place for you if you find comfort in just thinking about going home after school or work. Simply pick a comfortable place where you can stand, sit, and lie down and you are ready.

    B. *At home outside (backyard)*— Perhaps you prefer to be outside and you have a nice front or backyard area that you like. If so, you can take a mat, towel or blanket and do your flexibility exercises in your "new favorite spot" (weather permitting of course).

C. ***Local gym***—If you belong to a gym and exercise there, then consider adding a few minutes to your workout for stretching. Here are a few strategies for you to consider: (1) stretch after your CRE workout; (2) stretch in between sets and after your muscular fitness workout; (3) stretch after you warm up; (4) take your exercise prescription for flexibility with you and stretch as a total body workout rather than as a warm up or cool down; (5) sign up for a Yoga class and get your stretching done there;

D. ***At work***—Perhaps you work a long, hard day and by the time you come home you are tired, achy, and lack the motivation to do any physical activity. If that is your situation, then consider finding some time to stretch at work. You could come to work a few minutes early, stay a few minutes late or find some time in between (e.g., lunch hour, schedule 5-10 minutes for yourself to stretch). Finally, create a list of stretches that you can do at different times and just cross them out as you complete each, just like you would with your daily appointments, classes, etc.

E. ***Scenic place***—If you are someone who loves nature and is motivated to be in a beautiful, naturalistic setting, then consider a nice park, beach or aesthetically appealing location to do your stretches.

2. With whom do you like to stretch?

A. ***By yourself***—If you like to stretch alone then plan a time and place where you can be by yourself (e.g., early morning before work or school, lunch break, after work or school, before or after dinner, before bed time, at home, work, school, park, exercise facility during down time) to stretch. If you are very busy and have a full day of classes or appointments with few or no breaks in between, then you should consider scheduling an appointment with yourself a day or two in advance to stretch for a few minutes.

B. ***With a partner***—With a partner-If you are motivated to work on your flexibility, then you should consider enrolling in an exercise class. Believe it or not, many people enroll in exercise classes to find others with similar interests. Classes can often be found in these settings: (1) college or university activity program; (2) continuing education; (3) local Y or community center; (4) library; (5) private exercise facilities; Finally, if you are shy and feel uncomfortable going by yourself then how about enrolling one of your close friends, roommate(s), neighbors, co-workers or relatives to stretch with you?

   Once you find a partner to stretch with, make sure your schedules are compatible. Each of you should write time the days and times that you have free to stretch together. Once you have a match, then identify the location that you want to stretch together. Make the commitment to yourself as well as each other that once you write down your "flexibility schedule" you are no longer "flexible" to change it. Of course, emergencies do happen and therefore you should always have a back-up plan that if for any reason you cannot stick to your assigned schedule, you will immediately contact your partner and reschedule.

3. What ambiance motivates you the most to want to stretch?

   A. *Music*—If you like music, then create your own playlists designed strictly for listening to while stretching. This will help your mind and body relax and make it easier and more enjoyable for you to stretch.

   B. *Quiet*—If you prefer quiet, then find a place and time free from noise or distraction (bedroom after you wake up or right before you plan to go to sleep, at work before anyone else arrives, local park).

   C. *Television*—If you are a television buff and you have several favorite shows that you watch regularly, then maybe you should stretch during a segment of these shows or during the commercials.

   D. *Conversation*—If you like to talk then maybe you should stretch with someone while having a conversation. This can be done in person, face to face or even if you are on your phone or computer. Simply get into your stretching position, press speaker or skype and talk away. You'll be amazed at how much longer you might stretch when you are involved in a conversation vs. when you are alone, stretching by yourself.

4. Finally, if you are goal-oriented then set some SMAART flexibility goals (see below).

SETTING SMAART GOALS TO IMPROVE YOUR FLEXIBILITY

In order to create a high level of motivation and commitment to improve your flexibility, you need to set SMAART goals. You can use any of the four components of your exercise prescription to set your SMAART goals. Simply ask yourself any or all of the following: How many days should I work on my flexibility? What is my present tension point for the stretches I plan to do and what is my goal for how far I would like to be able stretch with each? How many seconds should I hold each stretch for? What flexibility technique(s) should I use and which flexibility exercises will work best for me? Let's use Stan as an example of how to set SMAART goals using F-I-T-T.

F Stan's goal is to stretch three times this week on Monday, Wednesday, & Friday at the campus exercise facility.

I Stan's goal is to reach his toes on the sitting toe touch stretch.

T Stan's goal is to stretch for 20 minutes this week and hold each stretch for at least 16 seconds.

T Stan's goal is to do two passive static stretches with a partner and four static stretches by himself. He will stretch the following muscle groups: (1) quadriceps, (2) hamstrings, (3) hip flexors; (4) glutes; (5) calves; (6) neck and (7) back.

As you can see, Stan has incorporated the SMAART principle in the following manner: He has identified *specific* muscle groups that he wants to work (e.g., quadriceps, hamstrings, hip flexors, etc.). His goals are clearly *measurable* in several ways: (1) stretch three times per week; (2) reach his toes on the toe touch stretch; (3) stretch for 20 minutes per week; (4) hold each stretch for 16 seconds; (5) perform a total of 6 different stretches per workout; He has an *action plan* of where the stretching will take place and what types of stretching will be done. His goals can easily be *adjusted* in the event that they will not be reached (e.g., three times to two times per week; stretch at home). His goals seem *realistic*, however, it may take Stan a week or two to see how close he is towards reaching his weekly goals and determine how realistic his goals really are. Finally, Stan has a *target date* of stretching for a total of 20 minutes this week. Now it's your turn to put into action what you know is so important to your overall fitness and health. So set your goals for flexibility and always remember to "STRETCH SMAART."

Another way to increase your motivation to improve your flexibility is to use the Stairway to Success. Figure 8.7 demonstrates how Debbie used the Stairway to Success to set goals for minutes in a single workout and a full week, and Figure 8.8 shows how Jeff used the Staircase to set goals for how long he wanted to hold a stretch. In the example used in Figure 8.8, Debbie started out stretching for 1 minute on January 15. Her long-term goal was to be able to stretch for 20 minutes by July 15. Every two weeks, Debbie set a short-term goal to improve her performance by stretching one to two minutes longer than she did in the previous week. Each time she reached her short-term goal, Debbie moved one step up the stairway, getting closer and closer to her long-term goal of stretching for 20 minutes. And before she knew it, Debbie's long-term dream goal of climbing up all of the stairs became nothing more than a single, short-term goal. Use Appendix 8E to create your own Stairway to Success goals to increase the length of time you would like to stretch each week.

In Figure 8.8, Jeff used the Stairway to Success to set a goal for how long he wanted to be able to hold a stretch. As of January 15, Jeff could only hold a stretch for 5 seconds while his long-term goal was to be able to hold a stretch for 30 seconds by 7/15. Jeff's first goal was to be able to hold a stretch for 6 seconds and he wanted to achieve that by 1/30. Each time Jeff achieved his short-term goal, he set a more challenging goal up the stairway until he eventually achieved his long-term goal of holding each of his stretches for 30 seconds each. Use Appendix 8F to create your own Stairway to Success goals if you want to improve holding each stretch longer.

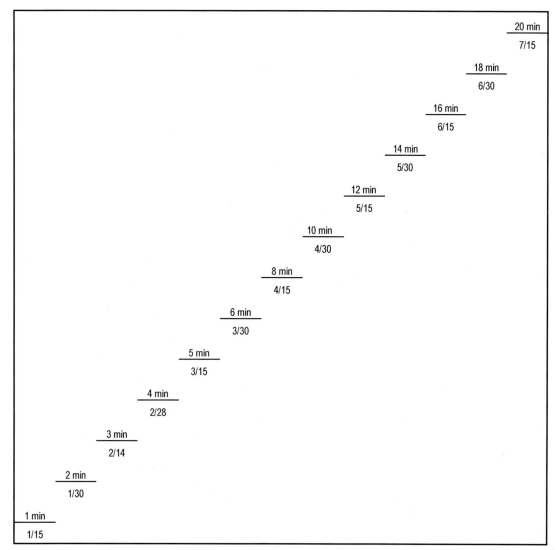

20 min
7/15

18 min
6/30

16 min
6/15

14 min
5/30

12 min
5/15

10 min
4/30

8 min
4/15

6 min
3/30

5 min
3/15

4 min
2/28

3 min
2/14

2 min
1/30

1 min
1/15

To use the Stairway to Success effectively, Debbie started out by using the bottom step to record her present performance (stretching for 1 min). Then she used the top step to set her long-term dream goal of stretching for 20 minutes. Then Debbie went back to the second step from the bottom to set her first short-term goal which was to   stretch for 2 minutes by 1/30. When Debbie reached that goal, she set a goal on the next step up and so on until she reached her long-term goal of stretching for 20 minutes by 7/15.

Figure 8.7—Stairway to Success for Minutes in a Workout

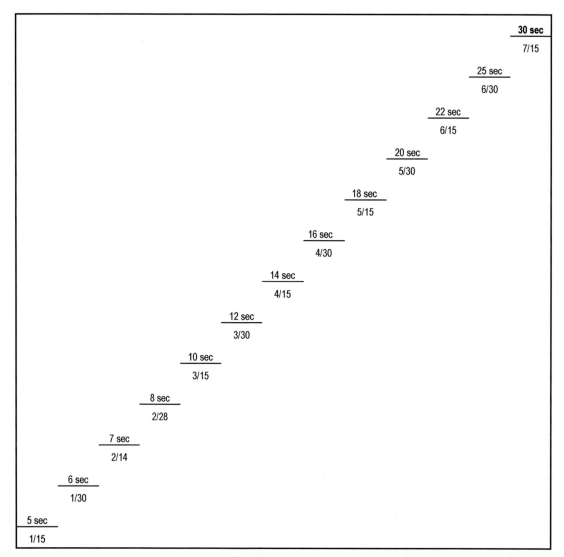

The bottom step is used to record Jeff's present number of seconds he could hold a stretch at the beginning of his flexibility program. (5 seconds on 1/15). The top represents Jeff's long-term goal of being able to hold a stretch for 30 seconds to be achieved by 7/15. The second step from the bottom is Jeff's first short term goal (hold a stretch for 6 seconds by 1/30). When Jeff reached that goal, he set a goal on the next step to hold a stretch for 7 seconds by 2/14 and so on until he reached his long-term goal of holding a stretch for 20 seconds by 7/15.

Figure 8.8—Stairway to Success for Seconds a Stretch is Held

INCORPORATING THE PRINCIPLES OF FITNESS INTO YOUR FLEXIBILITY PROGRAM

Warm Up Principle—Working on your flexibility means more than just stretching as a warm-up for other activities. To prepare your muscles to be stretched properly and efficiently, you have to warm them up first. Otherwise, you might feel discomfort while stretching and increase your chances of injuring yourself, too. An effective way to warm up before stretching is to activate "your working muscles"—the muscles you are planning to stretch. For leg muscles (hamstring, quadricep, calf, hip flexor), you can start out by selecting any large muscle group activity (e.g., walking, jogging, riding a bike) and do it at a light intensity for a few minutes. For your upper body (arms, chest, back, shoulders), you can model some of the resistance training exercises without weights (e.g., tricep extension, bench press, lat pull down, front raises) and move your body in the exact same way you would if you were lifting weights. This will warm up these areas and facilitate stretching.

Principle of Progression—To satisfy this principle for flexibility, you must specify how you will improve your flexibility during your workouts. You can use any of the four components from your exercise prescription to systematically show your progress. For example, you can increase your Frequency by going from two to three days per week. You can increase your Intensity by identifying your present tension point and challenging yourself to reach new tension points (e.g., stretching from your ankles to your toes on a seated toe touch stretch). You can improve Time by stretching for a longer period. For example, if you were able to hold your stretches for 8 seconds in Week 1, you can strive to hold for 10 seconds in Week 2. If you stretched for a total of 5 minutes in Week 1, you can increase to 6 minutes in Week 2. Finally, you can improve Type by adding more stretches or incorporating different flexibility techniques into your program. For instance, say you began with four different static stretches in Week 1. In Week 2, you can add another static stretch and one passive static stretch for a total of six stretches.

Principle of Individuality—Whether you decide to stretch by yourself, with a partner or in a small group or class, remember to focus on your own level of flexibility and not compare your performance with anybody else. Be proud of getting started and recognize that your progress is bound to happen provided you do one simple thing: Stick to your program.

Principle of Fun—There are several ways to incorporate fun into your flexibility workouts and they include: (1) finding a comfortable place to stretch (e.g., park, beach, backyard, pool, using a mat instead of the gym floor; (2) listening to music that makes you feel good while stretching; (3) stretching while watching your favorite TV shows; (4) stretching while talking or playing games on your cell phone; (5) with a partner or significant other; (6) taking a Yoga class with an awesome instructor; (7) stretching with your SMAART goals in mind;

Principle of Reversibility—To avoid going backwards and losing what you have gained, you have to make improving your flexibility a priority and stick to your program. That means focusing on when you will stretch (day and time), where you will stretch (e.g., home, office, gym), with whom you will stretch with (e.g., myself, workout partner or significant other, exercise class), and for how long will you stretch. If for any reason, you do not stick to your program, identify what stopped you and IMMEDIATELY incorporate a strategy to overcome your barrier(s) (e.g., set SMAART goals, change your environment, listen to different music, call a friend, etc.) and GET BACK INTO ACTION. Ideally, it is best if you can incorporate a few flexibility workouts per week into your schedule. However, if that is not practical for you, then consider incorporating stretching exercises into your CRE and MF exercise routines. For instance, before you begin your CRE or MF workouts, warm up by performing an aerobic activity for a few minutes at a light intensity (e.g., stationary bike, walking, jogging). Then

perform a few dynamic stretches. Not only will this make your muscles feel better, it will also improve the quality of your workout. Once you have completed your workout, you should stretch again using static, passive static or PNF stretches. This will decrease muscle soreness and tension caused by your exercise overload. While working on muscular fitness, you can also stretch in between sets to reduce any tension commonly caused by overloading your muscles. All you need to do is to go through the MF exercises that you just performed and use them as stretches. The only difference here is that you are elongating the motion and then holding the stretch for at least 10 seconds. See Figure 8.9 to review stretching during a MF workout.

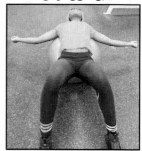

Figure 8.9
Seated Fly Stretch

Another suggestion to consider is to take a few minutes out of your daily schedule to stretch. For instance, if you work at a job that requires a lot of stationary position or if you are in school and sitting in classes all day (i.e., sitting at a desk, standing behind a register) then plan to stretch for one minute every hour. You can make a note for yourself "Get Up & Stretch" or "Reach the Sky." The key is to heighten your awareness about how important it is for you to first improve your flexibility and then maintain it by creating viable strategies of how, when and where you can address your flexibility needs on a day to day basis. This is certainly better then finishing your day feeling stress and tension in your body.

Principle of Specificity—First, make sure you know what stretches you intend to do for the muscles and joints that you want to stretch as well as what your tension point are for each of the stretches. Next, determine if you are going to stretch as a prelude to either your cardio-vascular or muscular fitness workout or if you are going to stretch as part of your flexibility workout. Finally, warm up properly by addressing the muscles that you plan to use in your workout and remember to always stretch to a point of tension and not pain.

EVALUATING THE SUCCESS OF YOUR FLEXIBILITY PROGRAM

Have you followed your exercise prescription for flexibility? How did your level of commitment change from before you started working on your flexibility until now? Were there any barriers that stopped you from improving your flexibility at any time during the four weeks of your flexibility program. What strategies did you incorporate to overcome these barriers and how successful were you in getting back into action? What improvements have you made from Weeks' 1 to 4? Use Appendix 8G to evaluate the success of your flexibility program.

If you did not improve your flexibility over the past four weeks, then you should determine what stopped you and then develop a plan of action to overcome your barrier(s) and get back on track. Simply understanding the importance of being more flexible is not enough. You MUST take action! You can use Appendix 8H to discover what, if anything is stopping you from improving your flexibility.

As long as you are highly committed to improving your flexibility, then you will continue to search for the all the ways your flexibility exercise prescription will fit into your life. Remember, commitment does not mean that you will always reach your goals. It does mean, however, that if you get stopped then you will identify exactly what's stopping you and incorporate strategies that help you to immediately get back into action and reach your goals. Please fill the questionnaire located in Appendix 8I, "Determining the Benefits of Working on Your Flexibility."

PREVENTING INJURIES

One of the most effective ways to reduce and prevent injuries is to work on your flexibility. There are several guidelines that you should incorporate in order to get the best stretch and reap the many benefits associated with good flexibility. They are:

1. Learn correct form while stretching
2. Warm up before stretching by getting your total body moving for a few minutes
3. Inhale before you start to stretch and slowly exhale as you move towards and hold at your tension point
4. Use flexibility as a workout rather than only a warm up or a cool down
5. Stretch after you cool down
6. Learn where your tension points are
7. Stretch to a point of tension, not pain
8. Stretch slowly and gently
9. Avoid overstretching
10. Avoid bouncing

This chapter introduced you to muscular flexibility and explained the importance of incorporating flexibility exercises into your lifestyle. A variety of flexibility assessments (e.g., formal and informal) and exercises have been introduced so that you can determine how flexible you are and assist you in designing a flexibility exercise prescription that is just right for you. In addition, several strategies are introduced to spice up your flexibility workouts and create a fun and productive atmosphere that will help motivate you to work on your flexibility.

Finally, guidelines to prevent injuries are listed to help you exercise safely. So be a little flexible and find the time to stretch it out!

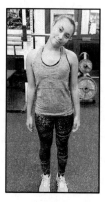
Lateral Head Tilt
(Neck)

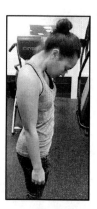
Chin to Chest
(Neck)

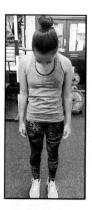
Chin to Chest
(Neck)

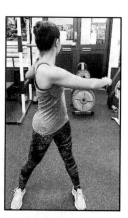
Trunk Rotation
(Upper Body)

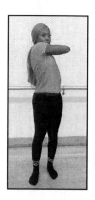
Wrap Around
(Upper Body)

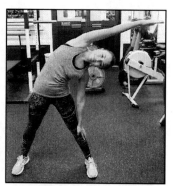
Side Bend (Shoulders, Obliques)
(Shoulders, Obliques)

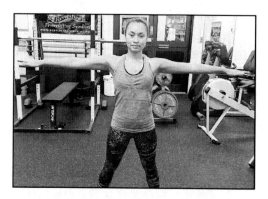
Lateral Raise
(Shoulders)

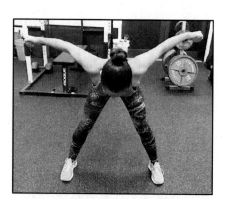
Bent over Lateral Raise
(Shoulders and Arms)

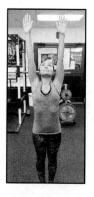
Touch the Sky
(Shoulders, Arms, Back)

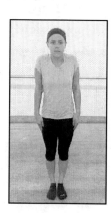
Shoulder Shrug
(Shoulders)

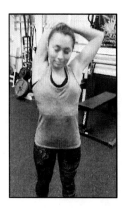 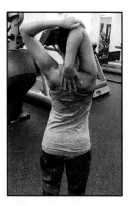 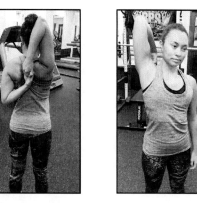

Press Arm Down behind Head
(Shoulders, Arms)

Interlocking Fingers
behind Back Shoulders, Arms
(Shoulders, Arms)

Tricep Stretch
(Triceps)

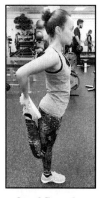 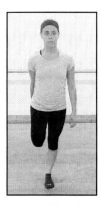 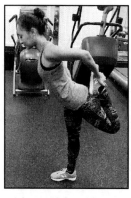 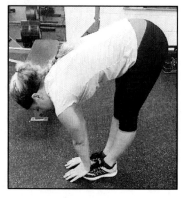

Quad Stretch
Side Angle

Quad Stretch

Advanced Quad Stretch

Standing Toe Touch
(Hamstrings, Lower Back)

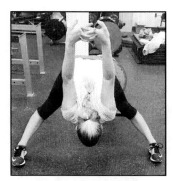 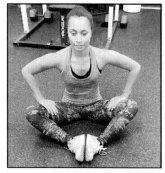 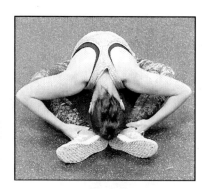

Standing Toe Touch
Fingers Interlaced

Butterfly
(Groin, Hip, Flexors, Abductors)

Butterfly
(Groin, Hip, Flexors, Abductors, Back)

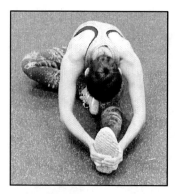

Modified Hurdler's Stretch

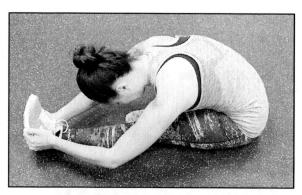

Modified Hurdler's Stretch Side Angle
(Hamstrings & Lower Back)

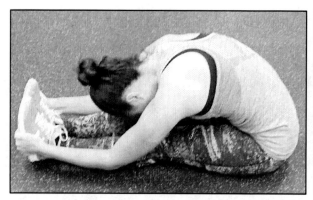

Seated Toe Touch Feet Together
(Hamstrings, Lower Back)

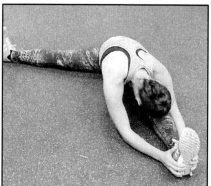

Seated Toe Touch Feet Apart
(Hamstrings, Groin, Lower Back)

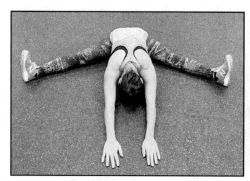

Seated Forward Reach
(Back, Hamstrings, Shoulders)

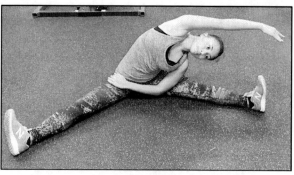

Sitting Side Stretch
(Hips, Shoulders, Obliques, Hamstrings, Lower Back))

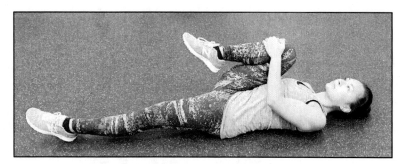

Knee to Chest Stretch
(Quadriceps, Lower Back)

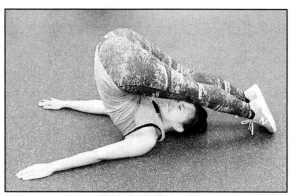

Lying Toes Behind Head Stretch
(Back Shoulders, Arms, Legs

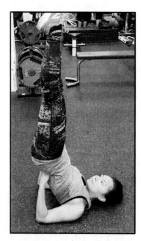

Toes to the Sky
(Back, Legs, Abdominals)

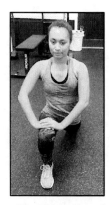

Hip Flexor Stretch
(Hip Flexors)

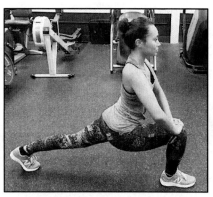

Hip Flexor Stretch Side Angle
(Hip Flexors)

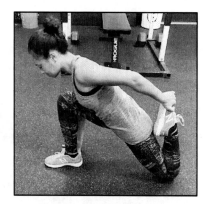

Kneeling Heel to Buttocks
(Hip Flexors, Quadriceps)

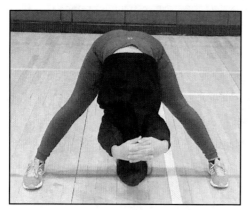

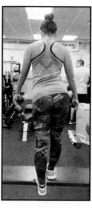

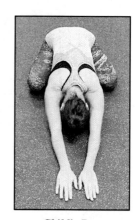

Head Down and Fingers Interlaced
(Hamstrings, Back, Shoulders, Arms)

Calf Stretch

Child's Pose
Total Body Stretch

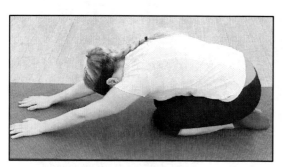

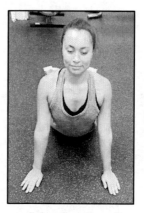

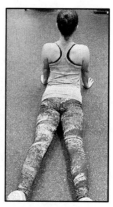

Child's Pose Side Angle

Cobra Core Stretch

Cobra Core Stretch
Back Angle

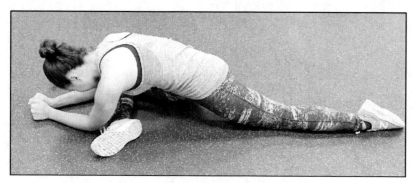

Pigeon Core Stretch

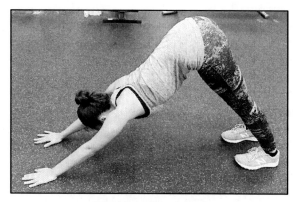

Down Dog Core Stretch

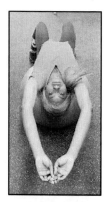

Upper Body Stretch on Ball

REVIEW QUESTIONS

1. Define flexibility.

2. List five benefits of being flexible and explain which one(s) mean the most to you?

3. Describe two ways to assess flexibility.

4. List four different flexibility techniques and explain the benefits and limitations of each?

5. What are some common problems people have when stretching?

6. What solutions can you offer to prevent these problems from occurring?

7. Explain the difference between warming up and stretching.

8. List three to five ways to spice up your flexibility program. Which one(s) work best for you and why?

9. Create two S-M-A-A-R-T Goals that can help you improve your flexibility?

10. Explain how you have incorporated the principles of fitness into your flexibility program?

11. What can you do to make your flexibility exercise program even more successful?

12. List four ways you can prevent injuries while stretching.

LAB ASSIGNMENT 8.1

Questions 1-10 should be answered prior to beginning your Flexibility Exercise Program.

1. How committed are you to improving your flexibility over the next four weeks?

   1   2   3   4   5   6   7   8   9
   extremely   extremely
   uncomfortable   comfortable

2. If you have a low level of commitment, what strategies will you incorporate to increase your level of commitment to improve your flexibility?

3. List your SMAART goals for improving your flexibility over the next four weeks?

S	
M	
A	
A	
R	
T	

4. Using the stairway to success, convert your SMAART goals into stairway goals over the next four weeks.

_____

_____

_____

_____

5. Develop an exercise prescription to improve your flexibility over the next 4 weeks.

	Week 1	Week 2	Week 3	Week 4
F				
I				
T				
T				

* For intensity—list each exercise and your present tension point in Week 1 and your desired tension points (where you are striving to get to in Weeks' 2-4. For Type, list the exercises you plan to use to improve your flexibility as well as the flexibility techniques (e.g., static, passive static, PNF) you are considering.

6. Explain how you will be satisfying the principle of progression over the next four weeks.

7. How do you plan to satisfy the warm up principle prior to working on your flexibility?

8. What strategies are you considering to incorporate the principle of fun into your flexibility workouts?

9. What strategies do you have planned to avoid the principle of reversibility?

Questions 10-13 should be answered after you have completed your 4-week Flexibility Exercise Prescription

10. What were the numerical results of your flexibility workouts over the past 4 weeks? Include: (1) frequency of times you worked on flexibility, (2) how your tension points changed, (3) how long you stretched and (4) if you increased the number of exercises that you did.

11. What effect did SMAART goals have on your motivation, performance and enjoyment of stretching?

12. Is there anything that stopped you from reaching your SMAART goals? If so, please explain. If not, then explain what you did to overcome your barriers and improve your flexibility.

13. How much fun did you have working on your flexibility? If you had fun then explain the strategies that you incorporated to enjoy working on flexibility. If you did not have fun, then explain what you plan to do over the next few weeks to make your flexibility workouts more enjoyable (e.g., listening to music, stretching with a partner, etc).

References and Recommended Readings

American College of Sports Medicine (1998). Position Stand: The recommended quantity and quality of exercise for developing and maintaining cardiorespiratory and muscular fitness and flexibility in healthy adults. *Medicine and Science in Sports and Exercise, 30*, 975-991.

Alter, M. (2004). *Science of stretching*. Third Edition. Human Kinetics Books. Champaign, Il. 6 good reasons you need to stretch

Blahnik, J. (2004). *Full-body flexibility*. Human Kinetics, Champaign, Il.

Bowles, H.R., Morrow, J.R., Jr., Leonard, B.L., Hawkins, M., & Couzelis, P.M. (2002). The association between physical activity behavior and commonly reported barriers in a worksite population. *Research Quarterly for Exercise and Sport, 73*, 464-470.

Bracko, M.R. (2002). Can stretching prior to exercise and sports improve performance and prevent injury? *ACSM's Health and Fitness Journal, 6*(5), 17-22.

Corbin, C., Welk, G., Corbin, W., & Welk, K. (2006). *Concepts of physical fitness: Active lifestyles for wellness,* pp 160 13th edition. McGraw Hill

Hoeger, W.K. & Hoeger, S.A. (2004). *Principles & labs for fitness and wellness* 7th edition. pp 226-246. Thomson:Wadsworth.

Knudsen, D.V. (2002). Stretchig during warm-up: Do we have enough evidence? *Journal of Physical Education, Recreation, and Dance, 70*, 271-277.

Kravitz, L. & Heyward, V. (1995). Flexibility training. *Fitness Management, 11* (2), 32-33, 36-38.

Liemohn, W.P. (2003). Exercise prescription for flexibility and low-back function. *In Health Fitness Instructor's Handbook.* 4th ed. E.T. Howley and B.D. Franks (eds). Human Kinetics: Champaign, IL.

McAtee, R.E. & Charland, J. (1993). Facilitated stretching, 2nd edition. Human Kinetics: Champaign, IL.

McAtee, R.E. & Charland, J. (2007). *Facilitated stretching*. Third Edition. Human Kinetics, Champaign, Il.

Millar, A.L. (2016). Improving flexibility and balance. www.acsm.org/public-information/articles/2016/10/07/improving-your-flexibility-and-balance.

Morrow, Jr, J.R., Krzewinski-Malone, J.A., Jackson, A.W., Bungun, T., & FitzGerald. S.J. (2004). American adults' knowledge of exercise recommendations. *Research Quarterly for Exercise and Sport, 75*, 3, 231-237.

Therien, S. (2015). What are the benefits of good flexibility? www.livestrong.com/article/332-519-what-are-the-benefits-of-good-flexibility/June 2, 2015.

www.shape.com/fitness/workouts/6-good-reasons-you-need-stretch.

APPENDIX 8A
INFORMALLY ASSESSING YOUR FLEXIBILITY

Flexibility Exercises	Area(s) Being Addressed	Tension Point Achieved	Length of Time Held	Level of Comfort	Level of Enjoyment
Lateral Head Tilt	Head & Neck				
Chin to Chest	Head & Neck				
Head to Ceiling	Head & Neck				
Trunk Rotation	Shoulders, Lower Back, Hips				
Touch the Sky	Shoulders, Back, Arms				
Lateral Raise	Shoulders				
Bent Over Lateral Raise	Shoulders, Back				
Self Hug	Shoulders, Arms				
Side Bend	Shoulders, Hips, Obliques				
Front Raise to the Sky	Shoulders, Lower Back, Arms				
Upper Body Towel Stretch	Shoulders, Arms, Back				
Bend Over, Interlock Hands	Shoulders, Arms, Lower Back, Hamstrings				
Triceps Stretch	Triceps, Shoulders				
Toes Behind Head	Lower Back, Shoulders, Arms, Legs, Abdominals				
Toes to the Sky	Total Body "Core Stretch"				
Chest Stretch	Chest, Arms, Back				
Standing Toe Touch Wide Base	Lower Back, Hamstrings				
Standing Toe Touch, Feet Together	Lower Back, Hamstrings				
Seated Toe Touch, Feet Spread Apart	Lower Back, Hamstrings				
Seated Tow Touch, Feet Together	Lower Back, Hamstrings				
Modified Hurdler's Stretch	Lower Back, Hamstrings				
Standing Quad Stretch	Quadriceps, Hip Flexors, Knees, Ankles				
Kneeling Quad Stretch	Quadriceps				
Single Knee to Chest	Lower Back & Hamstrings				
Double Knee to Chest	Upper & Lower Back & Hamstrings				
Butterfly	Inner thigh, Groin				
Standing Hip Flexor Stretch	Hip Flexors				
Kneeling Hip Flexor Stretch	Hip Flexors				
Standing on Bench	Calves				

Step Stretch	Calves				
Push the Wall	Calves, Hamstrings				
Cobra	Lower Back, Arms, Abdominals				
Pigeon	Total Body "Core" Stretch				
Down Dog	Total Body "Core" Stretch				
Child's Pose	Total Body "Core" Stretch				

To determine your level of comfort while performing each stretch during your informal flexibility assessment, please answer the following questions and place your answer in the column marked "Level of Comfort Experienced."

This exercise was comfortable

       1   2   3   4   5   6   7   8   9

   extremely   extremely

  uncomfortable   comfortable

To determine the level of enjoyment while performing each stretch during your informal flexibility assessment, please answer the following questions and place your answer in the column marked "Level of Enjoyment."

This exercise was enjoyable

       1   2   3   4   5   6   7   8   9

   not at all   very much

APPENDIX 8B
FLEXIBILITY EXERCISE PRESCRIPTION

	Week 1	Week 2	Week 3	Week 4
F	1-2-3-4-5-6-7	1-2-3-4-5-6-7	1-2-3-4-5-6-7	1-2-3-4-5-6-7
I–Include the names of the flexibility exercises that you plan to do and your present tension points for each in week 1 and your desired tension points in weeks 2-4				
T–include the number of stretches you will do each week and how long you plan to hold each stretch				
T–list the flexibility technique(s) that you will use (SS, PS, PNF).				

F—Circle the number of days that you plan to work on your flexibility.

APPENDIX 8C
FLEXIBILITY WORKOUT CARD

Flexibility Exercise		Day 1	Day 2	Day 3	Day 4	Day 5	Day 6	Day 7
	Sec Held Sets TP							
	Sec Held Sets TP							
	Sec Held Sets TP							
	Sec Held Sets TP							
	Sec Held Sets TP							
	Sec Held Sets TP							
	Sec Held Sets TP							
	Sec Held Sets TP							
	Sec Held Sets TP							
Goal	Sec Held Sets TP							

Sec Held—Record the number of seconds you hold each stretch in the sec held column;
Sets—Record the number of sets that you did for each of the exercises that you checked.
TP stands for tension point. Each time you stretch record your tension point.

APPENDIX 8D
MY TIME COMMITMENT TO FLEXIBILITY CHART
"Determining Your Days, Times and Minutes You are Committed to Flexibility

Time	M	T	W	Th	Fr	Sa	Su
6-8 AM	1 2 3 4 5 6 7 8 9 10 11 12 13 14 15 16 17 18 19 20 21 22 23 24 25 26 27 28 29 30	1 2 3 4 5 6 7 8 9 10 11 12 13 14 15 16 17 18 19 20 21 22 23 24 25 26 27 28 29 30	1 2 3 4 5 6 7 8 9 10 11 12 13 14 15 16 17 18 19 20 21 22 23 24 25 26 27 28 29 30	1 2 3 4 5 6 7 8 9 10 11 12 13 14 15 16 17 18 19 20 21 22 23 24 25 26 27 28 29 30	1 2 3 4 5 6 7 8 9 10 11 12 13 14 15 16 17 18 19 20 21 22 23 24 25 26 27 28 29 30	1 2 3 4 5 6 7 8 9 10 11 12 13 14 15 16 17 18 19 20 21 22 23 24 25 26 27 28 29 30	1 2 3 4 5 6 7 8 9 10 11 12 13 14 15 16 17 18 19 20 21 22 23 24 25 26 27 28 29 30
8-10 AM	1 2 3 4 5 6 7 8 9 10 11 12 13 14 15 16 17 18 19 20 21 22 23 24 25 26 27 28 29 30	1 2 3 4 5 6 7 8 9 10 11 12 13 14 15 16 17 18 19 20 21 22 23 24 25 26 27 28 29 30	1 2 3 4 5 6 7 8 9 10 11 12 13 14 15 16 17 18 19 20 21 22 23 24 25 26 27 28 29 30	1 2 3 4 5 6 7 8 9 10 11 12 13 14 15 16 17 18 19 20 21 22 23 24 25 26 27 28 29 30	1 2 3 4 5 6 7 8 9 10 11 12 13 14 15 16 17 18 19 20 21 22 23 24 25 26 27 28 29 30	1 2 3 4 5 6 7 8 9 10 11 12 13 14 15 16 17 18 19 20 21 22 23 24 25 26 27 28 29 30	1 2 3 4 5 6 7 8 9 10 11 12 13 14 15 16 17 18 19 20 21 22 23 24 25 26 27 28 29 30
10 AM 12 PM	1 2 3 4 5 6 7 8 9 10 11 12 13 14 15 16 17 18 19 20 21 22 23 24 25 26 27 28 29 30	1 2 3 4 5 6 7 8 9 10 11 12 13 14 15 16 17 18 19 20 21 22 23 24 25 26 27 28 29 30	1 2 3 4 5 6 7 8 9 10 11 12 13 14 15 16 17 18 19 20 21 22 23 24 25 26 27 28 29 30	1 2 3 4 5 6 7 8 9 10 11 12 13 14 15 16 17 18 19 20 21 22 23 24 25 26 27 28 29 30	1 2 3 4 5 6 7 8 9 10 11 12 13 14 15 16 17 18 19 20 21 22 23 24 25 26 27 28 29 30	1 2 3 4 5 6 7 8 9 10 11 12 13 14 15 16 17 18 19 20 21 22 23 24 25 26 27 28 29 30	1 2 3 4 5 6 7 8 9 10 11 12 13 14 15 16 17 18 19 20 21 22 23 24 25 26 27 28 29 30
12-2 PM	1 2 3 4 5 6 7 8 9 10 11 12 13 14 15 16 17 18 19 20 21 22 23 24 25 26 27 28 29 30	1 2 3 4 5 6 7 8 9 10 11 12 13 14 15 16 17 18 19 20 21 22 23 24 25 26 27 28 29 30	1 2 3 4 5 6 7 8 9 10 11 12 13 14 15 16 17 18 19 20 21 22 23 24 25 26 27 28 29 30	1 2 3 4 5 6 7 8 9 10 11 12 13 14 15 16 17 18 19 20 21 22 23 24 25 26 27 28 29 30	1 2 3 4 5 6 7 8 9 10 11 12 13 14 15 16 17 18 19 20 21 22 23 24 25 26 27 28 29 30	1 2 3 4 5 6 7 8 9 10 11 12 13 14 15 16 17 18 19 20 21 22 23 24 25 26 27 28 29 30	1 2 3 4 5 6 7 8 9 10 11 12 13 14 15 16 17 18 19 20 21 22 23 24 25 26 27 28 29 30
2-4 PM	1 2 3 4 5 6 7 8 9 10 11 12 13 14 15 16 17 18 19 20 21 22 23 24 25 26 27 28 29 30	1 2 3 4 5 6 7 8 9 10 11 12 13 14 15 16 17 18 19 20 21 22 23 24 25 26 27 28 29 30	1 2 3 4 5 6 7 8 9 10 11 12 13 14 15 16 17 18 19 20 21 22 23 24 25 26 27 28 29 30	1 2 3 4 5 6 7 8 9 10 11 12 13 14 15 16 17 18 19 20 21 22 23 24 25 26 27 28 29 30	1 2 3 4 5 6 7 8 9 10 11 12 13 14 15 16 17 18 19 20 21 22 23 24 25 26 27 28 29 30	1 2 3 4 5 6 7 8 9 10 11 12 13 14 15 16 17 18 19 20 21 22 23 24 25 26 27 28 29 30	1 2 3 4 5 6 7 8 9 10 11 12 13 14 15 16 17 18 19 20 21 22 23 24 25 26 27 28 29 30
4-6 PM	1 2 3 4 5 6 7 8 9 10 11 12 13 14 15 16 17 18 19 20 21 22 23 24 25 26 27 28 29 30	1 2 3 4 5 6 7 8 9 10 11 12 13 14 15 16 17 18 19 20 21 22 23 24 25 26 27 28 29 30	1 2 3 4 5 6 7 8 9 10 11 12 13 14 15 16 17 18 19 20 21 22 23 24 25 26 27 28 29 30	1 2 3 4 5 6 7 8 9 10 11 12 13 14 15 16 17 18 19 20 21 22 23 24 25 26 27 28 29 30	1 2 3 4 5 6 7 8 9 10 11 12 13 14 15 16 17 18 19 20 21 22 23 24 25 26 27 28 29 30	1 2 3 4 5 6 7 8 9 10 11 12 13 14 15 16 17 18 19 20 21 22 23 24 25 26 27 28 29 30	1 2 3 4 5 6 7 8 9 10 11 12 13 14 15 16 17 18 19 20 21 22 23 24 25 26 27 28 29 30
6-8 PM	1 2 3 4 5 6 7 8 9 10 11 12 13 14 15 16 17 18 19 20 21 22 23 24 25 26 27 28 29 30	1 2 3 4 5 6 7 8 9 10 11 12 13 14 15 16 17 18 19 20 21 22 23 24 25 26 27 28 29 30	1 2 3 4 5 6 7 8 9 10 11 12 13 14 15 16 17 18 19 20 21 22 23 24 25 26 27 28 29 30	1 2 3 4 5 6 7 8 9 10 11 12 13 14 15 16 17 18 19 20 21 22 23 24 25 26 27 28 29 30	1 2 3 4 5 6 7 8 9 10 11 12 13 14 15 16 17 18 19 20 21 22 23 24 25 26 27 28 29 30	1 2 3 4 5 6 7 8 9 10 11 12 13 14 15 16 17 18 19 20 21 22 23 24 25 26 27 28 29 30	1 2 3 4 5 6 7 8 9 10 11 12 13 14 15 16 17 18 19 20 21 22 23 24 25 26 27 28 29 30
8-10 PM	1 2 3 4 5 6 7 8 9 10 11 12 13 14 15 16 17 18 19 20 21 22 23 24 25 26 27 28 29 30	1 2 3 4 5 6 7 8 9 10 11 12 13 14 15 16 17 18 19 20 21 22 23 24 25 26 27 28 29 30	1 2 3 4 5 6 7 8 9 10 11 12 13 14 15 16 17 18 19 20 21 22 23 24 25 26 27 28 29 30	1 2 3 4 5 6 7 8 9 10 11 12 13 14 15 16 17 18 19 20 21 22 23 24 25 26 27 28 29 30	1 2 3 4 5 6 7 8 9 10 11 12 13 14 15 16 17 18 19 20 21 22 23 24 25 26 27 28 29 30	1 2 3 4 5 6 7 8 9 10 11 12 13 14 15 16 17 18 19 20 21 22 23 24 25 26 27 28 29 30	1 2 3 4 5 6 7 8 9 10 11 12 13 14 15 16 17 18 19 20 21 22 23 24 25 26 27 28 29 30
10 PM 12 AM	1 2 3 4 5 6 7 8 9 10 11 12 13 14 15 16 17 18 19 20 21 22 23 24 25 26 27 28 29 30	1 2 3 4 5 6 7 8 9 10 11 12 13 14 15 16 17 18 19 20 21 22 23 24 25 26 27 28 29 30	1 2 3 4 5 6 7 8 9 10 11 12 13 14 15 16 17 18 19 20 21 22 23 24 25 26 27 28 29 30	1 2 3 4 5 6 7 8 9 10 11 12 13 14 15 16 17 18 19 20 21 22 23 24 25 26 27 28 29 30	1 2 3 4 5 6 7 8 9 10 11 12 13 14 15 16 17 18 19 20 21 22 23 24 25 26 27 28 29 30	1 2 3 4 5 6 7 8 9 10 11 12 13 14 15 16 17 18 19 20 21 22 23 24 25 26 27 28 29 30	1 2 3 4 5 6 7 8 9 10 11 12 13 14 15 16 17 18 19 20 21 22 23 24 25 26 27 28 29 30

2-4 AM	1 2 3 4 5 6 7 8 9 10 11 12 13 14 15 16 17 18 19 20 21 22 23 24 25 26 27 28 29 30	1 2 3 4 5 6 7 8 9 10 11 12 13 14 15 16 17 18 19 20 21 22 23 24 25 26 27 28 29 30	1 2 3 4 5 6 7 8 9 10 11 12 13 14 15 16 17 18 19 20 21 22 23 24 25 26 27 28 29 30	1 2 3 4 5 6 7 8 9 10 11 12 13 14 15 16 17 18 19 20 21 22 23 24 25 26 27 28 29 30	1 2 3 4 5 6 7 8 9 10 11 12 13 14 15 16 17 18 19 20 21 22 23 24 25 26 27 28 29 30	1 2 3 4 5 6 7 8 9 10 11 12 13 14 15 16 17 18 19 20 21 22 23 24 25 26 27 28 29 30	1 2 3 4 5 6 7 8 9 10 11 12 13 14 15 16 17 18 19 20 21 22 23 24 25 26 27 28 29 30
4-6 AM	1 2 3 4 5 6 7 8 9 10 11 12 13 14 15 16 17 18 19 20 21 22 23 24 25 26 27 28 29 30	1 2 3 4 5 6 7 8 9 10 11 12 13 14 15 16 17 18 19 20 21 22 23 24 25 26 27 28 29 30	1 2 3 4 5 6 7 8 9 10 11 12 13 14 15 16 17 18 19 20 21 22 23 24 25 26 27 28 29 30	1 2 3 4 5 6 7 8 9 10 11 12 13 14 15 16 17 18 19 20 21 22 23 24 25 26 27 28 29 30	1 2 3 4 5 6 7 8 9 10 11 12 13 14 15 16 17 18 19 20 21 22 23 24 25 26 27 28 29 30	1 2 3 4 5 6 7 8 9 10 11 12 13 14 15 16 17 18 19 20 21 22 23 24 25 26 27 28 29 30	1 2 3 4 5 6 7 8 9 10 11 12 13 14 15 16 17 18 19 20 21 22 23 24 25 26 27 28 29 30

At the top of the chart, circle the specific day(s) of the week that you are committed towards working on your flexibility. Then in column 1 to circle the time(s) of the day that you are committed towards working on your flexibility. Finally, in the boxes corresponding to the day(s) and time(s) that you selected, circle the number of minutes that you are committed towards working on your flexibility.

APPENDIX 8E
STAIRWAY TO SUCCESS—LENGTH OF TIME PER WEEK

Start out by using the bottom step to record the present total of minutes you stretch for each day or week (e.g., 1 min). Then use the top step to record your dream goal of how many minutes you would like to stretch for 6 months from the date that you started stretching. Then go back to the second step from the bottom and set your first short-term goal of how many minutes you would like to stretch for approximately 1-2 weeks from your starting date. When you reach that goal, you can set your next short-term goal on the next step above and so on. If at any time you do not reach your short-term goal, determine what stopped you. Next incorporate the strategies you have learned to get back in action and climb the stairs toward your next goal. Finally, set a new target date.

APPENDIX 8F
STAIRWAY TO SUCCESS —LENGTH OF TIME STRETCH IS HELD

Start out by using the bottom step to record the present total of minutes you stretch for each day or week (e.g., 1 min). Then use the top step to record your dream goal of how many minutes you would like to stretch for 6 months from the date that you started stretching. Then go back to the second step from the bottom and set your first short-term goal of how many minutes you would like to stretch for approximately 1-2 weeks from your starting date. When you reach that goal, you can set your next short-term goal on the next step above and so on. If at any time you do not reach your short-term goal, determine what stopped you. Next incorporate the strategies you have learned to get back in action and climb the stairs toward your next goal. Finally, set a new target date.

APPENDIX 8G
EVALUATING THE SUCCESS OF YOUR FLEXIBILITY PROGRAM

1. Have you achieved success in the following areas?

   a. number of days you work on flexibility   YES   NO

   b. number of minutes stretched in a daily workout   YES   NO

   c. number of minutes stretched in a week   YES   NO

   d. number of exercises being incorporated into your flexibility workout   YES   NO

   e. reaching new tension points   YES   NO

2. Has you level of motivation to work on flexibility increased, decreased or remained the same during the past four weeks? Explain.

   INCREASED   DECREASED   REMAINED THE SAME

3. Compare how you felt on the days you worked on flexibility with the days you did not. Please explain in detail.

   FELT BETTER   FELT WORSE   FELT THE SAME

4. How did you feel about setting Stairway to Success Goals to improve your flexibility?

5. Describe the effect that your SMAART Goals had on your flexibility performance and enjoyment.

6. Has you level of commitment to improve your flexibility been affected by the last four weeks? Please explain.

   INCREASED   DECREASED   REMAINED THE SAME

7. What were the numerical results of your flexibility workouts over the past 4 weeks? Please include the following: (1) number of flexibility exercises that you performed, (2) number of days that you stretched; (3) number of minutes that you stretched; (4 how long you held each stretch.

Week	# of Flexibility Exercises Performed	# of Days Stretched	# of Minutes Stretched	Length of Time Each Stretch Was Held
1				
2				
3				
4				

APPENDIX 8H
WHAT IS STOPPING YOU?

Boredom   Doesn't fit into my schedule
No Results   Cannot find a partner
No Fun   Too painful
Inconvenient   Not sure what to do
Other

Circle all of the possible barriers you have discovered for not following your flexibility exercise prescription (FEP). Then take a few moments and create a strategy to overcome each of your identified barriers and *get back into action.* Remember, even if you commit to only one day per week, as long as it fits into your schedule then it's the right start for you.

Strategy 1 _____

_____

_____

Strategy 2 _____

_____

_____

Strategy 3 _____

_____

_____

Strategy 4 _____

_____

_____

Strategy 5 _____

_____

_____

APPENDIX 8I
DETERMINING THE BENEFITS OF WORKING ON YOUR FLEXIBILITY

1. After I stretch I feel   better   worse

2. Stretching is   relaxing   stressful

3. Stretching helps/does not help my productivity in other forms of exercise (e.g., CRE, MF)

4. Has stretching had any affect on my past or present injuries?

5. As a result of working on my flexibility over the past 1-2-3-4 weeks, I am more motivated to spend time stretching   yes   no

6. I enjoy stretching

1	2	3	4	5	6	7	8	9
Not at all								Very much

7. If I get stopped from sticking with my flexibility program, I will incorporate the following strategies to increase my commitment: (Circle all possibilities)

   enroll a partner to stretch with me

   set SMAART goals for frequency, intensity, time or type to keep me focused on stretching

   listen to music

   set aside time to stretch

   write down when I will stretch

   consider several places that motivate me to want to stretch (backyard, local park, gym, office, beach, shower, etc.).

   other

Chapter 9

Body Composition

OBJECTIVES

After reading this chapter, you will be able to:

- Define and assess body composition
- Distinguish among *underweight, overweight, overfat, obese* and *extreme obese*
- Learn strategies to improve body composition
- Determine your level of commitment to improve your body composition
- Recognize myths about improving your body composition

For many years, the traditional method of determining if you needed to gain or lose weight was to get on the scale to see how much you weighed and then compare your results with a standardized height-weight chart. If your weight exceeded the amount listed for your height, you were considered overweight and if your weight was below what was listed for your height, you were considered under-weight.

Unfortunately, this method creates several problems. First, the scale only determines total body weight and not what your body weight consists of (e.g., muscle, bones essential and storage fat, etc). Second, the height/weight charts are based on norms or averages of weight and height and even though you may be above or below the average, you are not necessarily in an unhealthy range. Finally, body weight scales do not distinguish between overweight vs. overfat. For example, people who are muscularly fit can get on a scale and exceed their rec-ommended body weight for height because they have more muscle then the average person of their height and muscle weighs more than body fat does (although it takes up a lot less space). However, what the scale neglects to tell you is your percent body fat and while the height/weight charts may tell you that you are overweight, you just might be overweight, yet under-fat. When determining whether you need to gain or lose weight, it is recommended that you first distinguish "weight" vs "fat." Then you should have your body composition assessed in conjunction with the scale. This will tell you what your total body weight consists of and help you decide if you need to lose or gain fat or muscle weight.

WHAT IS BODY COMPOSITION?

Body composition refers to what the body is comprised of. It consists of lean body mass and total body fat. Lean body mass is composed of muscle, bones, organs and connective tissues. Body fats consists of two types: (1) essential fat and (2) storage fat. Essential fat is needed for normal bodily functions and it is found in muscle, nerves, bones, intestines, heart liver and lungs. Storage fat is the fat stored in adipose tissue (just beneath the skin and around major organs of the body). This fat serves three basic functions:

1. as a secondary source of energy to be used during moderate to long bouts of exercise;

2. as an insulator to retain body heat and maintain a normal core body temperature;

3. as a cushion to absorb physical trauma to the body-imagine if you had the same amount of body fat around your brain, heart, lungs and other vital organs as you have around your elbow joint or knee cap. Even the slightest bit of contact to any of these organs could result in "ouch" serious injuries.

The amount of storage fat varies from person to person and is based on many factors including age, gender, heredity, diet, metabolism, and activity level. In general, excessive storage fat is often the result of consuming more food and beverage (input) then is expended (output) from metabolic functions and physical activity. Essential fat consists of approximately 3% of the total body weight in men and 12% of the total body weight in women. Women have a higher percentage of essential fat because part of their essential fat is sex-specific fat which is found in the breasts, uterus and other sex-related areas.

Body composition is an important component of health-related fitness. Having an optional amount of body fat will help you to live healthier, have more energy, and feel better about yourself. It will also lower your risk of chronic diseases (e.g., heart disease, cancer, stroke, diabetes, obesity, high blood pressure) that are linked to excessive amounts of body fat.

UNDERWEIGHT VS. OVERWEIGHT VS. OVER-FAT VS. OBESITY

Underweight refers to an extremely low body weight with a total percent body fat to be less than 8-12% for women and 3-5% for men. Underweight also refers to a body weight that is considered to be below the normal recommended weight for an individual's height, build and sex with a body mass index (BMI) of < 20 (www.wrongdiagnosis.com). While the prevalence of becoming underweight is less than becoming overweight or obese, having too little body fat can become dangerous and increase risks of certain illnesses including anemia, heart irregularities, osteoporosis, and anorexia nervosa www.wrongdiagnosis.com/u/underweight/ intro.htm). Some possible causes of becoming underweight are malnutrition, reduced or lost appetite, difficulty chewing, dental pain, excessive overtraining, digestive organ diseases, cancer, hyperthyrodiIsm, diabetes, and genetics).

Overweight is defined as having a total body weight that exceeds the recommended range for good health. As alluded to earlier, being overweight often refers to exceeding the standard of recommended body weight based on actual height. It does not necessarily mean that you are too fat and need to lose weight. For example, if the recommended body weight for your height is 150 pounds and you weigh 160 pounds, it simply means that you weigh 10 more pounds than the average of people who are your height. Hence, you are labeled overweight and not necessarily overfat. In fact, there are many athletes who fall into this category (e.g., football players, body builders, wrestlers). Emmit Smith, the NFL's all-time leading rusher is 5'10 and weighed 216 pounds at the height of his career. This weight is well over the recommended amount of weight for someone who is 5'10. However, if you were to examine the percentage of Mr. Smith's body fat, he would fall well within the recommended range, if not lower. The reason for Mr. Smith being overweight is his muscularity, not his amount of body fat.

Overfat refers to a condition of having too much body fat. According to experts, it is generally agreed that a healthy range of body fat falls between 12%-18% for men and 18%-22% for women. Of course, as age increases, the healthy range for body fat also increases. This is most often due to the percent of muscle weight that decreases as one ages (See Table 9.1 for ideal body fat percentages by age). It is interesting to note that you can be overfat without being overweight by simply being over the recommended amount of percent body fat for age while being at or under the recommended body weight for height.

Table 9.1
Ideal Body Fat Percentage by Age

Age	Men	Women
20	8.5	17.7
25	10.5	18.4
30	12.7	19.3
35	13.7	21.5
40	15.3	22.2
45	16.4	22.9
50	18.9	25.2
55	20.9	26.3
Obese	32% plus	26%

Obesity is a medical condition in which excess body fat has accumulated to the extent that it has an adverse effect on health (WHO,2006). Research has concluded that adult obesity exists when total body fat exceeds 25% in men and 30% in women. For children and youth, obesity is defined by having a body mass index (BMI) in the 95th percentile. Percentiles are determined by averaging the height and weight of children by age to determine average, below average and above average.

The Prevalence of Adult Obesity in the United States: 1960's to Present

Since the early 1960's, the prevalence of obesity in adults aged 20 and older has more than doubled increasing from 13.4% to 35.7% overall with men increasing from 10.7% to 33.9% and women increasing from 15.8% to 36.1% (See Table 9.2 to review trends in adult obesity). To determine the present state of adult obesity in the United States the CDC conducted two surveys: (1) the National Health and Nutrition Examination Survey (NHANES) and the National Health Interview Survey (NHIS) and discovered the following:

• More than two-thirds (68.8%) of adults are considered to be overweight and obese.

• Almost 3 in 4 men (74%) had overweight or obesity.

• Almost 2 in 3 women had overweight or obesity (64%).

• More than one-third (35.7%) of adults are considered to be obese (78.6 million).

• The prevalence of obesity is similar for men and women (36%).

• More than 1 in 20 adults (6.3%) have extreme obesity (at least 40% body fat).

• About 8% of women and 4% of men have extreme obesity.

• An estimated 600 million adults were classified as obese in 2015.

Prevalence of Adult Obesity: State by State

In addition to determining the prevalence of obesity by age, distinguishing adults from children, youth and adolescents, research has also investigated the prevalence of obesity by state. The primary purposes of this type of investigation are twofold: (1) to determine if there is consistency in adult obesity throughout the United States and (2) to ascertain if there is a pattern of distinct levels of obesity in different regions of the United States. The results for adults from 2003-2015 are as follows:

In 2003, there were nine states will a prevalence rate of adult obesity less than 20%, thirty-five states were between 20%-25% and seven states were between 25%-30%. In 2008, only one state (Colorado) had a prevalence rate of adult obesity less than 20%, twenty-eight states were over 25% and three states were over 30% (Alabama, Mississippi & West Virginia). In 2012, no states had a prevalence rate of obesity under 20%, forty states were over 25% (an increase of 12) and thirteen states were over 30% (an increase of 10). In 2015, no states had a prevalence rate of obesity under 20%, forty-two states were over 25% (14 more than 2008 & 2 more than 2012), twenty-three states were over 30% (20 more than 2008 & 10 more than 2012) and four states entered a new category of over 35% obesity (Alabama, Louisiana, Mississippi & West Virginia). (See Table 9.3 for State by State Prevalence Rates of Adult Obesity in the United States).

Table 9.2

Trends in Overweight, Obesity, and Extreme Obesity among Adults, United States:
Ages 20-74, 1960-2012

YEAR	Overweight	Obese	Extremely Obese
1960-1962	31.5	13.4	0.9
1971-1974	32.7	14.5	1.3
1976-1980	32.1	15.0	1.4
1988-1994	32.6	23.2	3.0
1999-2000	33.6	30.9	5.0
2001-2002	34.4	31.2	5.4
2003-2004	33.4	32.9	5.1
2005-2006	32.2	35.1	6.2
2007-2008	33.6	34.3	6.0
2009-2010	32.7	36.1	6.6
2011-2012	33.3	35.3	6.6

Trends in Overweight, Obesity, and Extreme Obesity Among Male Adults,
United States: Aged 20-74 1960-2012

YEAR	Overweight	Obese	Extremely Obese
1960-1962	38.7	10.7	0.3
1971-1974	41.7	12.1	0.6
1976-1980	39.9	12.7	0.4
1988-1994	40.3	20.5	1.8
1999-2000	39.2	27.7	3.3
2001-2002	41.5	28.3	3.9
2003-2004	39.4	31.7	3.0
2005-2006	39.7	33.8	4.3
2007-2008	39.4	32.5	4.4
2009-2010	38.0	35.9	4.6
2011-2012	37.3	33.9	4.5

Trends in Overweight, Obesity, and Extreme Obesity Among Female Adults,
United States: Aged 20-74 1960-2012

YEAR	Overweight	Obese	Extremely Obese
1960-1962	24.7	15.8	1.4
1971-1974	24.3	16.6	2.0
1976-1980	24.9	17.0	2.2
1988-1994	25.1	25.9	4.1
1999-2000	28.0	34.0	6.6
2001-2002	27.3	34.1	6.8
2003-2004	27.3	34.0	7.3
2005-2006	24.7	36.3	7.9
2007-2008	27.9	36.2	7.6
2009-2010	27.5	36.1	8.5
2011-2012	29.5	36.1	8.6

Table 3
State by State Prevalence Rates of Adults Obesity 2003-2015

State	2003 % of Obesity	2008 % of Obesity	2012 % of Obesity	2015 % of Obesity	Highest Obesity Rate
Alabama	28.4	30.1	33.0	**35.6**	2015
Alaska	23.5	27.3	25.7	**29.8**	2015
Arizona	20.1	23.3	27.1	**28.4**	2015
Arkansas	25.2	28.1	**34.5**	34.5	2012, 2015
California	23.2	23.1	**25.0**	24.2	2012
Colorado	16.0	18.4	**20.5**	20.2	2012
Connecticut	19.1	20.8	**25.6**	25.3	2012
Delaware	24.0	25.9	26.9	**29.7**	2015
District of Columbia	20.3	**22.1**	21.9	**22.1**	2008, 2015
Florida	19.9	23.3	25.2	**26.8**	2015
Georgia	25.2	27.5	29.1	**30.7**	2015
Hawaii	16.4	20.7	**23.6**	22.7	2012
Idaho	21.8	24.6	26.8	**28.6**	2015
Illinois	23.2	25.3	28.1	**30.8**	2015
Indiana	26.0	27.5	**31.4**	31.3	2012
Iowa	23.9	26.3	30.4	**32.1**	2015
Kansas	22.6	25.8	29.9	**34.2**	2015
Kentucky	25.6	28.4	31.3	**34.6**	2015
Louisiana	24.8	29.5	34.7	**36.2**	2015
Maine	19.9	23.7	28.4	**30.0**	2015
Maryland	21.9	25.2	27.6	**28.9**	2015
Massachusetts	16.8	20.9	22.9	**24.3**	2015
Michigan	25.2	27.7	31.1	**31.2**	2015
Minnesota	23.0	24.8	25.7	**26.1**	2015
Mississippi	28.1	31.7	34.6	**35.6**	2015
Missouri	23.6	27.4	29.6	**32.4**	2015
Montana	18.8	21.7	**24.3**	23.6	2012
Nebraska	23.9	26.5	28.6	**31.4**	2015
Nevada	21.2	23.6	26.2	**26.7**	2015
New Hampshire	20.2	23.6	**27.3**	26.3	2012
New Jersey	20.1	22.9	24.6	**25.6**	2015
New Mexico	20.2	24.0	27.1	**28.8**	2015
New York	20.9	23.5	23.6	**25.0**	2015
North Carolina	24.0	27.1	29.6	**30.1**	2015
North Dakota	23.7	25.9	29.7	**31.0**	2015
Ohio	24.9	26.9	30.1	**30.4**	2015
Oklahoma	24.4	28.1	32.2	**32.5**	2015
Oregon	21.5	25.0	**27.3**	26.5	2012
Pennsylvania	23.8	25.7	29.1	30.0	2015
Rhode Island	18.4	21.4	25.7	**27.3**	2015
South Carolina	24.5	29.2	31.6	**31.7**	2015
South Dakota	22.9	26.1	28.1	**29.9**	2015
Tennessee	25.0	29.0	31.1	**33.7**	2015
Texas	24.6	27.2	29.6	**30.4**	2015
Utah	20.8	21.8	**24.3**	24.1	2012
Vermont	19.6	21.1	23.7	**24.7**	2015

State	2003 % of Obesity	2008 % of Obesity	2012 % of Obesity	2015 % of Obesity	Highest Obesity Rate
Virginia	21.7	25.2	**27.4**	27.2	2012
Washington	21.7	24.5	26.8	**27.2**	2015
West Virginia	27.7	30.6	33.8	**35.1**	2015
Wisconsin	20.9	25.5	29.7	**29.8**	2015
Wyoming	20.1	24.0	24.6	**27.8**	2015
States With Highest % of Obesity From 2003-2015	0	1	11	**40**	
Average Prevalence of Childhood Obesity in the United States	1125.2 22.06	1289.5 25.28	1424.7 27.93	**1483.1 29.08**	

In summary, the research findings over the past fifty years on adult obesity is quite alarming to say the least. Dating back to 1962, about 13 percent of adults in the United States were categorized as obese and 1 percent extremely obese. These percentages gradually increased until the late 1970s, at which time they began to climb more rapidly until 2000 when they leveled off at around 31 percent obesity and 5 percent extreme obesity. By 2010, the percentage of adults who were obese increased to 36 percent and 6 percent were considered extremely obese (Ogden & Carroll, 2010).

Today, adult obesity is estimated to be at its' highest point ever at 38 percent. While states in the southeast and southwest (Alabama, Mississippi, Kentucky, West Virginia, Arkansas, Louisiana) have a higher obesity rate than the rest of the country, adult obesity has significantly risen in all 50 states and the District of Columbia, too. Is the prevalence of childhood obesity rapidly growing the United States, too? Let's take a look.

The Prevalence of Childhood Obesity in the United States: 1970's to Present

Over the past four decades, obesity rates have more than tripled among children and adolescents ages 2-19 years starting at about 5% in the early 1970's and escalating to over 17% by 2014-2015. The results of two surveys by the HANES and the NHIS revealed the following:

- About 31.8% are considered to be either overweight or obese.
- Approximately 16.9% are considered to be obese.
- About 1 in 3 boys (33%) and girls (30.4%) are considered to be overweight or obese.
- About 18.6% of boys and 15% of girls are considered to be obese.
- 8.9% of pre-school children ages 2-5 are obese.
- 17.5% of school children aged children ages 6-11 are obese.
- 20.5% of adolescents aged 12-19 are obese.
- About 13 million children (16.9%) in the United States ages 2-19 are obese.

While childhood obesity rates increased from an average of 14.3% in 2003 to 15.3%, in 2008, they remained the same from 2008 to 2011 and slightly decreased to just under 15% in 2015. Although recent data suggests that childhood obesity rates may be stabilizing, obesity as a public health concern has captured the interest of health care professionals, policymakers, schools, employers, and the media (Dabrowska, 2014). (See Table 9.4 to review trends in childhood obesity).

Table 9.4
Trends in Obesity among Children and Adolescents
Ages 2-19 Years in the United States

YEAR	Obese 2-19 years	Obese 2-5 years	Obese 6-11 years	Obese 12-19 years
1966-1970			4.2	4.6
1971-1974	5.2	5.0	4.0	6.1
1976-1980	5.5	5.0	6.5	5.0
1988-1994	10.0	7.2	11.3	10.5
1999-2000	13.9	10.3	15.1	14.8
2001-2002	15.4	10.6	16.2	16.7
2003-2004	17.1	13.9	18.8	17.4
2005-2006	15.4	10.7	15.1	17.8
2007-2008	16.8	10.1	19.6	18.1
2009-2010	16.9	12.1	18.0	18.4
2011-2012	16.9	8.4	17.7	20.5

Source: CDC/NHANES, National Health and Nutrition Examination Survey (2011, 2012)

Prevalence of Childhood Obesity: State by State

In 2003, the average childhood obesity rate across the United States was 14.3% with three states (Colorado, Utah & Wyoming) under 10%, thirty states between 10%-15%, fifteen states between 15%-20% and three states over 20% (District of Columbia, Kentucky and West Virginia). In 2008, the average childhood obesity rate increased to 15.3% with only one state below 10% (Oregon 9.6%). Twenty-six states were between 10%-15%, fifteen states were between 15%-20% and 9 states were over 20% (an increase of 6 from 2003). In 2011, Oregon remained the only state under 10% (9.9%), twenty-five states were between 10%-15%, nineteen states were between 15%-20% (an increase of 4 since 2008) and six states were between 20-25%. In 2015, there were two states (Oregon 8.7 & Colorado 8.9) that were under 10% obesity. Thirty-four states were between 10%-15% and 15 states were between 15% and 20%. Most important, thirty-six states had a decrease in childhood obesity from 2011 to 2015 and no states were over 20% (a decrease of 6 states in from 2011 and 9 states

Table 9.5
State by State Prevalence of Obesity Rates in Children Ages 2-18 2003-2015

State	2003 % of Obesity	2007 % of Obesity	**2011** **% of Obesity**	2014-2015 % of Obesity	Highest Obesity Rate
Alabama	16.7	17.9	**18.6**	17.0	2011
Alaska	11.1	14.1	14.0	**15.7**	2015
Arizona	12.2	17.8	**19.8**	14.7	2011
Arkansas	16.4	**20.4**	20.0	17.5	2007
California	13.2	15.0	15.1	**15.2**	2015
Colorado	9.9	**14.2**	10.9	8.9	2007
Connecticut	12.3	12.5	**15.0**	14.2	2011
Delaware	14.8	13.3	**16.9**	16.6	2011
District of Columbia	**22.8**	20.1	21.4	14.1	2003
Florida	14.4	**18.3**	13.4	12.8	2007
Georgia	16.4	**21.3**	16.5	14.1	2007
Hawaii	**13.3**	11.2	11.5	11.6	2003
Idaho	10.1	**11.8**	10.6	11.1	2007
Illinois	15.8	**20.7**	19.3	15.7	2007
Indiana	**15.6**	14.6	14.3	14.1	2003
Iowa	12.5	11.2	13.6	**13.8**	2015
Kansas	14.0	**16.2**	14.2	13.9	2007
Kentucky	20.6	**21.0**	19.7	17.2	2007
Louisiana	17.2	20.7	**21.1**	15.9	2011
Maine	12.7	12.9	12.5	**13.6**	2015
Maryland	13.3	13.6	**15.1**	14.4	2011
Massachusetts	13.6	13.3	**14.5**	14.0	2011
Michigan	14.4	12.4	**14.8**	14.2	2011
Minnesota	10.1	11.1	**14.0**	13.2	2011
Mississippi	17.8	**21.9**	21.7	18.4	2007
Missouri	**15.6**	13.6	13.5	13.2	2003
Montana	11.1	11.8	**14.3**	12.4	2011
Nebraska	11.9	**15.8**	13.8	14.6	2007
Nevada	12.4	15.2	**18.6**	14.3	2011
New Hampshire	12.9	12.8	**15.5**	14.3	2011
New Jersey	13.7	**15.4**	10.0	11.3	2007
New Mexico	16.8	**16.0**	14.4	14.2	2007
New York	15.3	**17.1**	14.5	14.0	2007
North Carolina	19.3	**18.6**	16.1	15.8	2007
North Dakota	12.1	11.4	**15.4**	14.6	2011
Ohio	14.2	**18.5**	17.4	14.5	2007
Oklahoma	15.4	16.4	**17.4**	16.2	2011
Oregon	**14.1**	9.6	9.9	12.4	2003
Pennsylvania	13.3	**15.0**	13.5	13.5	2007
Rhode Island	11.9	**14.4**	13.2	13.8	2007
South Carolina	18.9	15.3	**21.5**	16.9	2011
South Dakota	12.0	13.2	13.4	**14.1**	2015
Tennessee	20.0	**20.6**	20.5	18.0	2007

State	2003 % of Obesity	2007 % of Obesity	**2011 % of Obesity**	2014-2015 % of Obesity	Highest Obesity Rate
Texas	19.1	**20.4**	19.1	14.9	2007
Utah	8.5	11.4	**11.6**	8.7	2011
Vermont	11.3	**12.9**	11.3	12.6	2007
Virginia	13.8	**15.2**	14.3	15.8	2007
Washington	10.8	11.1	11.0	**12.2**	2015
West Virginia	20.9	**18.9**	18.5	17.9	2007
Wisconsin	13.5	13.1	**13.4**	13.2	2011
Wyoming	8.6	10.2	**10.7**	10.5	2011
States with Highest % of Obesity from 2003-2015	**5**	**22**	**18**	**6**	
Average Prevalence of Childhood Obesity in the United States	**14.09**	**15.32**	**15.32**	**14.17**	

Bold – indicates highest percent of obesity during all four time periods

from 2008). (See Table 9.5 for State by State Prevalence Rates of Childhood Obesity in the United States).

Overall, this certainly reflects the possibility that America is doing a better job at educating and implementing positive lifestyle habits such as eating healthier and exercising more for our childhood, youth and adolescent populations (ages 2-19), however, this doesn't seem to be the case for our adult world. Today, adult obesity remains at its' highest rate ever which has caused a massive increase in the costs of treating people with obesity and obesity-related illness including heart disease, stroke, and cancer.

THE COSTS OF OBESITY

Did you know that an obese person incurs an average of $1429 more in annual medical expenses than a person who is not obese? Were you aware that it costs employers $506 more per obese worker per year due to a higher illness rate, more medical visits, medication prescribed due to obesity, greater worker absenteeism and lower job productivity? On a larger scale, it is estimated that $147 to $210 billion is spent on added medical expenses related to obesity each year (Cawley & Meyerhoefer, 2012). In addition, obesity costs society an estimated $117 billion in direct (preventative, diagnostic and treatment services related to weight) and indirect (absenteeism, loss of future earnings due to premature death) costs.

Obesity is, was and will always will be the leading preventable cause of death in the United States and worldwide. However, the rate of obesity cannot change by itself. There has to be a cohesive effort from national, state, local and individuals to address the problems of obesity both on the adult as well as the childhood level and implement programs designed to enhance over public health.

PREVENTING OBESITY

There is no one single, simple solution to eliminating the obesity epidemic. Obesity has become a complex problem that requires a comprehensive, cohesive effort by policy makers, state and local organizations, businesses and community leaders, school, childcare and health care professionals and individuals to work together to transform communities into places that support and promote healthy lifestyle choices for all U.S. residents (Khan et al., 2009). Presently, the Centers for Disease Control and Prevention (CDC) has offered a variety of strategies to promote healthy living behaviors that prevent obesity through three separate, but related venues: (1) state and local programs; (2) community efforts and (3) healthy living strategies.

State and Local Programs

Presently, the CDC funds all 50 states and the District of Columbia over $14 million annually in order to advance the nation's chronic disease prevention and health promotion efforts of which $8.2 million is awarded to programs for the specific purpose of reducing obesity in high obesity areas (defined as counties that have more than 40% prevalence of adult obesity) across the United States. The money is offered to colleges and universities in the form of grants in order to help residents in communities with high obesity and less access to healthy food and physical activity options. The universities conduct intervention strategies through existing cooperative extension and outreach services at the county level, in targeted counties, to improve physical activity and nutrition, reduce obesity, and prevent and control diabetes, heart disease and stroke CDC, 2017).

In addition to the work done at the college and university level, all states are required to put into action key strategies in their states that include the following:

- Promote the adoption of food service guidelines and nutrition standards.

- Promote the adoption of physical activity in early child care centers, schools, and worksites.

The purpose of this is twofold: (1) to educate the country on eating healthy and (2) to increase the level of physical activity by offering a variety of facilities that are located close to home or work; The bottom line is this. The more accessible healthy food and physical activity are to a person the more likely they will give a try and hopefully adopt into their lifestyle.

Community Efforts

While it is imperative that all states receive funding for the purposes of preventing obesity and increasing physical activity, it is unrealistic to think that all communities in need have been and will continue to be adequately addressed. If that was the case, then the obesity rate in the United States would not continue to be on the rise. Healthier food and beverage choices would not be a luxury, but commonplace and at an affordable rate. Consequently, the CDC has made the following recommendations to local communities to prevent obesity:

1. **Communities should increase availability of healthier food and beverage choices in public service venues**. Presently, a policy exists to apply nutrition standards that are consistent with the dietary guidelines for Americans (USDHHS, USDA, 2005). Offering fruits, vegetables and water instead of candy, cake, fried foods and soda in public places including schools, after-school programs, child-care centers, community recreational facilities (parks, playgrounds, and swimming pools), city and county buildings, prisons and juvenile detention centers will allow people an opportunity to make healthier food and beverage choices. For example, including a salad bar in the schools, childcare facilities, hospitals and worksites is an excellent way to maximize healthy eating practices at an affordable rate. In addition, offering baked, grilled, boiled, broiled, low fat, fat-free and no sugar added instead of fried as well as fat free and low-fat options allows the individual to make healthier meal choices. Finally, offering a variety of fruits instead of the candy machine allows the individual to snack healthy, too.

2. **Communities should improve availability of affordable healthier food and beverage choices in public service venues.** Healthier foods are generally more expensive than unhealthy foods which has caused low income or financially challenged individuals to make food choices based on cost instead of health. This poses a significant barrier to purchasing and consuming healthier foods, particularly for low-income consumers. Therefore, the following strategies to improve the affordability of healthier foods and beverages should be implemented: (a) lowering prices of healthier foods and beverages; (b) providing discount coupons; (c) creating vouchers redeemable for heathier foods and (d) including bonuses tied to the purchase of healthier foods which can decrease costs of purchasing healthier foods in the future. Pricing strategies can include lowering the prices of healthier foods sold in vending machines and cafeterias and increasing the price of less healthy foods and beverages.

3. **Communities should improve geographic availability of supermarkets in underserved areas.** Supermarkets and full-service grocery stores have a larger selection of healthier food at lower prices compared with smaller grocery and convenience stores. However, research has demonstrated that low-income, minority, and rural communities have fewer supermarkets as compared with more affluent areas (Larson, Story & Nelson, 2008). Increasing the number of supermarkets in areas where they are unavailable or where availability is limited will increase access to healthy foods.

4. **Communities should provide incentives to food retailers to locate in and/or offer healthier food and beverage choices in underserved areas.** The availability of healthy foods and beverages are limited in underserved communities resulting in an increase in obesity due to poor eating habits. To address this issue, communities can provide incentives to food retailers (e.g., supermarkets, grocery stores, convenience stores and street vendors) to offer a greater variety of healthy foods and beverages). Incentives can include tax benefits and discounts, low interest loans and grants.

5. **Communities should improve availability of mechanisms for purchasing food from farms.** Mechanisms for purchasing food directly from farms include farmers' markets, farm stands, community-supported agriculture, "pick your own" and farm-to school-initiatives. By offering healthier foods like fresh fruit and vegetables directly to the consumer, availability is increased and the cost can be reduced making healthy foods more affordable.

6. **Communities should restrict availability of less healthy foods and beverages in public service venues.** Presently, the availability of unhealthy foods far exceeds the availability of health foods. In fact, if you were to tour colleges and universities across the United States you would easily find a wealth of fast food venues at one's disposal. The same cannot be said for heathy food places. Moreover, public places that house vending machines (e.g., schools, parks, courthouses, office buildings) often carry unhealthy choices like soda, candy and cookies. Consequently, the availability of less healthy foods and the unavailability of healthy foods is positively associated with an increase in unhealthy eating which often leads to obesity. Therefore, replacing unhealthy food options with healthy food options will promote people to make healthier choices. For example, schools can restrict the availability of less healthy foods by setting standards for the types of food sold, restricting access to vending machines that sell unhealthy foods and banning unhealthy snack foods as rewards in classrooms. The same can be done in other public venues including child care centers, community recreational facilities (parks, recreation centers, playgrounds, and swimming pools), city and county buildings, prisons and juvenile detention centers.

7. **Communities should institute smaller portion size options in public service venues.** Often times people consume the amount of food placed in a bag, box or plate thinking that one of each constitutes one serving. However, if you peruse the back of the label you will often see the nutritional value listed per serving and the number of servings in one bag, box or container may be more than one. Consequently, people may overeat by eating everything on their plate or finishing the entire bag so they can throw it out, unaware that they may have consumed two, three or four servings in just a few minutes. By reducing the portion sizes in a restaurant, the packaging of prepared foods or the amount a person learns to put on his or her plate will ultimately reduce overeating.

8. **Communities should limit advertisements of less healthy foods and beverages.** Research has demonstrated than more than half of television advertisements viewed by children and adolescents are food-related; the majority of them promote fast foods, unhealthy snacks, sweets, and sugar-sweetened beverages (Institute of Medicine, 2005). Television advertising has been determined to influence children to prefer and request high-calorie and low-nutrient foods and beverages (Institute of Medicine,

2005, 2006). Therefore, limiting advertisements of less healthy foods might decrease the attraction, purchase and consumption of such products.

9. **Communities should discourage the consumption of sugar-sweetened beverages.** Consumption of sugar-sweetened beverages (e.g., carbonated soft drinks, sports drinks, flavored sweetened milk, and fruit drinks) has increased dramatically in children and youth since the 1970s and is associated with higher daily caloric intake and greater risk of obesity. While consumption of sugar-sweetened beverages occurs most often in the home, schools and child care centers also contribute to the problem either by serving sugar-sweetened beverages or by allowing children to purchase sugar-sweetened beverages from vending machines (CDC, 2006). Policies that restrict the availability of sugar-sweetened beverages in schools and child care center might discourage the consumption of high-caloric beverages among children and adolescents. Moreover, including healthier beverage choices like water in place of unhealthier beverage choices will encourage children and youth to drink healthy.

10. **Communities should require physical education in schools**. The National Association for Sport and Physical Education (NASPE) and the American Heart Association (AHA) recommend that all elementary school students should participate in at least 150 minutes of physical education (PE) per week and that all middle and high school students should participate in at least 225 minutes of PE per week for an entire school year (NASPE & AHA, 2006). While many states mandate some level of PE in schools, the extent to whether these requirements are enforced remains unclear. Moreover, many states have reduced or eliminated the amount of PE in their schools due to budget cuts and pressure to emphasize a higher academic standard. Ironically, a Community Guide review identified no evidence that time spent in PE classes harms academic performance (CDC, 2005). On the contrary, Physical Education has traditionally been considered an essential part of curricula to promote a range of benefits including general health, cognitive development, motor skills and social behavior (Baily et al., 2009; Pate, O'Neill & McIver, 2011). In fact, research has consistently demonstrated that both aerobic and resistance training are equally important for maintaining brain and cognitive health and having a healthy heart and lungs may be one of the most important factors for middle school students to make good grades in math and reading (Mercola, 2012). A review of 14 studies from the past few decades revealed that children who participate in physical activity also tend to benefit in the classroom (Topek, 2012). According to the NY Times, as schools everywhere strive to improve the academic performance of their students, many have cut physical education and recess periods to leave more time for sedentary classroom instruction. A report from the Institute of Medicine revealed just how shortsighted this trend can be. They found that exercise can significantly improve children's cognitive abilities and their academic performance as well as their health. According to the Institute of Medicine, there is a growing body of evidence suggesting children who are more active

are better able to focus their attention, are quicker to perform simple tasks, and have better working memories and problem-solving skills than less active children. They also perform better on standardized tests. Consequently, physical activity should be a core educational concern, not a disposable option.

11. **Communities should increase time opportunities for extracurricular physical activity.** Increasing the amount of physical activity in school-based PE classes has demonstrated to be effective in increasing fitness among children. However, just because PE class may be required, it does not necessarily mean that all students are as physically active as they could or should be during that time. Problems such as overcrowded classes, lack of time to change in proper attire, lack of equipment and inadequate space have all contributed to children not getting enough physical activity on a daily basis. Therefore, it is imperative that extracurricular physical activity outside of school hours are implemented to complement required PE class and to help prevent obesity in children and youth. This strategy focuses on offering noncompetitive physical activity opportunities such as games and dance classes available through community and after-school programs that excludes tryouts and welcomes all.

12. **Communities should create safe environments for physical activity.** One reason why parents may not allow their children to participate in physical activity in local parks and recreation facilities may be due to unsafe conditions either due to a lack of professional supervision or poorly maintained and outdated equipment. By offering physical activity programs that are supervised and taught by physical educators and recreation specialists and making sure facilities and equipment pass inspection and are deemed safe and appropriate for use, children can learn and master a variety of physical activities in a safe manner (swimming, gymnastics, dance, martial arts, etc.).

13. **Communities should improve access to outdoor recreational facilities.** Recreation facilities provide space for community members to engage in physical activity and include places such as parks, outdoor sports fields and facilities, walking and biking trails, public pools, and community playgrounds. Accessibility to these places depends on a number of factors such as proximity to schools or homes, cost, hours of operation, and overall ease of access. Improving the accessibility to these recreation facilities might increase physical activity among children and adolescents.

14. **Communities should enhance infrastructure supporting biking.** Enhancing infrastructure by creating bike lanes, bike racks, shared-use paths and routes on existing and new roads can increase the frequency of physical activity for utilitarian purposes (e.g., commuting to work and schools, errands).

15. **Communities should enhance infrastructure supporting walking.** Well-developed infrastructure supporting walking is an important element associated with physical activity in both children and adults. Interventions aimed at supporting infrastructure for walking include paved sidewalks and streets, improved street lighting, speed

humps and timed traffic lights. Creating a safe, inviting and convenient environment can increase the frequency and enjoyment of walking either for physically activity or exercise.

16. **Communities should enhance personal safety in areas where persons are or could be physically active**. Personal safety is affected by crime rates and other non-traffic-related hazards that exist in communities. Improving community safety might affect parents' decisions to allow their children to play and walk outside. Interventions to improve safety include police presence, decreasing the number of abandon buildings and homes, and improving street lighting.

17. **Communities should participate in community coalitions or partnerships to address obesity**. Community coalitions consist of public-and-private-sector organizations that work together with individual citizens to achieve a common goal through the coordinated use of resources, leadership, and action (IOM, 2005). For example, potential stakeholders in community coalitions aimed at obesity might include health-care professionals, local and state public health agencies, industries (building and construction, restaurant, food and beverage, and entertainment), the media, educational institutions, government (including transportation and parks and recreation departments), youth-related and faith-based organizations, nonprofit organizations and foundations, and employers. The effectiveness of community coalitions stems from the multiple perspectives, talents, and expertise that are brought together toward a common goal. Most important, coalitions build a sense of community that enhances residents' engagement in community life that provides a vehicle for community empowerment. For example, research on tobacco control has demonstrated that the presence of antismoking community coalitions might be effective in lowering the rates of cigarette use. Consequently, it is plausible that community coalitions who seek to prevent obesity might be successful by improving physical activity and nutrition in their local areas.

HEALTHY LIVING STRATEGIES

The key to achieving and maintaining a healthy weight is not a quick-fix solution. It is a lifestyle commitment that includes healthy eating and regular physical activity and exercise.

The first step is awareness. For people to live a healthy life they must be aware of what a healthy life consists of. Here are 8 strategies that can help you live healthy:

1. Let's start with something simple, your body weight. Do you know how much you weigh or how much you should weigh? Get on the scale and find out.

2. Have your body composition measured. This will determine your percent body fat and let you know if you have too much, too little or the perfect amount of body fat.

3. Become familiar with MyPlate and begin to adopt healthy eating habits that include learning how many calories you consume per day and per meal, what the calories consist of in terms of simple and complex carbohydrates, saturated and unsaturated fats, proteins, sodium and artificial ingredients.

4. Count the fruits and vegetables you consume on a daily basis and plan to eat at least one fruit and vegetable every day and preferably more as this becomes part of your daily routine.

5. Become aware of how much water you drink on a daily basis. Begin to drink more water by making sure it is accessible to you. For example, buy water in bulk, by the case. Then plan to take a bottle of water with you before you start your day and include drinking water with every meal. It's so simple!!

6. Plan your meals—this means knowing what you will eat, when you will eat, where you will eat, how much you will eat and how long it will take you to eat your meals; Start buying healthy foods and beverages and replace them with your unhealthy foods and beverages.

7. Determine how physically active and fit you are. How many days per week are you exercising? How many minutes per workout? Do you address all the components of health-related fitness? If not, discover the barriers that are stopping you and begin to incorporate strategies to overcome your barriers and get started.

These are just a few strategies designed to improve your health. Hopefully, you will use at least one and preferably more to incorporate them into your life.

8. Utilize Social Support Interventions—these programs have been created to help participants identify barriers to physical activity and eating healthy and create solutions using a variety of social networks including men, women, different age groups, people who are inactive, community and worksite programs, universities, etc. For example, the Boston Health commission created the neighborhood walk program by organizing 56 walking groups in 7 racially diverse neighborhoods. Opportunities for local residents to join neighbors in a community walk at least once per week for 30-60 minutes. Each group has a walking leader who coordinates the activity by mapping out the walking course, promoting the walk, distributing walk logs and providing incentives to participants. A post walk survey is completed to get feedback on the walk, route, frequency of walks, changes in physical activity, and recommendations for the future. This makes all participants feel important. Imagine if every community in the United States had this? Would you or your family participate if your local community sponsored a walking group?

ASSESSING BODY COMPOSITION

Assessing body composition is a more accurate way of measuring your percent body fat and determining if you need to lose, gain or maintain present body weight that the bathroom scale. Four of the most popular methods of assessing body fat are (1) skinfold calipers (2) underwater weighing (3) bioelectrical impedance and (4) girth measurements.

1. ***Skinfold measurements***—involves using calipers to measure the thickness of skinfolds at usually three, four or seven different sites or parts of the body. Some experts recommend measuring two to three sites (e.g., triceps-suprailium-thigh for women and chest-abdomen-thigh for men) and then incorporating the measurements into a formula to determine overall body fat. However, failure to measure skinfold at other sites (e.g., calf, back) will only increase the margin of error and make it difficult to accurately predict the amount of estimated body fat on an individual's entire body. Therefore, it is recommended that you should assess body fat using multiple sites throughout the body and use the actual measurements rather than a formula to determine body fat. This will reduce the margin of error and help you to more accurately monitor your body fat. (See Figure 9.1 to familiarize yourself with sites that can be used to assess body composition).

Strengths—Assessing body fat using skinfold calipers is a relatively quick and simple procedure to implement and with a little practice it can be conducted properly and in a variety of settings including: (1) at home; (2) school nurse's office, laboratory or gymnasium; (3) local youth center and (4) public or private exercise facilities; In addition, calipers are inexpensive (about $10 per pair) and easy to locate.

Limitations—There is an estimated margin of error of 3-4 percent when using a formula with limited (2-3) sites measured. In addition, the margin of error can increase if test administrations do not have adequate experience using calipers and have difficulty distinguishing actual body fat from skin.

Procedures for Assessing Body Fat using Skinfold Calipers

1. Consider using the following sites to measure body fat. For men, chest, abdomen, thigh, tricep, calf, back. For women, thigh, triceps, suprailium, calf, and back.
2. Using the thumb and index finger, gently grasp the thickness of each skin from each site
3. Place the caliper about ½ inch below your fingers and hold for three seconds.
4. Measure each site 3X and record to the nearest one-half millimeter.
5. Record the averages of the two closest readings.
6. Plan to measure each site every month and compare the actual results (measurements in millimeters) rather than a formula to estimate percent body fat. This will reduce the margin of error and more accurately determine improvement.

MALES   FEMALES

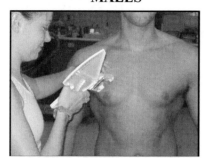

Chest

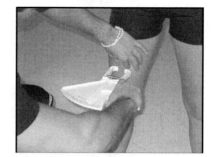

Thigh

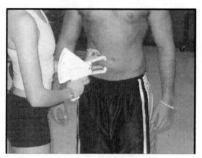

Abdomen

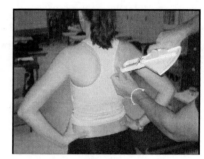

Back

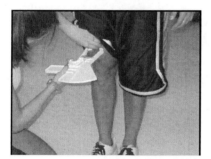

Thigh

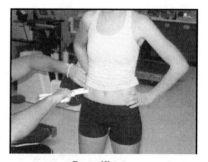

Suprailium

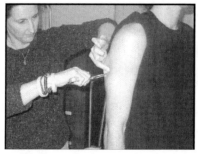

Tricep

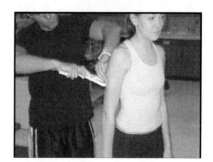

Tricep

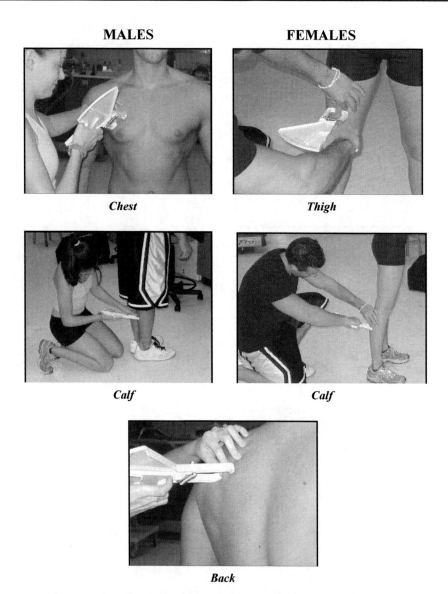

MALES   **FEMALES**

Chest   *Thigh*

Calf   *Calf*

Back

Figure 9.1—Assessing Body Composition Using Skinfold Calipers

2. ***Underwater weighing***—is considered the standard for assessing body composition and is general agreed to be the most accurate of all body composition assessments. In this procedure, an individual's normal body weight is taken outside of water and then compared to his or her body weight while submerged and weighed underwater. The percentages of fat and fat-free weight are calculated from body density. Since fat floats and muscle sinks, people with more body fat will weigh less under water while lean people will weigh more.

Strengths—Underwater weighing is a highly accurate method for assessing body composition with a low percentage of error.

Limitations—Underwater weighing requires the expertise of a well-trained technician who knows how to administer this assessment and analyze the data properly. The equipment needed can be quite expensive and the overall process is rather time consuming, thus limiting the practicality when used in large sample (exercise class; sports' teams). Moreover, not everyone feels comfortable in the water and may become anxious about the thought of being submerged under water.

Procedures for Using Underwater Weighing

1. Minimal clothing should be used since that can affect measures of body weight.
2. The individual is first weighed on dry land.
3. Then the individual will be placed into a large tank of water.
4. While sitting on a special scale, the individual is lowered underwater and asked to expel all air from lungs and remain motionless while the water weight is measured.
5. Procedure is repeated three times and then averaged.
6. A special calculation is then used to determine lean weight from fat weight and calculate a person's percentage of body fat.

3. *Bioelectrical impedance*—determines percent body fat by placing electrodes on the body and measuring the resistance of a small amount of electrical current that runs through the body. Since lean tissue has more water around it than body fat, it is a better conductor and less resistant to electrical current than fat. It conducts electrical impulses quicker than fatty tissue and so a faster response time is correlated with a leaner physique. Individuals with a large amount of body fat and adipose tissue (the fat that is just underneath the skin) have less water content and therefore are a poorer conductor of electrical current.

Strengths—Bioelectrical impedance is a fairly accurate method of assessment and it can be done quickly and relatively inexpensively.

Limitations—The accuracy of measurements can be greatly affected by hydration levels (individuals must avoid becoming overhydrated or underhydrated since the amount of water in the body can bias the overall results), meal times (what you eat, how much you eat and when you eat can skew results) and workouts (taking a reading directly after exercise can lead to a lower body fat reading). In addition, individuals may become anxious with the thought of allowing electrical current to run through their body (Duvall, 2017).

Procedures for Using Bioelectrical Impedance

At one time there was one method for assessing body composition using bioelectrical impedance. Today, however, there has been a flow of different devices to assess body fat using bioelectrical impedance including certain body weight scales. Therefore, it is recommended that you investigate the variety of methods for assessing body composition using bioelectrical impedance in order to determine your interest.

4.   ***Girth Measurements***—are circumference measurements at standard anatomical sites around the body measured with a tape measure. Girth measurements can be used to determine body size and composition and to monitor changes in these parameters (www.Topend sports.com).

Strengths—Girth measurements provide quick and reliable information that can be used to track changes in body shape and size over time;

Limitations—provides little information about the fat and fat free components of the body.

Procedures for Using Girth Measurements

1.   Mark sites to be measured
2.   Use a flexible metal tape measure and pen to mark the skin
3.   Make sure tape is not too tight or too loose
4.   Tape should be lying horizontal and flat on the skin
5.   Common sites to be measured include: head-neck-arm relaxed-arm flexed-forearm-wrist-chest-waist-hip-thigh-calf-ankle.

5.   **Body Mass Index (BMI)**—is a value derived from an individual's height and weight. BMI is an attempt to quantify the amount of tissue mass (muscle, fat, and bone) in an individual and then categorize that person as either being underweight, normal weight, overweight or obese based on that value. The BMI is defined as the body mass divided by the square of the body height and is universally express in units of kilograms. BMI is not a direct measure of body fat, however, research has indicated that BMI correlates well with direct measures of body fat. BMI percentiles are determined using population-based growth charts developed by the CDC that show age and sex specific BMI. The BMI is used to compare the individual based on height, weight, age and sex compared to their respective referenced populations. In children, a BMI over the 95th percentile of the age and sex-specific BMI is considered an indicator of possible obesity. It is important to note that not all children with a high BMI are overweight or obese. Some children could be heavier due to extra muscle mass, not extra body fat. BMI is widely used in clinical and school settings because it is considered a reliable, easy and inexpensive way to screen individuals over the age of two for possible weight problems.

IMPROVING YOUR BODY COMPOSITION

To improve your body composition, you should start off by first becoming more physically active and exercising by participating in cardiorespiratory, muscular fitness, and flexibility programs. Chapters' 6-8 include exercise programs that are specifically designed to meet your health-related fitness needs while determining your level of commitment to be physically fit and improve in these areas. Once you determine exactly what exercises you will do, how many days per week you will exercise, how much time you will devote to each workout, where you will work out and whom you will work out with, the next step is to focus on eating healthy. I encourage you to use the strategies outlined in Chapter 10 appropriately titled "Eating Healthy" and learn how to analyze your dietary habits and make healthy choices. Here are some strategies for you to consider when you want to change your body composition.

CHANGING YOUR BODY COMPOSITION

Losing Fat—If you want to lose fat, then you have to expend more energy than you consume. That means increasing your physical activity on a daily basis (e.g., walking instead of driving, taking the stairs instead of the elevator, exercising at least three times per week) and eating properly. The goal is not only to lose fat weight, but to keep it off permanently. As long as you continue to stay physically active and eat healthy, then losing fat weight and keeping it off will become a realistic goal.

Gaining Weight—If you want to gain weight, you have two choices: (1) eat more calories than you expend or (2) build muscle. If you plan on eating more calories, make sure that your percent body fat is below the recommended amount (10-12% for women and 5-8% for men) and focus on eating more based off of the nutritional guidelines outlined in the MyPlate section of Chapter 10. If you want to build muscle in order to gain weight then you need to work more on strengthening your muscles to give you the added weight you desire. That means working out with a higher weight (at least 70%-90% of your one-rep max) and performing between 2-8 reps per set.

Although many people choose to exercise in order to lose weight, it is important to remember that this may not always be a realistic goal. As you get older your metabolism will naturally slow down and losing weight can become more challenging. Therefore, your focus should be on being more physically active and eating healthy. Doing so will make you feel better and thus help to you see all the physical improvements that are certain to occur from participating in this type of lifestyle.

DETERMINING YOUR COMMITMENT TO HAVE A HEALTHY BODY COMPOSITION

On a scale of 1-9 (check commitment scale), circle your level of commitment towards having a healthy body composition.

	1	2	3	4	5	6	7	8	9
Low commitment				Moderate Commitment				High Commitment	

If you selected anything less than 7, then there is probably something stopping you from making a full commitment. Therefore, you should identify what your barriers are. Then, incorporate the strategies discussed in Chapter 10 to improve your dietary habits, design an exercise program that fits into your life (Chapters' 6-8) and set SMAART goals (Chapter 3) that will motivate you to overcome your barriers and have fun while improving your health-related fitness.

Recognizing Myths about How to Improve Body Composition

There are many myths about how to lose fat and tone muscles with minimum to no work involved. Unfortunately, some people believe these myths and become disheartened when the claims made about the product or method proves to be false. Here are a few of the more popular myths about exercise and body composition followed by a realistic explanation of what you can do to achieve your health-related fitness goals.

1. ***Doing abdominal work like sit ups turns stomach fat into muscle*** —Wouldn't it be great if you do a few reps of sit ups and turn that unwanted stomach fat into washboard abs? This procedure is more commonly known as "Spot Reducing" which is based on the belief that you can reduce body fat from designated places on the body. Unfortunately, this is not possible for several reasons. First, you cannot turn fat into muscle. Fat is fat and muscle is muscle. In order to see toned muscles, you have to first get rid of the fat and that happens from eating properly and working on your cardiovascular endurance and muscular fitness. Second, there is no exercise that guarantees you will lose fat from a certain area on your body. Just like when you overeat, you do not know exactly where the body fat will be stored. When you exercise, you cannot accurately assume that fat as energy will come only from the place(s) that you want. However, the tendency is that if you have an area of your body where you tend to have a higher portion of body fat, there is a good chance that when your energy expenditure exceeds your energy input, some of the fat that is used for energy will come from that area.

   Reality: What you need to do! First, eat healthy and make sure you do not overeat. Next, increase your CRE by first exercising for longer amounts of time each week. Once you can achieve 20-30 minutes of continuous activity, you can then choose to either increase intensity and/or going for longer amounts of time. This will help you expend more and more calories. Finally, work on toning your major muscle groups. This will make your body look better and increase your metabolism which will help to expend more calories at rest.

2. ***Skipping meals helps me lose weight***—That could be true. If you skip meals and are consuming fewer calories in a day than you expend then you will lose weight. However, if you are not physically active and you are losing in excess of two or more pounds per week, then the weight you are losing is most probably coming from water,

not fat. In time, you will have to replace the water or you will become dehydrated. It is also important to point out that skipping meals does not guarantee that you will lose weight, especially if you overeat during your other meals or consume a significant portion of your caloric intake later in the day and evening. If you are physically active and exercise and you skip meals then the quality of your workouts will decrease. Over time, you will not have enough energy in your body to help you overload during your workouts and thus your physical improvements (e.g., exercising for longer amounts of time, increasing intensity) will diminish.

Reality: What you need to do— Instead of skipping meals, how about planning your meal(s) the night before and choosing healthier foods with the right portion sizes! Overall, this will provide you with more energy throughout the day which will inevitably result in a greater amount of energy expenditure—burning off more calories to help you get rid of unwanted and excessive body fat.

3. ***Lifting weights creates big muscles for women***—While there are some women that train competitively for body building and power lifting and have developed large muscles, it is important to note that these women train significantly harder and put significantly more time and effort into their workouts than is recommended for most women who simply want to get fit and stay fit and improve their physical appearance by toning their muscles. In addition, it is important for you to know that women do not have enough of the male hormone, testosterone to allow for producing large muscle growth.

Reality: What you need to do! Women should give weight training a try by working on the major muscle groups a few times per week. All you need to do is choose 2-3 exercises per body part and perform 1-2 sets per exercise lifting approximately 50-60% of your max or (12-15 reps per set). This regimen will help women to tone and define their muscles, not make them grow large. See Chapter 7 for a list of possible muscular fitness programs designed specifically for you.

4. ***Eating more protein will get me bigger muscles and improve my health***—While protein does serve a role in repairing muscle tissue, eating too much of it will not create bigger muscles unless you work on improving your muscular strength. In fact, according to medical experts, a diet in which protein makes up more than 30% of your daily caloric intake could cause more harm than good. As your caloric intake of protein increases over 30% it causes a buildup of toxic ketones which can overwork kidneys by having to flush these ketones from your body. As your kidneys rid your body of these toxic ketones, you can lose a significant amount of water, which puts you at risk of dehydration, particularly if you exercise heavily (Butterfield as cited by Cole-Peralta, (2007 & Nelson, 2002).

Another problem with excessive protein intake is that it can increase storage fat build up and thus increase risk of coronary heart disease. Finally, if you increase protein intake and deplete yourself of complex carbohydrates you can overwork the dietary system and increase the risk of illness. For more information on the risks of consuming too much protein please read Cousens, G at www.creationsmagazine.com/articles/c108/counsens.html.

Reality: Stick to eating a well-balanced diet. This will give your body as much protein as it needs to perform the role that it is meant to (approximately 15-25% of your caloric intake). If you want bigger muscles then work on improving your muscular strength by lifting 70% or more of your max and performing 2-8 reps per set.

5. ***No pain, no gain!*** Some people think that in order to improve the way their body looks they must feel pain during their workouts. Thankfully, this is not true. You do not need to nor should you want to feel pain during exercise. In fact, feeling pain may be a sign that you might be exercising improperly and/or overdoing it and thus increasing your chance of injury.

Reality: Overload your body so that you feel tension, not pain. Recognize the signs and systems of overloading each system during workouts. For example, know what your heart rate should be during aerobic activity. You should always be able to talk and you should never be out of breath. During muscular fitness training, you should feel tension in the working muscles during lifting that eases up in between sets. Finally, during flexibility exercises, you should feel tension while stretching that decreases in intensity the longer the stretch is held for. Once you recognize how to create tension rather than pain, you will see that there are enormous gains without pain!

6. ***Being skinny means you are physically fit***—Having a low percent body fat or looking thin does not necessarily mean you are physically fit especially if you became thin only from dieting and you are not physically active. Through dieting, you have addressed one important component of health-related fitness (body composition), however, you may have neglected the other important components (cardiorespiratory endurance, muscular fitness, flexibility).

Reality: Focus more on being physically fit by exercising regularly and overloading the components of health-related fitness such as cardiorespiratory endurance, muscular fitness, flexibility, and eating healthy. Then if you become skinny, it will be for the right reasons.

7. ***Muscle turns to fat when you stop exercising***—Although it is common to gain weight when you stop exercising for extended periods of time, it is not because the muscle has turned to fat. When muscles are not being overloaded or when they are used in a reduced capacity, they can lose size as well as shape. If you start overeating you will increase the amount of stored fat, resulting in what looks like fat replacing muscle.

Reality: Once again, stay physically active and eat healthy. In times when you are not able to stick to your exercise program, work on being as physically active as possible (e.g., walking instead of driving to local places, doing a few toning exercises before going to bed). Plan to get at least one workout in per week during this time period in order to maintain your present level of fitness. Avoid overeating especially now that you have reduced your exercise frequency and time and your metabolism may have slowed down a bit. Most important, work on a new plan of action that helps you to fit exercise back into your life.

In conclusion, you now know what body composition is and how to assess your own body composition to determine if you are in a healthy range. You have been introduced to the myths about how to improve body composition, as well as being provided with a wealth of strategies to improve body composition. Remember the old phrase, "You are what you eat!" Well, if you want to be, look and feel physically fit and live a healthy lifestyle then you have to make sure that you eat healthy and exercise properly. So just how committed are you towards living a healthy lifestyle? Hopefully, by now you are extremely committed. If not, then go back to chapter 1 and start again!

REVIEW QUESTIONS

1. What is the problem with using height/weight charts to determine if you need to lose or gain weight?

2. Define body composition.

3. What is the difference between essential fat and storage fat?

4. What are the three roles that fat plays in the body?

5. Describe the differences between someone who is overfat from someone who is overweight?

6. Define obesity and explain what can be done to avoid being obese?

7. Compare and contrast 5 ways that you can assess body composition and discuss the strengths and limitations of each approach.

8. Which body composition technique do you like most, least, and why?

9. Discuss the procedure for assessing body composition using skinfold calipers.

10. Explain why you are better off using actual measurements rather than a formula to determine actual body composition.

11. What suggestions can you offer someone who wanted to improve his/her body composition?

12. List at least two strategies that you will consider using to maximize your commitment to have a healthy body composition.

13. Discuss at least three myths about how to improve body composition.

14. What suggestions can you offer someone who believes in these myths?

LAB ASSIGNMENT 9.1

Your assignment is to find an advertisement via the internet, newspaper, magazine, commercial, or infomercial on any of the following topics: (1) losing body weight; (2) turning body fat into muscle; (3) diets; (4) nutritional supplements; (5) exercise equipment that promotes significant changes in the body;

1. Determine how accurate the information being presented is?

2. Is the information being advertised consistent with the research. Please be sure to cite research to support your position.

3. If you were to conduct your own infomercial on body composition, list five important facts that you would like to communicate to your audience.

4. Explain three strategies that you would recommend to help people obtain the proper percent of body fat.

5. Describe the proper method for using skinfold calipers.

REFERENCES AND RECOMMENDED READINGS

American Dietetic Association www.eatright.org

American Obesity Association (2006). www.obesity.org

Bailey, R., Armour, K., Kirk, D., Jess, M., Pickup, I., & Standford, R. (2009). The Bera physical education and sport pedagogy special interest group. The educational benefits claimed for P.E. and school sport: an academic review. Research papers education 24 (1), 1-27.

Bray, G. (1993). The nutrient balance approach to obesity. *Nutrition Today, 28,* 13-18.

Cawley, J. & Meyerhoefer, C. (2012). The medical care costs of obesity: An instrumental variables approach. *Journal of Health Economics, 31*(1): 219-230.

Cawley, J., Rizzo, J.A. & Haas, K. (2007). Occupation-specific absenteeism costs associated with obesity and morbid obesity. *Journal of Occupational and Environmental Medicine, 49*(12): 1317-1324.

Centers for Disease Control and Prevention (2017). CDC 24/7: Saving lives, protecting people. www.cdc.gov/nccdphp/dnpao/state-local-program/high-obesity-program.html.

Centers for Disease Control and Prevention (2006). Does drinking beverages with added sugars increase the risk of overweight? Atlanta, GA: U.S. Department of Health and Human Services, CDC.

Centers for Disease Control and Prevention, (2005). The guide to community preventative services: what works to promote health? New York, NY: Oxford University Press.

Clark, N. (1991). How to gain weight healthfully. *Physician and Sportsmedicine 19*, 53.

Clarkson, P.M. (1998). The skinny on weight loss supplements and drugs: Winning the war against fat. *ACSM's Health and Fitness Journal*: 18

Counsens, G. www.creationsmagazine.com/articles/c108/counsens.html.

Dabrowska, A. (2014). Childhood overweight and obesity: Data brief. Congressional Research Service. www.crs.gov.

Duvall, J. (2017). The 6 best ways to measure body fat percentage. Dailyburn.com/life/health/how-to-measure-body-fat-percentages/January 12, 2017.

Exercise AC (2009). Ace lifestyle and weight management consultant manual, The ultimate Resource for fitness professionals. American Council on Exercise.

Flegal, K.M., Carroll, M.D., Kit, B.K., Ogden, C.L. (2012). Prevalence of obesity and trends in the distribution of body mass index among United States adults, 1999-2010. Journal of the American Medical Association. 307(5): 491-497.

Fryar, C.D., Carroll, M.D. & Ogden, C.L. (2004). Prevalence of overweight, obesity, and extreme obesity among adults: United States, 1960-1962 through 2011-2012.

Gates, D., Scoop, P., Brehm, B. et al., (2008). Obesity and presenteeism: The impact of body mass index on workplace productivity. *Journal of Occupation and Environmental Medicine, 50*(1): 39-45.

Hedley, A.A., Ogden, C.L., Johnson, C.L., Carroll, M.D., Curtin, L.R., & Flegal, K.M. (2004). Prevalence of overweight and obesity among US children, adolescents, and adults, 1999-2002. *Journal of the American Medical Association, 292*: 2847-2850.

Institute of Medicine (2005). Food marketing to children and youth: threat or opportunity? Washington, DC: The National Academies Press.

Institute of Medicine (2005). Preventing childhood obesity: health in the balance. Washington, DC: The National Academies Press.

Jackson, A.C. & Pollock, R.L. (1978). Generalized equations for predicting body density of men. *British Journal of Nutrition, 40*, 497-504.

Jackson, A.C., Pollock, R.L., & Ward, N. (1980). Generalized equations for predicting body density of women. *Medicine and Science in Sports and Exercise, 12*, 175-182.

Kassirer, J.P., & Angell, M. (1998). Losing weight-An il-fated new year's resolution. *New England Journal of Medicine, 338*, 52-54.

Khan, L.K., Sobush, K., Keener, D., Goodman, K.,, Lowry, A., Kakierek, J. & Zaro, S. (2009). Recommended community strategies and measurements to prevent obesity in the United States. *Morbidity and Mortality Weekly Report, 58*, 7, 1-30.

Klarenbach, S., Padwal, R., Chuck, A., & Jacobs, P. (2006). Population-based analysis of obesity and workforce participation. *Obesity, 14,* 920-927.

Larson, N.I., Story, M.T. & Nelson, M.C. (2008). Neighborhood environments: disparities in access to healthy foods in the U.S. *American Journal of Preventative Medicine, 36,* 75-81.

Lichtenstein, A.H., Appel, L.J., Brands, M., Carnethon, M., Daniels, S., Franch, H.A., Franklin, B., Kris-Etherton, P., Harris, W.S., Howards, B., Karanja, N., Lefevre, M., Rudel, L., Sacks, F., Van Horn, L., Winston, M., & Wylie-Rosett, J. (2006). Diet and lifestyle recommendations revision 2006. A scientific study from the American Heart Association Nutrition Committee, *Circulation, 114*, 82-96.

Mercola, J. (2012). Physical fitness in childhood linked to higher reading and math scores. www.fitnss.mercola.com/sites/fitness/archive/2012/09/28/physical-activity-improves- academic-performance; aspx.

Mokdad, A.H., Ford, E.S., Bowman, B.A., Dietz, W.H., Vinicor, F., Bales, V.S., & Marks, J.S. (2003). Prevalence of obesity, diabetes, and obesity-related health risk factors. *Journal of the American Medical Association, 289,76*-79.

National Association for Sport and Physical Education and American Heart Association (2006). Shape of the nation report: status of physical education in the USA. Reston, VA: National Association for Sport and Physical Education.

Nelson, M. (2202). Will eating more protein help your body gain muscle? www.medicine.-net.com

New York Times Editorial Board (2013). Exercise and academic performance. www.nytimes.com/2013/05/25/opinion/exercise-and-academic-perofrmance.html.

Ogden, C.L., Carroll, M.D., Curtin, L.R., McDowell, M.A., Tabak, C. J. Tabak, Flegal, K.M. (2006). Prevalence of overweight and obesity in the United States, 1999-2004. *Journal of the American Medical Association, 295,* 1549-1555.

Ogden, C.L., Carroll, Fryar, C.D., & Flegal, K.M. (2015). Prevalence of obesity among adults and youth: United States, 2011-2014. NCHS Data Brief NO. 219, November, 2015. www.cdc.gov/nchs/data/databriefs/db219.pdf.

Ogden, C.L., Carroll, M.D., & Kit, B. (2014). Prevalence of childhood and adult obesity in the United States, 2011-2012. *JAMA, 311*, 8 806-814.

Ogden, C.L. & Carroll, M.D. (2010). Prevalence of overweight, obesity, and extreme obesity among adults: United States, trends 1960-1962 through 2007-2008. NCHS Health E-Stat. Hyattsville, MD: National Center for Health Statistics.

Pardo Silva, M.C., De Laet, C., Nusselder, W.J., Mamum, A.A. & Peeters, A. (2006). Adult obesity and the number of years lived with and without cardiovascular disease. *Obesity*, *14,* 1264-1273.

Pate, R.R., O'Neill, J.R., & McIver, K.L. (2011). Physical activity and health: does physical education matter? *Quest, 63*: 19-35.

Peralta, K.C. (2007). How much protein should you eat? www.americanchronicle.com/-articles/view/Article.asp?articleID=25079

Statistics related to overweight and obesity: Economic costs related to overweight and obesity. Weight Control Information Network, 2006.

Thompson, D. & Wolf, A.M. (2001). "The medical-care cost burden of obesity", *Obesity Reviews, 2* (3), 189-197.

Topek. B. (2012). Strong evidence of link between physical activity, academic success. www.blogs.edweek.org/edweek/schooled_in_sports/2012/strong_evidence_of_link_betw een_physical_activity_academic_success.

Trogdon, J.G., Finkelstein, E.A., Feagan, C.W. & Cohen, J.W. (2012). State-and-payer-specific estimates of annual medical expenses attributable to obesity. Obesity (Silver Spring). Jan; 20 (1) 214-20.

U.S. Department of Health and Human Services, U.S. Department of Agriculture (2005). Dietary guidelines for Americans. 6th ed. Washington, DC: US Government Printing Office; 2005.

U.S. Department of Health and Human Services (2001). The Surgeon General's call to action to Prevent and decrease overweight and obesity. (Rockville, MD): U.S. Department of Health and Human Service, Office of the Surgeon General. Available from: US GPO, Washington.

WHO (2016). Obesity and overweight. www.who.org??

WHO, 2006. pp. 6

www.builtlean.com/2010/08/03/ideal-body-fat-percentage-chart/#fn-1368-1.

www.cdc.gov/nchs/data/hestat/obesity_adult_11_12/obesity_adult_11_12.htm

www.cdc.gov./apps.need.a-quick-assessment-of-child-and-teen-BMI.

www.choosemyplate.gov

www.heart.org/HEARTORG/HealthyLiving/WeightMAnagement/Obesity/Obesity-
    Information_UCM_307908_Article.jsp#.WYDRZdPytmA.

www.niddk.nih.gov/health/information-statistics/overweight-obesity. (www.rueters.com).

www.Topendsports.com

www.wikipedia.org/wiki/Obesity_in_the_United_States.

www.mypyramid.gov

www.obesity.org/subs/fastfacts/obesityyouth.shtml)

www.rueters.com

Chapter 10
Improving Your Nutritional Habits By Eating and Drinking Healthy

OBJECTIVES

After this chapter, you will be able to:

- identify what poor eating is and what motivates you to eat this way
- learn what healthy eating really is
- distinguish between the Old and New Food Guide Pyramids and the Healthy Plate
- learn the functions of the six basic nutrients
- implement strategies to improve your nutritional habits
- determine your level of commitment to healthy eating
- set S-M-A-A-R-T goals to improve your nutritional habits
- evaluate the success of your present nutritional habits

- "I don't have time."
- "I'm just not hungry for breakfast."
- "I have to have my coffee in the morning."
- "It just doesn't taste as good without the extra cheese."
- "I never eat lunch."
- "I eat whenever I'm hungry."
- "But I'm hungry late at night."
- "I can't stop eating when I'm hungry."
- "It looks too good to pass up."
- "Just one more and then I'll stop."

Years ago, many people believed that eating a good meal meant eating a lot of food and the more you ate, the better the meal. Back then, many adults simply did not know what a healthy meal consisted of and terms like "balanced diet," "fat free food," "complex carbs," "plant-based," "polyunsaturated" were rarely heard. Today, one hears these and other related words or phrases every day. The fact is most people today know how to eat healthy, yet they choose not to. The bottom line here is that it's always easier to put off today what you can plan for tomorrow than to make the commitment to get started today and actually follow through at that very moment.

If you go back a few hundred years ago and follow it up to the to the turn of the 20th century, you will learn that the main sources of food came from hunting and farming. Simply put, if you didn't hunt for your food or plant it on your own land, you could starve. Consequently, starvation was a main cause of death back then. Today, however, that is not the case. In fact, in many parts of the U.S. it is the exact opposite. As a result of the industrial and technological revolutions, the problem has shifted from having a lack of food to consuming too much of it. Presently, most people can go to the supermarket or local grocery store and in less than an hour take home enough food to last at least a week. All they have to be able to do is afford it and if they can't there's always a choice of fast food restaurants around that are often more financially affordable and usually open for longer hours to accommodate individuals with busy schedules. Subsequently, for many people eating fast food has shifted from a novelty to a lifestyle. According to the U.S. Department of Health and Human Services, two-thirds of adults in the United States (ages 20 and older) are overweight and over 30 percent are considered obese. Alarmingly, this number is not limited to only adults. The percent of young people (ages 6-19) who are overweight has tripled since 1980 (over 9 million) to over 16 percent resulting in an increased risk for many lifestyle illnesses (e.g., heart disease, cancer, obesity, atherosclerosis, high blood pressure, diabetes) (1-http://www.cdc.gov/nccdphp/dnpa/obesity.).

Today, there is a wealth of information at our disposal about how to eat healthy and maintain proper body weight. Courses in nutrition, fitness and wellness are offered in many different public and private sectors ranging from the university and collegiate level to local exercise facilities, libraries and community centers. Moreover, how to eat healthy and develop proper nutritional habits are taught in health classes as early as elementary school.

Unfortunately, this has not decreased poor eating habits. On the contrary, eating poorly continues to grow at frightening rates resulting in Americans consuming too many total calories per day. This has caused adult obesity to rise to an all-time high of over 36 percent.

Two important questions for you to answer are:

1. Do you know how to eat healthy?
2. Do you eat healthy?

If you are like most people, then your answers are that you probably know how to eat healthy, but sometimes or even often times, you do not. The next question is why? Why is it that you know how to eat healthy and yet you choose not to?

WHY DO PEOPLE EAT POORLY?

Most people know that fruits and vegetables are healthier than candy and cookies. They know that baked, grilled, broiled and boiled are better than fried. They know that drinking water is better than drinking soda or alcohol. They know that eating breakfast is better than snacking a few minutes before bedtime. Yet, if you ask someone you know if he/she eats healthy, for every one person that says "yes," I bet you will find at least one person and probably more that says "no."

The fact is that people eat poorly because they are more motivated to eat that way than they are to eat healthy. They would rather give in to their cravings for the foods and drinks that they love (e.g., fast foods, candy, cake, soda), regardless of how unhealthy they are because they have become attached to eating this way. Consequently, this often results in people rationalizing or explaining their motives to eat poorly in order to reduce the guilt that is commonly associated with poor eating. Does this ring a bell for you? Here are a few common reasons that people give for eating poorly.

1. ***Poor Planning/Not enough time***—One of the most popular reasons for eating poorly is the "misconception" that eating healthy takes more time than eating poorly. Many people eat "on the run," and prioritize convenience over health benefits by getting something that is easily accessible and quick more so than finding something with more nutritional value. Hence, the choice often becomes to eat fast food more than healthy food.

2. ***Develop poor dietary habits from an early age***—If you grew up eating poorly then you may have acquired some bad habits (e.g., overeating, eating too many foods high in fat content, snacking on candy, eating late at night, skipping meals). Moreover, you may have become attached to these foods and find it hard to be without them (e.g., soda coffee, cheese, butter, french fries, ice cream, fast foods, candy).

3. ***Attraction to Food Ads***—How often have you seen a famous person or an attractive model endorsing a food product? You go to the supermarket and you see a product that you like with a picture of a celebrity or model on the cover. This somehow persuades you to buy the product without reading the label to determine its ingredients. (Like purchasing this product is going to make you rich and famous and look like the celebrity on the label or having someone famous advertise this product makes is healthier).

4. ***Emotional attachment***—Some people search for their favorite "unhealthy foods" and often overeat when they are stressed out or upset. For these people, food helps them to temporarily over-come negative mood states and replace them with a feeling of

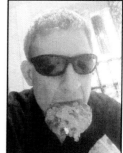

satisfaction by eating what they crave, no matter how low in nutritional value. Unfortunately, this doesn't last very long and the wind up is that the individual has now exacerbated his/her negative emotions and often feels guilty, angry and frustrated for succumbing to poor nutritional habits.

5. ***Psychological hunger***—Sometimes you may think you are hungry when you really 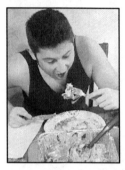 are not; you prompt yourself to satisfy a psychological instinct (e.g., just one more piece) and ignore physical cues (e.g., I am full). For example, you may be full from a meal, yet continue to eat because there is still more food on your plate. You may think you are hungry in places that you frequently store food (e.g., car, living room, bedroom, classroom, briefcase, book bag), regardless of whether or not you have just eaten. When you watch TV and see commercials for foods that you like, you may become tempted to eat even though are aren't hungry.

6. ***Eat too fast***— When you are in a rush and you only have a few minutes to eat, the tendency is to "eat too fast." Did you know that it takes the brain about 20 minutes to get a message from the stomach that the stomach is getting full? Since many people eat their meals in under 20 minutes, there is a strong chance that they may overeat without realizing it because the stomach has not sent the message to the brain that it is full yet. Then around the 20-minute mark the message has been received resulting in an immediate change of thought from "I am starved" to "I feel bloated and ate too much."

7. ***Lack of motivation***—Some people simply do not care if they eat healthy. They are more motivated to eat what they want, whenever they want and as much as they want then they are to be health conscious, especially if they perceive themselves to have a good physique and like the way they look. Consequently, they have developed a "myth of invincibility" and convince themselves to believe that as long as they look good on the outside they are healthy and nothing bad could ever happen to them despite how they might actually feel on the inside.

8. ***Blaming others***—Sometimes, people do not take responsibility for their poor nutritional choices and blame others. For example, "it's mom's fault for making it." "My friends all wanted fast food and encouraged me to eat it." "Everyone around me eats this way and I just couldn't say no." What you may not realize is that it is your choice to eat poorly. Nobody makes you eat what you don't want to and so blaming others for your poor eating habits is only a temporary mechanism to reduce your guilt which will inevitably prolong your actions to eat healthier.

EATING HEALTHY

Everywhere you look—television, newspapers, magazines, billboards—you can find advertisements about the latest fad diet or food. But in spite of all the hype, eating healthy today is no different than it was years ago. Nutritionists are still recommending that a diet that embraces complex carbohydrates consisting of fruits, vegetables and whole grains, along with proteins from both animal and plant-based sources and low amounts of fats, particularly saturated fats continue to be the healthiest way of eating.

The Old Food Guide Pyramid

With the prevalence of obesity among adults in the United States rising at a staggering pace from 13.4% in 1960-1962 to 30.9% in 1999-2000, the U.S. Department of Agriculture (USDA) developed the Food Guide Pyramid in 1992 which illustrated the recommended number of servings for five major food groups (See Figure 10.1 for the Old Food Guide Pyramid). According to the USDA, adults should be getting 6-11 servings per day of bread, whole grain cereal, rice and pasta, 2-5 servings per day of vegetables, 2-4 servings of fruits, 2-3 servings per day of milk, yogurt, cheeses, meat, poultry, fish, dry beans, eggs and nuts, and fats, oils and sweets in limited amounts and servings (U.S. Department of Health and Human Services, Department of Agriculture, 2000).

What complicated the Food Guide Pyramid was the definition of a serving size. For example, 1 piece of bread, 1/2 cup of cooked rice or pasta, ¾ of a cup of juice, 2 to 3 ounces of cooked lean meat, and 1 ounce of cereal were all considered to be one serving. However, most people determine one serving to be the size of one full plate of food and one full glass or cup of beverage. What they do not always realize is that the amount of food on their plate and drink in their glass or cup often exceeds one real serving. In addition, if condiments like butter, sauce, sugar or oils are being used to prepare or add flavor to foods then additional calories are being added to your foods.

The main problem with the Food Guide Pyramid was that it was not being used. For whatever reason, most Americans simply did not follow the recommended guidelines. According to the Harvard School of Public Health, the information in the Old Food Guide Pyramid didn't point to healthy eating because its blueprint was based on shaky scientific evidence which barely changed over the years to reflect major advances in understanding the connection between diet and health (www.hsph.harvard.edu/nutrition source/pyramids.html). Perhaps the Old Food Guide Pyramid was not practical for people to adopt on a consistent basis. 6-11 of this, 3-5 of that, one serving size means this, another serving size means that. All this could have made it too hard to follow. Another possibility is that the Food Guide Pyramid was not being advertised enough in the right places (e.g., restaurants, supermarkets, school cafeteria). Consequently, what people may have learned in the past about eating healthy was quickly forgotten and replaced with the same old eating habits (e.g., consuming too many calories; consuming too much fat; skipping meals; eating late at night). For more information on the Old and New Food Guide Pyramids, you can look at www.foodguidepyramid and www.health.harvard.edu/press.

The New Food Guide Pyramid

In 2005, the U.S. government unveiled the New Food Guide Pyramid designed to address nutritional needs by shifting from one program fits all to 12 new individualized food pyramids based on one's level of physical activity (http://www.health.gov/dietary guide lines/dga 2005 document). While the Old Food Guide Pyramid was horizontally based, the New Food Guide Pyramid was designed vertically and color coded into the following categories: (1) orange = grains; (2) green = vegetables; (3) red = fruits; (4) yellow = oils; (5) blue = milk products and (6) purple = lean meats; (See Figure 10.2 for the New Food Guide Pyramid). As you can see, the bands are different sizes with the larger bands represented by the food groups needed most to eat healthy (whole grains, vegetables and fruits). With 12 different nutritional programs, there certainly is a better chance that you might find one that fits your needs and helps you incorporate some of these guidelines into your lifestyle. It certainly beats the "one size fits all" approach of the Old Food Guide Pyramid.

Unfortunately, the New Good Guide Pyramid was unsuccessful in improving the dietary habits of Americans. The obesity rate continued to rise to over 34%. Perhaps the format was somewhat impractical just like the Old Food Guide Pyramid. In retrospect, having to remember colors for nutrients and determine which of the 12 programs worked best seemed a bit unrealistic for a population that had grown accustomed to eating spontaneously and not caring about the nutritional value of their choices.

My Plate

My Plate is the current nutritional guideline published by the USDA Center for Nutrition Policy and Promotion depicting a place setting with a plate and glass divided into five food groups. It replaced the USDA's New Food Guide Pyramid in 2011, ending 19 years of USDA food pyramid guidelines (www.choosemyplate.gov/). My Plate illustrates the five food groups that are the building blocks for a healthy diet using a plate as an image of a place setting so you can think about what goes on your plate, cup or bowl. My Plate is divided into four sections of approximately 30 percent grains, 40 percent vegetables, 10% fruits and 20 percent protein, accompanied by a smaller circle representing dairy, such as a glass of milk or a yogurt cup (www.wikipedia.org/wiki/MYPlate). In unveiling My Plate, First Lady Michelle Obama said, "Parents don't have the time to measure out exactly three ounces of chicken or look up how much rice or broccoli is in a serving. ... But we do have time to take a look at our kids' plates. ... It's as simple as that (Sweet, 2011). See Figure 10.3 to view MyPlate.

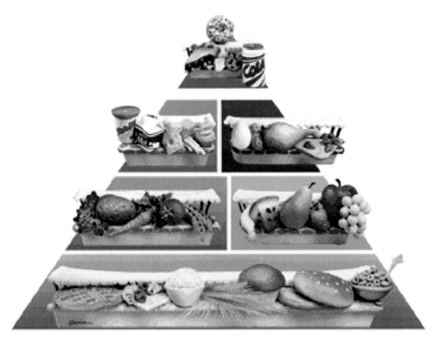

Figure 10.1—Old Food Group Pyramid

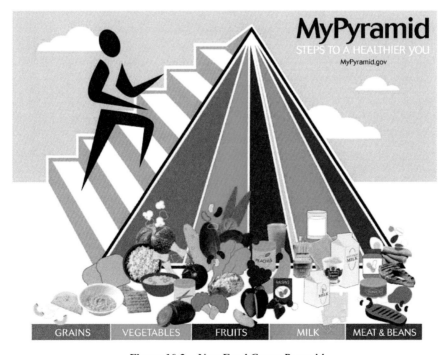

Figure 10.2—New Food Group Pyramid

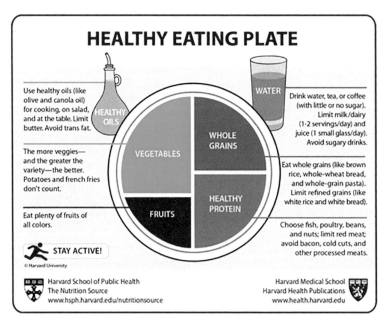

Figure 10.3—(My Plate)

SIX ESSENTIAL NUTRIENTS

There are approximately 45-50 nutrients in food that are necessary for the body's growth, development, maintenance, repair and overall good health. They are classified into the following six categories: (1) carbohydrates; (2) fats; (3) proteins; (4) vitamins; (5) minerals; and (6) water. These 6 nutrients can be broken down into two more categories: **macronutrients** and **micronutrients**. *Macronutrients* consist of carbohydrates, fats, and proteins, all of which are needed to provide energy for daily functions and for the building, repairing and maintenance of body tissues and organs. *Micronutrients* consist of vitamins and minerals and are needed in smaller amounts to regulate the functioning of the body's cells.

Carbohydrates—There are three major types of carbohydrates: (1) sugars more commonly known as simple carbohydrates; (2) starches, more common known as complex carbohydrates 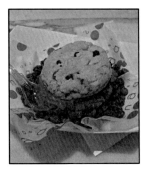 and (3) fiber. Simple carbohydrates have little nutritional value and are found in products like soda, cakes and candy. Complex carbohydrates are the most important nutrient and are equivalent to "premium octane gasoline." They help the body run more efficiently by providing the quickest source of energy. You can find complex carbohydrates in fruits, vegetables, whole grain breads, rice and pasta. Fiber is an indigestible carbohydrate that moves through the intestinal tract and provides bulk for feces in the large intestine, which in turn facilitates elimination. Fiber decreases the risk of cardiovascular disease and cancer and may also lower the risk of coronary heart disease. You can find fiber in fruits, legumes, oats, barley, wheat bran cereals, grains and vegetables.

Complex carbohydrates are our primary source of energy because the body is able to convert these nutrients faster than any other nutrients. When we consume carbohydrates, water is attached to it making it heavy and unable to stay that way for long. Therefore, it is just waiting to be used up. Of course, if you consume too many calories from carbohydrates, whatever is not used winds up being stored as fat. It is recommended that approximately 50-60% of your daily caloric intake come from complex carbohydrates (with no more than 10% coming from simple carbohydrates).

Isn't it interesting how many products today are advertising "low carb," "no carb" or "carb smart" as a mechanism to increase sales? Did you know that these products were made with few or no carbohydrates to begin with? They are simply being advertised to jump on the new

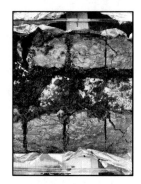

fad that "carbs" are bad. What they do not tell you is that the body relies mostly on carbohydrates as its main source of energy especially during intense activity. In fact, the brain's major source of fuel comes in the form of glucose which comes from the breakdown of carbohydrates. Without an adequate diet of complex carbohydrates, the body is forced to use other nutrients to do their job resulting in the body overworking itself and being forced to slow down considerably due to a lack of readily available energy. For example, if you planned on running for 30-40 minutes and you consumed mostly proteins and fats with very little complex carbohydrates for the past few days, you would probably find it very difficult to complete your run. After a few minutes of running, your body would exhaust its primary source of energy (complex carbohydrates), thus making it more difficult to keep running. You may be able to push it for a little while longer, but without the complex carbohydrates in your system to fuel your workout, you would have to slow down considerably and most probably stop before the 30-40 minutes were completed.

Fats—Fats serve the following needs. First, they protect our vital organs and here's an example of just how important that is. Have you ever banged your knee? Ouch! The main reason for that pain and discomfort is because there is so little body fat around your knee cap to absorb the shock from contact. Now imagine if you had the same around of body fat around your heart, brain, lungs or kidneys? Double Ouch! One little bang here or there and it can cause major problems. Second, fats help to keep your body insulated and your body temperature regulated. Without fat for insulation, body temperature could become unregulated resulting in the possibility of hypothermia when it gets cold and heat exhaustion and heat stroke when the body gets too hot. Third, fats add flavor to help you enjoy the taste of food. Finally, fats serve as the body's secondary source of energy and begin to be used for energy when you exercise for long periods of time. For example, if you consumed about 300 calories of complex carbohydrates and you are planning to exercise for a long period of time (e.g., 45 minutes or more), after 20-30 minutes, the body's readily available supply of complex carbohydrates may become depleted. Yet, what enables you to keep going is your body's ability to convert the fat that you recently ate along with some of your stored fat (the fat we all want to get rid of) to energy. An interesting way to view fats is to think of them as stored ice cubes. When you want a cold drink, you use ice with your beverage. The ice by itself will do little to quench your thirst, unless of course you want to wait an hour and let the ice melt. However, ice cools your drink more quickly, and a cold drink satisfies your thirst more efficiently. Fats in small amounts combined with carbohydrates gives the body two sources of energy that allow for longer and more efficient durations of activity.

Fats come in two forms—**saturated** and **unsaturated**. Saturated fats are found primarily in animal sources, including red meats, poultry, dairy products including egg yolks, milk and cheese as well as certain vegetable sources such as coconut and palm oils. Saturated fats are usually in a solid form and are used by the body to manufacture cholesterol. They do not melt at room temperature and therefore are not easily broken down by the body. Saturated fats are considered to be unhealthy and linked to cardiovascular disease, breast, colon, and prostate cancer and obesity. Unsaturated fats consist of two kinds: (1) **monosaturated** and (2) **poly-unsaturated**. *Monosaturated* fats come primarily from vegetable sources such as olive, peanut, and canola oil. *Polyunsaturated* fats also come primarily from vegetable sources including cottonseed, soybean, safflower, sunflower and corn oils as well as cold water fish including mackerel and salmon. Both types of unsaturated fat usually come in liquid form and are considered to be healthier than saturated fat because they reduce cholesterol and can be broken down by the body and used for energy when needed. Since fats do not carry water, they can be stored in the body for long periods of time. At one time, the average American consumed over 45% of their daily caloric intake from fats. Today, however, that percentage has dropped to approximately 30%-38%. A main reason for this stems from research findings by the USDA, CDC, NIH and other health-based organizations about the relationship between a high fat based diet and lifestyle illnesses (e.g., heart disease, diabetes, obesity). This sparked a significant amount of media attention that heightened the awareness of the American population to make healthier dietary choices. Moreover, this prompted many food companies who sell products high in fats to expand their selections of foods to include reduced, low, or fat free (e.g., milk, salad dressing, ice cream, meat, poultry) choices. Consequently, America has made a conscious effort to consume less fat in their daily caloric intake. The USDA recommends that calories from fat sources should be no more that 30% with saturated fats reduced to under 10%.

Proteins—Proteins are an important nutrient found in meats, fish, poultry, eggs, milk, cheese, and soy. Proteins serve many vital functions including: (1) enabling tissue growth, maintaining and regulating bodily processes; (2) forming integral body parts including skin, tendons, ligaments, membranes, muscles, organs and bones; (3) building up of the immune system; (4) helping the body maintain fluids; (5) transporting needed substances (e.g., oxygen, minerals) and (6) providing some fuel for the body's energy needs. As an energy source, proteins rank third behind carbohydrates and fats. They are only needed for energy when the body becomes depleted of both carbohydrates and fats. For example, during times of starvation the body is forced to break down the protein in the body and use it for energy to survive because carbohydrates and fats have been depleted. Consuming large quantities of protein in place of complex carbohydrates will only force the body to use it for a job it was not meant to do. Consequently, the body will wind up overworking itself and eventually break down and function inefficiently.

According to Pendick (2015), the recommended dietary allowance (RDA) for protein is 0.8 grams of protein per kilogram of body weight. To determine your RDA for protein, you can multiply your body weight in pounds by 0.36. For example, if you are a 20-year-old male who weighs 175 lbs. you would need 63 grams of protein a day. If you are a 120 lb. female, then you would need 43 grams of protein a day. According to research, it is generally recommended that a healthy diet consists of consuming approximately 15%-25% of total caloric intake from proteins, although you may need a little more depending on your age, sex and physical activity/fitness level.

Vitamins—Vitamins are organic molecules needed in small amounts to perform several bodily functions including growth, development, and metabolism. Vitamins are classified into two types: water soluble and fat soluble. Vitamins B and C are water soluble which means they dissolve in the blood and are carried to the cells. When not used, these vitamins can be excreted from the body by the kidneys. Vitamins A, D, E, and K are fat soluble which means they are stored and dissolved in fat and can stay in the body longer than water soluble vitamins. As a result, fat soluble vitamins should be taken in small quantities, otherwise they can become toxic. Since most vitamins cannot be manufactured by the body, they should be consumed on a daily basis.

Minerals—Minerals are elements needed in small amounts to help regulate a variety of bodily functions including: (1) aiding in the growth and maintenance of body tissue; (2) conduction of nerve impulses; (3) muscular contractions; (4) enzyme function; (5) water balance and (6) structural functioning of bones and teeth. The major minerals that the body needs include: calcium, phosphorous, magnesium, sodium, potassium, and chloride. The trace minerals that the body needs are selenium, iron, fluoride, copper, iodine, and zinc. When you eat a balanced diet, you generally consume the majority of the minerals needed. See Table 10.1 for a list of foods containing essential vitamins and minerals.

Water—It is generally agreed that water is the single most important nutrient with approximately 50-70 percent of a person's weight being composed of water. Without water, the body cannot survive. Water is needed to: (1) transport all nutrients throughout the body; (2) carry away waste; (3) help regulate body temperature and (4) assist in the absorption and digestion of food. Each day the body loses about 2 to 3 quarts of water and in vigorous exercise and hot weather water loss is even greater. It is recommended that you drink at least 8-10 8-ounce servings of water daily.

Table 10.1
Foods Containing Essential Vitamins and Minerals

Nutrients	
Fat Soluble Vitamins	**Where to Find**
Vitamin A	Liver, cheese, milk, yellow, orange and deep green vegetables and fruits
Vitamin D	Fortified milk, fish oils, salmon, tuna, egg yolks
Vitamin E	Vegetable oils, whole grain breads and cereals, nuts and seeds, yellow and green leafy vegetables
Vitamin K	Green leafy vegetables, eggs, cabbage, peas, potatoes, cauliflower
Water Soluble Vitamins	
Vitamin B (biotin, Folate, Niacin, Thiamin Pantothenic Acid, Roboflavin, Vitmain B6, Vitamin B12	Cereals, yeast, egg yolks, soy, flour, liver, green leafy vegetables, breads, fish, potatoes
Vitamin C	Fruits and vegetables
Minerals	**Where to Find**
Calcium	Milk and milk products, yogurt, tofu, cheese, fortified orange juice, bread, green leafy vegetables, dried beans, sardines, salmon
Copper	Seafood, meats, beans, nuts, whole grains
Iron	Meats and poultry, seafood, eggs, dried peas and beans, nuts, whole and enriched grains, green leafy vegetables, dried fruit
Phosphorous	Milk, fish, meats, eggs, whole grains, dried beans and peas, cereal.
Zinc	Milk, meat, seafood, liver, whole grains, nuts, eggs, dried beans
Magnesium	Milk, green leafy vegetables, seafood, whole grains, nuts, legumes, soybeans
Sodium	Salt, meat, processed foods
Potassium	Milk, bananas, legumes, orange juice, whole grains, potatoes, dried fruit
Selenium	Meat, seafood, eggs, whole grains

MEASURING YOUR NUTRITIONAL INTAKE

The amount of energy present in food is measured in terms of calories. Technically, a calorie is the amount of energy needed to raise the temperature of 1 gram of water one-degree Celsius. The more calories a food has, the more "potential energy" it has. Unfortunately, we do not get full from the number of calories or potential energy that food or drink possesses. We get full from the volume or weight of the food or beverage consumed. For example, if you ate two Pop Tarts consisting of approximately 210 calories each (420 overall) you may not be as full as if you consumed a handful of carrots, 2 apples and a banana equaling about 170 calories. Yet, if you ate a 20-ounce steak, you would get fuller than if you ate a 12-ounce steak.

There are 4 calories in 1 gram of carbohydrates, 9 calories in 1 gram of fat and 4 calories in 1 gram of protein. Therefore, you can eat 2.25 times more carbohydrates and proteins than fat for the same number of calories. In other words, fat has more "potential energy" to be used. However, potential energy does not mean that it is readily available or that you will even use it. As you learned in the previous section, fat is our secondary source of energy and is best used with carbohydrates. If you do not eat enough carbohydrates, the fats will wind up sitting in your body and not be used efficiently (ice cubes without water). Nutrition experts generally agree that approximately 50-60 percent of your diet should consist of carbohydrates with no more than 10 percent coming from simple carbohydrates (sugars, candy, cake, etc.), 15%-25 percent should come from fats (predominately monounsaturated and polyunsaturated) and 15-25 percent should come from proteins. Of course, if you are physically active and you exercise, then you may need a little more carbohydrates for aerobic activities and protein for muscular fitness activities.

Energy Balance Equation

A simple way to determine if you need to lose or gain weight is to use the energy balance equation which consists of two components:

1. ***Energy output***—everything you do that requires energy (e.g., exercising, keeping your heart rate beating properly, keeping your body temperature regulated);
2. ***Energy input***—everything that you eat and drink; When your energy output exceeds your energy input, you lose weight and when your energy input exceeds your energy output, you gain weight.

Metabolism

Your metabolism is what determines the amount of energy you will expend to keep your life sustaining systems going (respiration, circulation, digestion, temperature regulation). The faster your metabolism, the more calories you will expend at rest.

If your goal is to lose weight, the first step is to increase your energy output by becoming more physically active. Start out slow and each week commit to doing just a little bit more (e.g., an extra minute or two of cardio; a few more reps or sets to your muscular fitness workout).

The next step is to take better control of what you eat. Determine how many calories you eat per day and what the calories consist of in terms of percentages of fat (saturated and un-saturated), carbohydrates (simple and complex), proteins, sodium, artificial ingredients, etc. This will help you to become more aware of the nutritional value of your foods and beverages. Generally, you should avoid consuming foods that contain more than 30% of the calories from fat (particularly saturated fat), are loaded with simple sugars, and contain large quantities of artificial ingredients. Finally, learn what your energy balance equation is and incorporate some of the strategies listed in the next section into your daily eating habits.

STRATEGIES TO EAT HEALTHIER

If you are truly committed to eating healthy, then you should consider incorporating a few of the following strategies to help you improve. The key is to choose the strategy that fits you.

1. ***Plan your meals***—Rather than waiting until you are hungry, you should plan your meal(s) a few hours to one day in advance. Choose what you are going to eat, when, where, how much, etc. For example, if you typically start out early in the morning and skip breakfast, then the night before you can plan what you will eat for tomorrow's breakfast (e.g., cereal, oatmeal, whole wheat toast, fruit). By planning your meal(s) in advance, you become less susceptible to skipping meals, binge eating or finding that fast food place to satisfy those hunger pains.

2. ***Do not feel compelled to clean your plate***—As you begin to feel full, you should stop eating, regardless of how much food is left on your plate. Sometimes, the focus becomes on finishing what is left on the plate rather than stopping because you are full. Consequently, you may overeat. By concentrating on how full you are getting, you are less likely to keep eating even though your plate still has food on it. If you want, just save the leftovers for lunch the next day.

3. ***Make second helpings hard to get***—Rather than put all the food on the table when you are eating, fill your plate before you sit down and leave the remaining food in a place where it came from (e.g., the stove, oven, counter, refrigerator). If you want a second serving, you will have to leave the table to get it. I bet that might change your mind from eating more.

4. ***Restrict eating to designated places***—To reduce the likelihood of overeating, restrict your eating to one or two designated places (e.g., kitchen, cafeteria) and don't put food in other places (e.g., your bedroom, living room, den, study or reading area, car). Eventually, you will not get hungry in places where you no longer keep food.

5. ***Shop from a list and be full***—Did you ever notice that you tend to buy more food when you shop hungry than when you are full? Everything looks so good on the cover or box when you're hungry and the more food you see, the hungrier you get and the more food you want to buy. Therefore, when you need to buy food, always remember to do three things: (1) shop from a list; (2) buy only the food on the list and (3) eat

before you go shopping. This can help you to resist the temptation of buying food based on hunger rather than health.

6. ***Fork up Fork Down***—One of the most common ways of eating is what is called the "Shovel Method." You put a fork full of food in your mouth and before you swallow it, you take another fork full of food and put that in your mouth so you can push the first batch down. The shovel method results in you eating too much food, too fast. Instead, consider putting your fork down on your plate until you completely chew and swallow the food that you first put in your mouth. This new method will slow your rate of eating and make it easier to identify when you are getting full.

7. ***20-minutes-per-meal rule***—As you learned earlier in this chapter, it takes about 20 minutes for your brain to get the message from your stomach that you are getting full. Eating a meal in less than 20 minutes often leads to overeating so taking longer to consume an entire meal will help you recognize when you are feeling full and reduce the chances of consuming too much food at one time.

8. ***Healthy snacks***—To reduce the temptation of snacking poorly, surround yourself with healthy snacks (fruits, vegetables). Take them with you and when you begin to feel hungry, you have them right there. Eventually, this will reduce the temptation of going to the candy machine when you think you need a little snack to tide you over for a few hours.

9. ***Moderation***—If you truly love some foods that are not so healthy, it is okay to have them once in a while as long as you display some portion control. For example, it is ok to have a piece of candy instead of an entire bag or box, a handful of chips rather than an entire large bag or a cup of ice cream instead of huge bowl. The key is moderation, both in portion sizes as well as the frequency of times you consume these foods. Most important, do not feel guilty about having these treats. Instead, enjoy it and recognize that it is perfectly fine to have them once in a while.

10. ***Drink Water***—Instead of drinking your calories with sodas or fruit drinks, plan to drink water. If you have difficulty replacing soda with water, then consider trying it once a day. Once you have achieved this then set a goal to do it twice per day, then three times, etc. Before you know it, you'll be drinking more water than soda and looking forward to it, too.

11. ***Use smaller plates***—Using smaller plates makes the portion sizes seem larger and makes you think there is a lot more food on your plate than there really is. This may help you to feel fuller and reduce the amount of food you may consume in one meal.

12. ***Avoid skipping meals***—When people skip meals, they often think they are entitled to eat whatever they want and as much of it as they choose simply because they are hungry. It is easy to convince yourself that it has been so long since your last meal that it is more important to resolve hunger pains regardless of its' nutritional value rather than to eat healthy. By planning your meals in advance and taking healthy snacks with

you, you will minimize skipping meals and reduce your chances of rationalizing why it's ok to eat poorly instead of eating healthy.

DETERMINING YOUR LEVEL OF COMMITMENT TO IMPROVE YOUR NUTRITIONAL HABITS

How committed are you to eating and drinking healthy? Are there any strategies listed above that motivate you to improve your dietary habits? If so, which one(s)? Remember that commitment starts from a desire to accomplish something and it is not about whether you have succeeded or failed in the past. For example, if you wanted to start eating healthy and you planned to incorporate positive nutritional habits into your daily schedule, yet for some reason you did one or more of the following:

(1) you skipped breakfast

(2) you had fast food for lunch

(3) you didn't eat any fruits or vegetables today

(4) you snacked on candy late at night.

Does that mean that you are no longer committed to eating healthy? Not necessarily! It may simply mean that you made a poor choice. Something may have stopped you from making those positive changes. Perhaps you forgot about your newly discovered commitment or maybe your poor eating habits just got the best of you. If you indeed, are truly committed to improving your eating habits, you will analyze what stopped you from sticking to your commitment to eat healthy and focus on creating other strategies that may be more realistic for you to fit into your lifestyle. Most important, stay in action. For instance, plan tonight what you will eat for breakfast tomorrow so this way you will not skip it in the morning. Maybe you can make your lunch tonight too or plan where you will eat to avoid eating fast food. Finally, you might want to consider taking a few healthy snacks with you (e.g. your favorite fruit and vegetable) so you can erase the temptation to eat candy in between or in place of your meals.

In sum, your commitment to start improving your nutritional habits is reflected in the strategies that you have considered to overcome the barriers that stopped you (e.g., eating breakfast, making your lunch, taking fruits with you for snacks) as well as the actions that you take. So take a few seconds and answer the following question:

How committed are you to eating and drinking healthy?
Circle the number that best represents how committed you are to eat and drink healthy. You can fill this out daily or weekly.

1   2   3   4   5   6   7   8   9

SETTING S-M-A-A-R-T GOALS
TO IMPROVE YOUR DIETARY HABITS

In chapters 6-8, you learned how to use S-M-A-A-R-T goals to improve your cardio-respiratory endurance, muscular fitness, and flexibility. Now it is time to set S-M-A-A-R-T goals to improve your nutritional habits. So, instead of just thinking about why you eat poorly or that you need to improve, let's "EAT SMAART." Below is an example of how to use SMAART goals to improve your nutritional habits.

S—*Specifically* determine what you want to improve (e.g., eating more fruits and vegetables; reducing caloric intake).

M—Set goal(s) that you can ***measure*** (e.g., total number of calories consumed on a daily basis; percent of calories coming from carbohydrates, proteins, fats; the number of meals you will plan each day; the number of glasses of water or fruits or vegetables you will consume in a day)? For example, if you normally skip meals, you can plan one meal a day in advance (e.g., I will have a tuna sandwich for lunch at 1 PM). If you do not eat enough fruits or vegetables, you can plan ahead and determine when you will. For example, you will eat a fruit in between breakfast and lunch and then have a salad for lunch. If you overeat, you can reduce your portion sizes. If you eat too fast, you can time your meals and concentrate on eating more slowly (e.g., I will take 30 minutes to eat my lunch). Whatever your goal is, you want to have an action that will direct your efforts toward reaching it.

A—If you know that you are not going to reach your goal, then you have to make an ***adjustment***. For example, if your goal was to replace soda with water one time per day and it is already Day 4 and you have not had any water this week, then you can adjust your goal by committing to drinking water one time over the next 3 days. Adjusting your goal allows you to focus on making improvements rather than giving up when you know that you cannot reach the original goal(s) set.

R—To make sure your goals are ***realistic*** you should set goals that are within your reach and based on your present nutritional habits. Therefore, it is recommended that you use the dietary log in Appendix 10A to jot down everything you consume over a four to seven-day period. This will help you to determine just how many calories you consume on a daily basis and more importantly it will help you break down exactly when you consume the majority of your calories and what your calories consist of in terms of carbohydrates, proteins, fats, artificial ingredients, etc. For example, maybe you eat candy every day so you set a goal to replace candy with fruit twice this week. Perhaps you are addicted to soda and drink at least three glasses per day. A realistic goal for you might be to replace soda with water once per day. Finally, maybe you eat the majority of your meals spontaneously and recognize that it often leads to poor dietary choices so you set a goal to plan one meal per day. Setting realistic goals will help you to make the transition from unhealthy to healthy in a way that works for you.

T—Establish a ***target date*** to reach your goals. You can set short-term goals that focus on your desired accomplishments on a daily to weekly basis or long-term goals that emphasize something that you want to achieve at least one to several months from when you get started. For example, say you consume fast food at least five times per week and you snack on fattening products every night until you go to sleep. You drink 2-3 cans of soda per day and use butter at least twice per day on items such as muffins, bread, and vegetables. Your meals are 80 percent spontaneous and only 20 percent planned, and too often your dietary analysis indicates that you eat more than 3000 calories per day, 50 percent of which comes from fat. In the short-term you may set a goal to replace one of your highly fattening foods for something lower in fat as well as calories (e.g., replace muffin with butter for a bowl of oatmeal twice this week). In the long-term you may set a goal to reduce your daily caloric intake from 3000 to 2000 calories per day, eat 3-5 fruits and vegetables per day and replace butter for jelly three months from the day you get started. Table 10.2 provides an example of how to set Nutritiously SMAART goals. You can use Appendix 10B to set your own Nutritiously SMAART Goals.

In addition to setting SMAART goals, you can also set Stairway to Success goals to improve your dietary habits just like those your created in Chapters' 6-8 for CRE, MF and Flexibility (Table 10.3 shows how Lindsay used the Stairway to Success).

Table 10.2
Setting Nutritional SMAARAT Goals

	SMAART Goal #1	SMAART Goal #2
S	Eating healthier by planning my meals.	Drink healthier by replacing soda with water.
M	Plan 5 meals this week	Drink 4 glasses of water per day
A	I will prepare some meals the night before and go shopping on the weekend and buy granola cereal to have for breakfast.	Buy a case of water bottles and pack one or two water bottles in your work or school bag.
A	If I do not reach my goal, I will put up post-its in my car and on my cell phone to remind me to plan my meals.	If I forget to bring water with me, I will drink water from the fountain on my break.
R	I usually plan 2-3 meals per week so getting to 5 is certainly realistic.	I usually drink about 2 glasses of water per day so this goal is realistic.
T	I will reach my goal by the end of this week.	I will reach my goal by the end of this week.

So here we have Lindsay, a sophomore in college who never eats breakfast and she wants to improve her dietary habits. On the bottom of the stairs there is a zero "0" for the number of times Lindsay currently eats breakfast. On the top of the stairs is Lindsay's long-term goal to eat breakfast 6-7 days per week 12 weeks from the day she starts. Then on the second step up from the bottom is Lindsay's first short-term goal which is to eat breakfast once in her first week. So, what are your short-term and long-term nutritional goals? Consider using the stairway to success. If it worked for Lindsay, it can work for you, too. Please use Appendix 10B to create your own Nutritional Stairway to Success.

Table 10.3
Staircase Goals for Improving Nutritional Habits

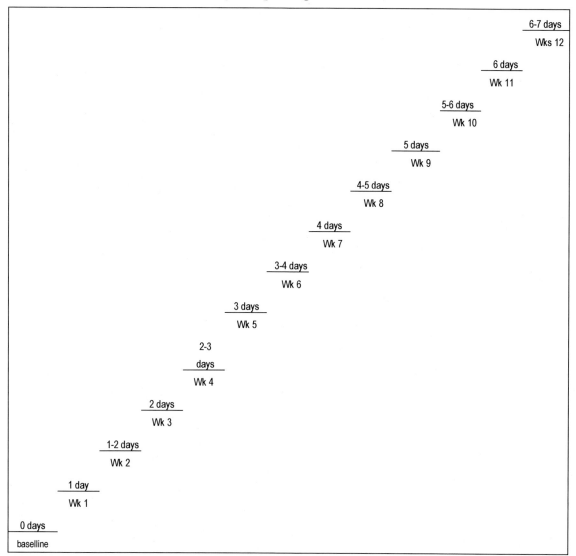

On the bottom of the stairs is a zero "0" for the number of times Lindsay currently eats breakfast. On the top of the stairs is Lindsay's long-term goal to eat breakfast 6-7 days per week four months after the day she starts. On the second step up from the bottom is Lindsay's first short-term goal which is to eat breakfast once in her first week. So, what are your short-term and long-term nutritional goals? Consider using the stairway to success. If it worked for Lindsay, it can work for you, too.

EVALUATING THE SUCCESS OF YOUR NUTRITIONAL HABITS

So how successful were you? What changes did you make to improve your dietary habits? Are you planning more meals? If so, how has that improved your eating? Have you replaced any unhealthy foods and beverages for healthier choices? If so, what changes have you made? Are you drinking more water? If so, how much water are you drinking on a daily basis? How conscious are you about what you eat? How much do you eat each day? How fast do you eat? Where do you eat? When do you eat?

Whatever results you have achieved, you should praise yourself for the effort that you expended no matter how little you may think that is. If you were successful, then continue to utilize the same strategies that have been working for you and maybe you are now ready to make another change to improve your dietary habits (e.g., replacing a different unhealthy food you eat with a healthier alternative, drinking one more glass or water per day or adding a vegetable to your dinner). If you were not successful, then you need to identify the barrier(s) that stopped you and create a different strategy to get you right back into action. Remember, staying in action will reinforce your commitment to improve your dietary habits and before you know it, you will have created strategies that work for you so that eating healthy will become part of your everyday life.

REVIEW QUESTIONS

1. List five reasons why people eat poorly.
2. Define healthy eating.
3. Describe the differences between the old and new Food Guide Pyramids and the healthy plate.
4. Which of the three nutritional programs do you like best and why?
5. List the six essential nutrients and explain the functions of each.
6. Explain the difference between a macronutrient and a micronutrient.
7. Why is water the most important nutrient?
8. Approximately what percent of your diet should come from carbohydrates, fats and proteins?
9. How many calories are there in one gram of carbohydrates, fats, and proteins?
10. Define the components of an energy balance equation (EBE).
11. List five strategies that you can use to eat healthier.
12. How committed are you to use at least one or more of these strategies?
13. Explain the purposes of using SMAART goals to improve your nutritional habits. List at least one SMAART goal that you have to improve your present nutritional habits.

LAB ASSIGNMENT 10.1
ANALYZING YOUR DIETARY CONSUMPTION

1. Using the dietary recall log in Appendix 10A, write down everything you eat and drink over a one-week period. Include the type of food that you consumed and how it was prepared (e.g., raw, baked, grilled, fried) since that can affect the quality of the meal as well as total number of calories. Pay careful attention to the portion sizes that you intake since many times the portion size of the label is less than the portion size consumed. Consequently, you may be consuming more calories than you think. You can determine caloric intake by reading the nutrition labels of everything you consume as well as familiarizing yourself with a variety of nutritional information sources located in the reference section at the end of this chapter.

2. Under column 1 labeled "Meal" include the time that you had that particular meal.

3. Under the column 2 labeled "Planned/Spontaneous" determine if your meal was planned or spontaneous. A planned meal is a meal where you know what you are going to eat at least a few hours in advance. A spontaneous meal is defined as eating when you get hungry, not knowing in advance what you will eat.

4. In column 3 labeled, "Length of time for meal" record how long each meal takes from the time you first started eating and drinking until your last bite and sip.

5. When the week is up, answer the following questions.

   a. How many calories did you consume each day?

Day 1	Day 2	Day 3	Day 4	Day 5	Day 6	Day 7

   b. When did you consume the majority of your calories?

   breakfast   lunch   dinner   snack

   c. How many calories did you consume for breakfast? lunch? dinner? snack?

Breakfast	Lunch	Dinner	Snack

   d. What percentage of your daily caloric intake came from carbohydrates, proteins, and fats?

   carbohydrates = _____ % + proteins = _____ % + fats = _____ % = 100%

e. Using the "Nutritional Awareness Chart," list all of the foods and beverages that are either too high in fat (over 30% of total calories comprised of fat; more than 20% total fat calories comprised of saturated fat), too high in simple sugars and/or have low or no nutritional value.

f. Rank each of the foods and beverages listed from question 5e on a scale of 1 (must have on a daily basis) to 9 (can do without) under the column listed unhealthy intake.

Nutritional Awareness Chart

Foods with over 30% of calories from fat	Foods & Drinks High in Simple Sugars	Foods & Drinks with little or no nutritional value	Ranking (1 must have it on a daily basis) to (9) I can do without it
			1 2 3 4 5 6 7 8 9
			1 2 3 4 5 6 7 8 9
			1 2 3 4 5 6 7 8 9
			1 2 3 4 5 6 7 8 9
			1 2 3 4 5 6 7 8 9
			1 2 3 4 5 6 7 8 9

g. Using the information listed above do you think you eat healthy? If so, explain why? If not, explain why not?

LAB ASSIGNMENT 10.2

1. Using the Healthy Alternative Chart, list the unhealthy foods or beverages that you have consumed over the past week and the frequency of times you had it. Then include a healthy alternative that you might consider to replace the unhealthy product (e.g., water for soda; jelly for butter, grilled chicken for fried chicken) over the next week.

Healthy Alternative Chart

Unhealthy Food or Beverage	Frequency of Times Consumed over the Past Week	Healthy Alternative

2. How committed are you to improving your nutritional habits and replacing at least one or more unhealthy food(s) and/or beverage(s) for healthy alternatives listed above?

So where are you on the commitment scale?

1	2	3	4	5	6	7

Not committed   Extremely committed

3. List 1-3 strategies that you will incorporate to improve your dietary habits this week?

_____

_____

_____

4. How motivated are you to incorporate these strategies into your nutritional plan this week?

So where are you on the commitment scale?

1	2	3	4	5	6	7

Not committed   Extremely committed

5. Are there anything stopping you from incorporating these new strategies? If so, list each and include a strategy to overcome these barriers.

6. After the week is up, evaluate the success of your eating habits.

a. Did you adopt the healthy alternative(s) into your dietary habits this week? If so, how often and how do you feel about your accomplishment(s)? If not, explain why?

                YES   NO

b. How do you feel about your accomplishments?

c. What do you have planned next week to improve your dietary habits?

REFERENCES AND RECOMMENDED READINGS

Beck, J. (2016). More than half of what Americans eat is ultra-processed. www.the atlantic.com/health/archive, March 10, 2016.

Bouchard, C., Bray, G.A., & Hubbard, V.S. (1990). "Basic and Clinical Aspects of Regional Fat Distribution. *American Journal of Clinical Nutrition*, 52, 946-950.

Duffy, R.L. (2002). ADA Complete Food and Nutrition Guide, 2nd ed. Chicago, IL: American Dietetic Association: An excellent review of current nutrition information.

Flegal, K.M., Carroll, M.D., Ogden, C.L., Curtain, L.R. (2010). Prevalence and trends in obesity among United States adults, 1999-2008. *JAMSA*, January 20, 2010; 303 (3) 235-241.

Ford, E.S., Zhao, G., Tsai, J. (2011). Trends in obesity and abdominal obesity among adults in the United States from 1999-2008. *International Journal of Obesity, 35*, 736-743.

Ford, E.S., Li, C., Zhao, G., Pearson, W.S. & Capewell, S. (2009). Trends in the prevalence of low risk factor burden for cardiovascular disease among United States adults. Circulation, September 29, 2009; 120 (13): 1181-8.

Food and Nutrition Board, Institute of Medicine, 2002. *Dietary reference intakes for Energy, Carbohydrates, Fiber, Fat, Fatty Acids, Cholesterol, Protein, and Amino Acids.* Washing -ton, D.C. National Academic Press.

FDA Center for Food Safety and Applied Nutrition. Provides information about topics such as food additives, food labels, and food borne illness.

Ogden, C.L., Carroll, M.D., Curtain, L.R., McDowell, M.A., Tabak, C.J., & Flegal, K.M. (2006). Prevalence of overweight and obesity in the United States from 1999-2004. *JAMA, 295*:1549-1555.

Pendick, D. (2015). How much protein do you need every day? www.harvard.edu/blog/ how-much-protein-do-you-need-every-day-201506188096. Samper-Tement, R. & Al Snih, S. (2012). Obesity in older adults: Epidemiology and implications for disability. www.ncbi.nim.hih.gov/pmc/articles/pmc3278274/

Sweet, L. (2011). "Michelle Obama hypes icon switch: Bye food pyramid, hello food plate. Transcript"(http://blogs.suntimes.com/sweet/2011/06/michelle_obama_hypes_icon_swit. html). *Chicago Sun Times*. Retrieved 6 June 2011.

"USDA's MyPlate" (http://www.choosemyplate.gov/). *United States Department of Agriculture.* Retrieved 2 June 2011.

U.S. Department of Health and Human Services, Department of Agriculture, *Nutrition and your health Dietary Guidelines for Americans,* Home and Garden Bulletin NP. 232 (Washington , DC:DHHS, 2000).

U.S. Department of Health and Human Services, Department of Agriculture, Center for Nutrition Policy and Information, 1996, Food Guide Pyramid, USDA Home and Garden Bulletin no. 252

Wilmore, J.H. (1994). Exercise and weight control: Myths, misconceptions, and quackery. ACSM, Indianapolis, IN, June 1994.

Wong, S.H.S., & Chung, S. (2003). Glycemic index: An educational tool for health and fitness professionals? *ACSM's Health and Fitness Journal*, November/December.

www.cdc.gov/nccdphp/dnpa/obesity = #1 reference cited...

www.cdc.gov guidelines/dga 2005 document

www.fitday.com

www.foodguidepyramid

www.health.gov/dietary guidelines/dga 2005 document

www.health.harvard.edu/press.

(www.usda.gov; www.uhealthcare.com/topics/weight/weightcontrol).

www.healthfitcounter.com

www.hhs.gov

(www.hsph.harvard.edu/nutrition source/pyramids.html)

www.my-calorie-counter.com

www.nutritionexplorations.org/educators/pyramid-main-asp

www.usda.gov.com

(www.usda.gov; www.uhealthcare.com/topics/weight/weightcontrol).

www.wikipedia.org/wiki/MYPlate.

APPENDIX 10A

Meal	Planned or Spontaneous	Length of Time for Meal	What else were you doing besides eating?	Total Calories	Carb Cals	Fat Cals	Protein Cals
Breakfast							
Lunch							
Dinner							
Snack							

APPENDIX 10B
STAIRCASE GOALS FOR IMPROVING NUTRITIONAL HABITS

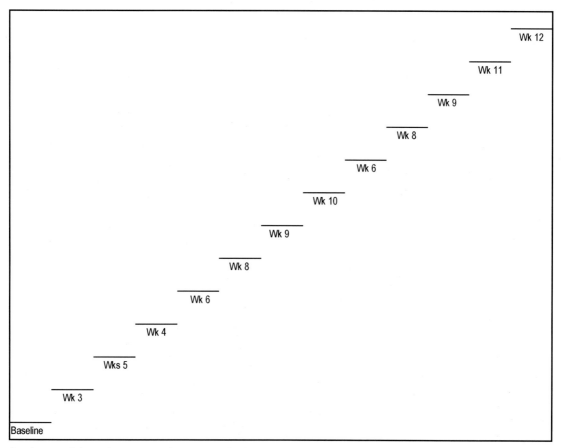

On the top of the stairs, put your long-term nutritional dream goal (e.g., eating fruits ___ times per day, drinking water ___ times per day, planning your meals ___ times per day). On the bottom of the stairs put your baseline and what you are presently doing. On the step just above your baseline, put your first short-term goal. Once you reach that goal, you can set a goal on the next step up and so on.

Chapter 11

Cognitive Strategies: Maximizing Your Thoughts During Exercise

OBJECTIVES

After reading this chapter, you will be able to:

- Define cognitive strategies
- Incorporate association, dissociation, positive self-talk and imagery into your exercise program
- Evaluate the effectiveness of using cognitive strategies to enhance your exercise enjoyment, motivation, and performance
- Determine your level of commitment to use different cognitive strategies during exercise

An important part of your exercise program involves your thoughts or cognitions—what you focus your attention on during exercise (Weinberg & Gould, 2003). If you find exercise boring and unenjoyable, then the thoughts in your mind will probably be negative which will diminish your motivation and incentive to exercise in the long term. However, if you like to exercise and enjoy what you are doing then your mind will be filled with positive thoughts which will increase your motivation to find the time to fit exercise into your life.

One of the most popular reasons for not exercising is because it is perceived to be boring. Whether the feeling of boredom is related to the activity itself (e.g., doing the same workout repeatedly), the exercise environment, (being in the same place and not liking the surroundings, e.g., dark, cold, old equipment, overcrowded facility), the people around you (feeling uncomfortable because you think that you do not have anything in common with the them), focusing more on differences than similarities (age, gender, fitness level, education) many people stop exercising because they do not like it and it is boring to them.

In this chapter, you will learn what cognitive strategies are and how to incorporate them into your exercise program in order to create an empowering atmosphere that will increase your enjoyment and desire to make exercise an integral part of your life. So rather than wish exercise was more enjoyable, now you can plan to make it happen!

WHAT ARE COGNITIVE STRATEGIES?

Cognitive strategies are structured ways of thinking that are designed to enhance concentration skills for the purposes of increasing performance and/or enjoyment in exercise and sport. In essence, cognitive strategies are ways to program your thoughts. This chapter introduces four different cognitive strategies: (1) association; (2) dissociation; (3) positive self-talk and (4) imagery and it explains how to use each strategy in order to maximize exercise performance, enjoyment, and safety during your workouts. The thinking starts now!

Association is defined as concentrating on the relevant or related aspects of the activity or exercise (e.g., how your muscles feel, your breathing rate, pacing, technique) that you are engaged in. For example, if you are going for a run, associating would involve focusing on important factors related to running (e.g., heart rate, breathing pattern, pace, form, muscular tension, how your body feels, how much energy you believe you have in order to complete the desired distance or time). If you are working on muscular fitness, association would involve concentrating on proper form, correct breathing, how your muscles feel from one rep to the next and knowing how much strength it will take to complete a given set. Finally, associating while working on flexibility would involve concentrating on proper form, stretching to your tension point, breathing slowly, determining how long you will hold a stretch for and being aware if and when you could stretch a little further.

Dissociation is defined as concentrating on the irrelevant or unrelated aspects of the activity or exercise for which you are engaged in. Dissociation is designed to take your mind off of exercise and onto things that you enjoy, thus enhancing your overall exercise experience. For example, dissociating while exercising may include listening to music while going for a run, watching television while stretching, reading in between sets of lifting weights, and talking with an exercise partner during CRE, MF or flexibility activities. With each strategy, your mind becomes centered on information unrelated to exercise (e.g., music, talking, television, reading, conversation, texting, etc.).

Whether you realize it or not, you are always associating or dissociating during exercise. The challenge is knowing how and when to use both strategies in order to gain the maximum benefits. Three factors to consider when deciding whether you should associate or dissociate during exercise are: (1) safety; (2) performance and (3) enjoyment.

Safety—For individuals who are first starting out and getting accustomed to the demands of exercise, association should be the cognitive strategy used. By listening to your body and focusing on using proper technique, determining the right pace and knowing how and when to increase or decrease the time and intensity, you will decrease your chances of injury, prevent undo fatigue, and ultimately increase your performance/fitness level.

Performance— According to research, association has been found to increase performance more than dissociation in high level competition including triathlons (Werner, 2003), competitive running (LaCaille, Masters & Health, 2004, Morgan & Pollack, 1977; Masters & Ogles, 1988; Nietfeld, 2003), swimming (Couture, Jerome, & Tihanyi, 1999), and rowing (Scott, Scott, Bedic, & Dowd, 1999). If you are primarily motivated to improve your exercise performance, (e.g., run faster, lift more weight stretch further) then you should focus more on associating by concentrating on the demands of the exercise and how your body is adapting to it.

For example, when running, you should know what pace works best for you, when you need to conserve your energy and slow down as well as when to pick up the pace to run faster. When lifting weights, you should focus on how many reps you want to do, how your muscles feel during each rep and how much strength it will take to get it done. Finally, for flexibility, you should know where your tension point is and concentrate on holding the stretch for a prescribed amount of time that will improve your range of motion in the desired area(s). So, if you want to increase your performance then associate by thinking about what you want to do and then do it.

Enjoyment—One of the most effective ways to increase your enjoyment is to combine exercise with other activities that you like to do. For example, listening to your favorite music while you go for your walk, run, or bike ride, reading an interesting book while riding your stationary bicycle, or working out with a friend and engaging in a friendly conversation can all take your mind off of your exercise activity and onto something with a greater perceived enjoyment. Interestingly, research has found that dissociation has been favored during practice or recreational activity and it has led to higher levels of exercise enjoyment, tranquility, better attendance and greater compliance of exercise than association (Martin, et al., 1984; Lacaille, et al., 2004). In other words, by focusing on things that stimulate you (e.g., music, television, conversation), you will pay less attention to the things you may not like while exercising (repetitiveness, fatigue, muscular tension) and thus enjoy exercising more.

INCORPORATING ASSOCIATION AND DISSOCIATION INTO YOUR EXERCISE PROGRAM

Association

Association should be used when you are familiarizing yourself with an activity or exercise and you need to learn and/or focus on the proper form and technique (e.g., bodily position), the demands of the exercise (e.g., muscular tension, heart rate, pace) and how your body responds to these demands (e.g., fatigue, feeling energized). For example, when you first begin to exercise, you should focus on making sure you are doing the exercise properly and pay attention to how your body feels. Are you comfortable? If you are using equipment like a bicycle, are you seated in the correct position? If you are on a treadmill, are you going at the right pace? How do your legs feel? How is your breathing? If you are lifting weights, are you sitting or standing properly? Is your body weight centered? Is the fulcrum/range of motion lever inserted in the correct position, creating the proper range of motion? When stretching, are you properly warmed up? Is your body in the correct position for each stretch? What is your tension point and how long do you plan on holding a stretch for?

Associating During CRE Activity

Here is a list of guidelines used to determine how and when to associate during CRE activity.

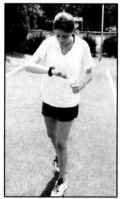

1. ***Familiarize yourself with the demands of the activity***—This involves learning how to do the exercise(s) properly. If you are exercising indoors then you need to learn how to use the equipment properly (e.g., treadmill, bike, elyptical, stairmaster), learning your proper pace, where your heart rate is and should be and where you should feel muscular tension. If you are exercising outdoors then you need to be aware of the environment (e.g., terrain, hills, weather) since they can all play a significant role in the quality and comfort of your workout.

2. ***Make sure your body is warmed up and ready***—Listen to your body to determine when you are warmed up and ready to begin exercise overload. Concentrate on how your muscles feel. Are you able to move around freely or do you still feel tight? Are you breathing comfortably or is your breathing labored?

3. ***Set the right pace***—Start off going slow and think about how your body feels. Pay specific attention to how you are breathing and the muscular tension you are experiencing, particularly in the lower extremities (quadriceps, hamstring, calves, hip flexors, ankles).

4. ***Making sure your heart rate is in the correct zone***—Every few minutes, you should monitor your heart rate to make sure that you are working at the right intensity. If your heart rate is too high (above your training zone) you will be breathing heavily and need to slow down and if your heart rate is too low (below your training zone) the exercise will feel too easy and then you can speed up. If you do not have access to a heart rate monitor, you can do the "talk test." Simply start talking aloud. If you are having trouble speaking, it can be a sign that you are breathing too heavy, so slow down. If can can talk without laboring then you are most likely going at a comfortable pace so keep talking (I mean going)!

5. ***Identifying how much energy you have***—At the beginning and every few minutes during your workout, you should check in with yourself to see how you are feeling and determine how much energy you have. You always want to feel like your perceived amount of energy can match or exceed the energy demands of your workout. This will make you feel more comfortable during your workout and allow you to increase the time, intensity or possibly both if you so desire. If the energy demands of the activity are greater than your perceived amount of energy, then you know it is time to slow down or stop.

6. *To increase performance*—If your primary goal is to increase your CRE performance (e.g., training for races or competition), association can help you to focus on pacing yourself properly, knowing how and when to conserve energy (slow down) or expend more energy (pick up the pace and go faster), control your breathing and maximize proper form (e.g., stride, balance).

Dissociating During CRE Activity

With CRE activity, the exercises you perform are rhythmic in nature and generally can be learned within a short period of time. Once you learn the proper form, pace and rhythm, you can begin to dissociate if you like. In fact, you will probably enjoy your CRE exercises more when you dissociate since you will be able to decide what you want to think about rather than focusing on how much longer you have to go or how bored you may be getting. Here are a list of guidelines used to determine when and how to dissociate during CRE activity.

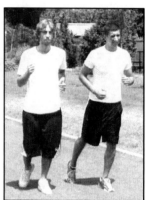

1. *Know What & How to Do*—Once you become familiar with the types of exercise(s) that you enjoy doing and you know how to do them properly, you can plan to dissociate by incorporating other activities that you enjoy into your workouts (e.g., listening to music, talking with a friend, watching TV, texting, playing games on your phone). Today, there are many exercise facilities with entertainment areas that include movies, music and television which are designed to help the individual take their mind off of exercise and enhance the cardio-exercise experience.

2. *Feel Comfortable*—Once you feel comfortable during your aerobic activities and you no longer have to think about what to do (e.g., pacing and proper form are automatic), you can incorporate dissociation into your workout.

3. *Replace Boredom for Fun*—If you find your workouts boring and monotonous and you have lost your desire to exercise on a regular basis, the time has come to make exercising more fun. Listed below are several dissociative strategies to consider.

- Listen to music
- Exercise with a friend
- Read
- Watch TV or a movie
- Play a video game
- Use the time to plan your day on your PDA
- Talk on the telephone.
- Text Messages
- Surf the Net or e-mail on your cell phone

Associating During Muscular Fitness Training

Associating is a very important technique when working on muscular fitness. The intensity of this type of training is greater than CRE or flexibility exercise and as a result there is greater risk of injury. Therefore, it is important for you to know what to focus on (e.g., concentrating on the correct form, choosing the correct weight, controlling and balancing the weight properly, breathing properly, knowing how many reps you will to do, etc.). Here are some guidelines for how and when to associate during muscular fitness training.

Warming Up— When you first get started, you should warm up your body by doing a few minutes of aerobic activity followed by a "warm up" set of the exercise that you plan to start

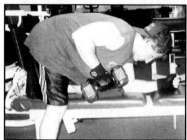

your muscular fitness workout with. Use a "light" or "no weight" and perform approximately 12-15 reps. During this time, you should concentrate on how your body feels as you prepare to raise the weight for your first set and get ready for exercise overload. If you plan to do different body parts in your workout then you should do a warm up set each time you address a new muscle group that has not been worked on thus far in your workout.

Using Correct Form—Each exercise requires that you use the correct form which means starting at the correct position, knowing how to lift weight properly, using your full range of motion, and controlling the weight on the exertion (lifting) and resting (putting the weight back to the stack, rack, floor or initial starting point), phases.

Listening to your body—While lifting, you need to know what your body is capable of doing and not doing. Listening to your body can help you recognize when you might be able to do a few more reps, as well as when you are at your limit and need to stop.

Lifting to the Full Range of Motion—Each exercise that you do requires that your lift goes to the full range of motion. That means that you should be concentrating on fully extending and contracting on every repetition. When using machines, you must know where to place the fulcrum (the knob that determines range of motion).

Breathing Properly-An important part of muscular fitness is breathing properly. Therefore, part of associating during muscular fitness training involves concentrating on your breathing. You should be inhaling before you start lifting and when you are in the resting phase. Then upon the lift or beginning of your exertion phase you should be exhaling. This will keep the flow of breathing consistent and more comfortable.

Counting Your Reps– Each repetition should take between 3 and 5 seconds to complete. One to 2 seconds should be devoted to the exertion phase (lifting the weight) and 3-4 seconds should be devoted to the resting phase (bringing the weight back to its' initial starting point). Concentrating on counting how long each phase of each rep will take will help you to properly overload your muscles and get a better workout. Once you finish your set, you should evaluate how your body feels. Are your muscles feeling tight, sore, and fatigued, or are you invigorated and strong? Concentrating on how your muscles feel will provide you with important information about how you will proceed with the rest of your workout. For example, if you feel tired, but want to continue, you may need to more time to rest in between sets, reduce the weight on the next set of the same exercise, or select a different exercise or body part to work on next. Conversely, if you think you can do more, then you may decide to increase the weight on the next set, decrease rest time in between sets or add an extra set or exercise in order to create a more challenging workout.

Dissociating During Muscular Fitness Training

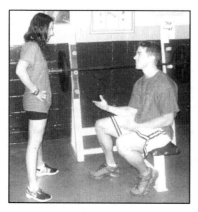

The only time you should be dissociating during muscular fitness training is in between sets or exercises. It is simply too dangerous and unsafe to take your mind off of what you are doing while working on your muscular fitness. However, once you have become used to how your body feels and you are familiar with the demands of each exercise that you do, you can begin to dissociate in between sets by listening to music, reading, talking to someone in between sets or using a journal to write down any thoughts that may enter your mind. Just remember that once your rest time has been completed, it is time to associate and begin concentrating on your next set.

Associating During Flexibility Training

The same rules apply for using association and dissociation during flexibility training as for CRE and MFT. First, you have to know how to stretch safely and therefore, you should always start off associating to make sure your body is ready to be stretched. So, ask yourself the following two questions: (1) Are you warmed up before you stretch? (2) Are your muscles ready to be stretched? If you answer "NO" to either question, then you are not ready to stretch yet and so you may need a few more minutes to warm up. If you answered "YES" to both questions, then you are ready to stretch so begin by concentrating and stretching to your tension point. Remember, your tension point is the furthest area that you can hold a stretch. Once you are there then you have the following options: (1) continue to associate by focusing on the tension that you are feeling and holding for a prescribed amount of time; (2) breathe rhythmically by inhaling before you begin your stretch and exhaling while you are stretching to your tension point and holding; (3) focusing on achieving a new tension point by reaching just a little bit further every few seconds.

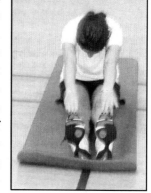

Dissociating During Flexibility Training

Once you have learned the correct way to stretch and you have identified your proper tension points, you can take your mind off of the tension you are feeling and begin to dissociate. Here are a few ideas about how and when to dissociate during flexibility training.

Listen to Music—Some people find stretching boring and a perfect way to spice up your flexibility program is with a little music that makes you feel good. Simply put the music on in the background to establish an environment that creates a positive, yet relaxing mood state.

Stretch with a Partner—Stretching with a partner can help you take your mind off of any negative thoughts associated with stretching and onto more pleasant thoughts. For example, if you are both competitive and enjoy challenging one another, you can make stretching into a

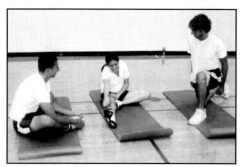 friendly, competitive game by seeing who can hold a stretch longer and/or further. Perhaps you are having some difficulty reaching your true tension or holding a stretch for more than a few seconds by yourself. Incorporating the use of a partner to do some passive static stretches while having her/him talk to you while stretching may help you redirect your thoughts from associating on the physical stress of stretching by yourself to dissociating and carrying on a conversation that has nothing to do with stretching (e.g., school, sports, family, relationships, vacations, TV, movies, music, etc.).

Watching Television—An excellent way to dissociate while stretching is to watch television during certain parts of the show (e.g., commercials, first five minutes) and take your mind off how your body feels. After a few minutes, your body should feel better and help you to stretch for longer periods of time.

Social Media-Once you are able to hold a stretch for at least 20 seconds, you can use your cell phone to take your mind off of stretching and onto things you enjoy like texting a friend, surfing the web, playing a game or maybe just doing some research for an upcoming paper or assignment that you have coming up.

The way you communicate with yourself prior to, during, and after exercise can have a huge influence on how well you perform and how much you enjoy exercise. For example, if you talk negatively to yourself about exercise (e.g., "I don't like this," "I'm not good at this" "I will never see results," "This is so boring"), it is likely that at some point in the near future you will find a reason not to exercise. After all, why would you want to find time to exercise when you are thinking negatively about it. However, if you talk positively to yourself about exercise and remind yourself of the many benefits associated with exercise and how good it makes you feel then you will be more motivated to do it. You will perform at a higher level and get the most out of it. Don't you agree? You better!

The following section focuses on how to use cognitive strategy #3, **"Positive Self-Talk"** during exercise.

SELF-TALK: FROM NEGATIVE TO POSITIVE

Self-talk is the act of talking to oneself, either silently or aloud in the form of thoughts, words, phrases or internal conversation. According to Psychologist, Susan Kraus Whitbourne, self-talk provides opinions and evaluations on what you're doing as you're doing it. Self talk is your inner voice, equivalent of sports announcers commenting on a player's successes or failures on the playing field. The only difference is with sports commentary, the athlete doesn't here what is being said. However, you always hear your internal voice and when that voice is upbeat and self-validating, the results will boost your productivity. However, when the voice is critical and harsh, the effects can be emotionally debilitating (Kraus Whitbourne, 2013). For example, have you ever had negative thoughts about exercise (or lack there-of) and your mind was filled with commentary like "What's the use of exercising? I never see results. I always quit. It's so boring. I'm not good at this anymore. I'm not as fit as my friends. I don't want to embarrass myself."

Believe it or not, self-talk is a very common process. In fact, most people are in constant communication with themselves all day long, involved in some type of mental chatter that unfortunately, is often filled with negative thoughts and emotions including anger, frustration, and guilt. In essence, your inner voice is validating your thoughts of frustration, embarrassment and upset resulting in you becoming more motivated not to exercise than to exercise which will inevitably lead to even more frustration and upset as time goes on, not to mention increasing your risk of lifestyle illness as you get older. Now imagine if you transformed the negative self-talk into positive self-talk by praising yourself for getting started and/or staying in action to live a healthy lifestyle. You begin to say to yourself "I'm so ready to get started. I am so proud of myself for signing up for Dr. Frierman's Fitness for Life class. I am really going to enjoy going to the gym.

It is important for you to recognize that your actions are inspired by your thoughts. If you are going to think negatively then your actions are going to reflect that in a negative capacity (e.g., no exercise, eat poorly). However, if you change the way you think from negative to positive, you can begin to transform the actions you take from "not doing or trying to do" to "doing and succeeding." This will help you to achieve personal growth and development across a variety of dimensions including mentally, emotionally and/or spiritually.

Positive Self-Talk

Positive self-talk is an internal dialogue that emphasizes increasing energy, effort, and positive attitude (Weinberg & Gould, 2003). It inspires you to focus on what you can do and have total control over rather than what you want to avoid. Although it sounds, simple, positive self-talk involves more than just saying you will do something. It's a process that takes some practice. Here are two similar, but different approaches to using positive self-talk: (1) Lim's 7 Steps to Positive Self-Talk and (2) Mike's 6 Rules for Positive Self-Talk.

Lim's 7 Steps to Positive Self-Talk

1. ***Eliminate Internal Negative Chatter***—The first step is to be aware of your thoughts that run through your mind. Everyone has a voice inside their head that constantly talks to us, often in a negative tone (e.g., I don't want to exercise; I'll never see the results I want; I'm wasting my time). Without awareness of these negative thoughts, you will continue to let them dictate your actions like an unconscious or automatic validation which will create negative habits (e.g., eat poorly; become sedentary). By being aware of your internal voice, you can bring them out to the open to deal with. Of course, the longer you have lived with negative self-talk, the more challenging it may become to switch to positive self-talk on a regular basis. For example, if you have a long history of starting to exercise and stopping, not seeing the results that you want, eating healthy then poorly then healthy then poorly, your inner chatter would be filled with talk of "It won't work" "Why bother, I'm not good at this." Your actions or "lack thereof" will only confirm your inner chatter of negativity. "I told you it wouldn't work." "I'm too out of shape." "I'll never see results." This will only decrease your self-esteem and make it even more difficult to lead a healthy lifestyle since you are always putting yourself down and confirming it with your negative chatter and negative actions. Key phrases for you to identify to make yourself more aware of the negative internal chatter is "I can't" or "It's too hard." "I have no time" or "I'm lazy." Focusing on these phrases will prevent you from achieving your health-related fitness goals. Therefore, your first step upon identifying your internal negative chatter is to use a cue word or phrase like "Stop" or "Cancel" and then transform the negative phrases in your mind (e.g., "I can or I will) into positive phrases by saying "I can" or "I will." This will help you to become more of a positive thinker by focusing on what you will do rather than on not believing in yourself due to past experiences of failure.

2. ***Positive Affirmations***—Affirmations are positive statements of a desired outcome or goal. They are usually short, believable and focused. By repeating them over and over again, you build inroads into your subconscious mind, opening up the possibility of a new state of thoughts. An important step when repeating affirmations is that you need to read your affirmations aloud with feeling. The mere reading of the words bears no consequence unless you put some emotions behind them. Of significant fact is that your subconscious mind takes any orders given in complete faith and after repeated self-talk. So the daily practice of repeating affirmations is important. (I can do this. I can do this. I really can do this)!

3. ***Positive Scripts***—One thing that you may observe is how easy it is for your mind to build negative thoughts upon negative thoughts. The chatter not only does not stop, but it spins around until it traps and limits you. Instead of spinning a negative story, make it positive story. Spin an uplifting story that runs like a movie script that has a positive outcome and imagine yourself in it. The longer you can tell this story to yourself, the

better. It is also best if you can make this story one about having all of your goals achieved. When you do this, you start to internalize your goals and dreams, as if they are something that you have already achieved. For example, imagine if you are like Rocky Balboa running up the steps to success at the Philadelphia Museum of Art (more commonly known as the Rocky steps), Diana Nyad swimming over 100 miles from Cuba to Florida or you crossing the finish line in a race that you have never run before.

4. ***Replace Negative Influences with Positive Ones***—It is important that you identify external negative factors in your life which may be holding your thoughts hostage and preventing you from exercising and/or living a healthy lifestyle. For instance, your mental state can become toxic by being around friends who are negative. If they eat poorly and do not exercise, then it is likely that you may follow in the same pattern. If you are not vigilant enough, you will start to adopt their thoughts as your own. Hence, be alert to what your negative influences are. If they come from certain friends, limit your exposure to them as much as you can. Refrain from discussing your plans with people who will be unsupportive of your dreams and goals. Instead surround yourself with thoughts and actions from people who will empower you. From being uninspired and de-motivated, you will begin to feel uplifted and driven to greater self-growth. The positive energy that they vibrate will start affecting the self-talk that you engage in as well. Therefore, ask around home, work or school if there is anyone interested in starting to exercise. Perhaps consider taking an exercise class (fitness for life, weight training, yoga, swimming) or joining a gym with a colleague, friend, co-worker or family member.

5. ***Present Tense Messages***—You may find yourself daunted by the many things you need to do in order to reach your goals. It may seem a bit overwhelming to think about reaching your fitness goals, especially if it has been a long while since you were in good physical condition and exercising on a regular basis. Your mind gets caught up in an endless stream of worry. What may be helpful is to concentrate on steps you can take in the "present." If you find yourself becoming stuck, stop and say, "What can I do right now?" Change your internal talk from a future anxiety ridden one to one that is about the more manageable present. You cannot control what will happen in the future, but you can take the necessary steps now that will build a better tomorrow. Taking the necessary steps require you to focus your thoughts and inner talk on "The Now." "I will exercise today and I feel great about it."

6. ***Confront Fears*** Fear is often what holds you back from your success. You are scared of taking chances because you fear losing the security that you have become accustomed to. You try to convince yourself that you are happy in your current state when in fact, you are not. Your self-talk may sound positive in your attempt to lie to yourself. But somehow, there is an inner knowing that you are short changing yourself. Ask yourself what you are afraid of. What can be the worst that can happen? For instance, you may be uncomfortable going to a public exercise facility that is filled

with mirrors and so you convince yourself that you don't need to exercise in these places or anywhere else. As times goes by, you start thinking about the need to exercise and get stopped by your fears. Here is what you can do.

Take a step-by-step approach in breaking down your fears and see if there is any way for you to look at things more positively. When you confront your fears, you will often realize that the worst-case scenario is not as bad as you think. In fact, the benefits of change are worth the risk. Your inner talk begins to change at this point. You will look forward to exercise whether it is in the gym or at home because you have learned to overcome your fears by focusing on the benefits of exercise and living a healthy lifestyle rather than your made-up story about why you didn't exercise.

7. ***Focus on Enjoyable Moments***—It is much easier to have a positive attitude if you focus on the enjoyable moments in life rather than the difficult ones. While there will inevitably be challenges, you need to remember that life consists of ups and downs and the good times are forged through the bad. So choose to fill your mind with positive images and thoughts. Make it a conscious habit. Simply bring your mind back every time it goes astray in its thoughts. For a start, you can be grateful for having the ability to exercise and lead a healthy lifestyle (Lim, 2008).

Conclusion

Replacing self-talk from negative to positive is not going to happen overnight. If your mind has ingrained habits of thinking negatively, it will take some work and time. However, if and when you find yourself struggling, unable to achieve your goals and talking yourself down, then you should grit your teeth and commit to the process of change. By following the above tips to positive self-talk, you will experience an improvement in the quality of your life. The rewards are plentiful with greater happiness, peace and joy. Best of all, you will feel empowered. With the change in energy, you are more likely to reach your highest potential and achieve success (Lim, 2008).

Mike's 6 Rules for Creating Positive Self-Talk

Another way to use positive self-talk comes from Mike (1987) who created the following 6 simple rules:
1. keep your phrases short and specific
2. use the first person and the present tense
3. construct positive phrases
4. say your phrases with meaning and intention
5. speak kindly to yourself
6. repeat phrases often

Table 11.1 displays how to use Mike's 6 rules of positive self-talk during exercise. You can use Appendix 11A to transform your negative thoughts into positive thoughts.

Table 11.1
Using Mike's 6 rules of Positive Self-Talk during Exercise

1	keep your phrases short and specific	I can do this. I got this.
2	use the first person and the present tense	"I"…
3	construct positive phrases	I can do this. I'm awesome! I can do this.
4	say your phrases with meaning and intention	I CAN DO THIS!
5	speak kindly to yourself	I can do this. I'm doing great. Way to go. Keep going!
6	repeat phrases often	I CAN DO THIS! I CAN DO THIS! I CAN DO THIS! I CAN DO THIS!

Related to positive self-talk is a technique called ***Thought Stopping***. Thought stopping is a process whereby you identify negative thoughts and then use a cue or trigger to stop the thought and clear your mind. For example, how often have you started exercising and discovered your mind was filled with negative thoughts like, "I don't want to do this right now," "I'm not in the mood to exercise," This is boring," only to feel guilty and upset later in the day that you allowed these negative thoughts to stop you from exercising.

Transforming Negative Self-Talk to Positive Self-Talk

The first step towards transforming negative thoughts into positive thoughts is to recognize that you are talking or thinking negatively to yourself. The next step is to use a cue word or phrase like "Stop" "Move on" or "Keep Going." You can also use a trigger, a quick gesture like clapping your hands, snapping your fingers, or tapping your thigh. The cue can help you stop your negative thoughts. The final step involves selecting a positive cue or phrase that will redirect your thoughts and energy onto what you want to accomplish while exercising (e.g., I can do this; This is great; I got this; I'm unstoppable).

While it is certainly common for people to have negative thoughts about exercising either before (e.g., I don't feel like exercising today, I'm not in the mood to exercise) or during exercise (this is boring, I don't want to keep going, I'm tired), recognizing negative thought patterns and immediately putting a stop to them and then transforming the negative into positive self-statements is a powerful way to increase exercise performance and enjoyment. Table 11.2 displays an example of how to transform negative thoughts into positive thoughts. Using Appendix 11A, your assignment now is to list any negative thoughts that you may have about exercise in the left-hand column and in the right-hand column list a cue word or phrase that transforms your negative self-talk into positive self-talk.

Table 11.2
Transforming Negative Self-Talk into Positive Self-Talk

I can't do this.	I will do this.
I'm too tired to exercise today.	Exercise will energize me.
This is boring.	This is exciting.
I don't have time to exercise today.	I may take to exercise.
I'm too lazy to exercise	I'm awesome when I exercise.
I don't want to exercise.	I want to exercise.
I never see results.	I create the results I want.
I hate working out in this place.	I love working out in this place.
I's not fair that I have to do this.	I want to do this.
I'll never be as fit as I used to be.	I'm in better shape today than yesterday.
It's not working.	I make it work.
I don't like this.	I love this.

USING IMAGERY WITH EXERCISE

The fourth and final cognitive strategy for you to use with exercise is called ***Imagery***. Imagery is defined as creating or recreating an experience in the mind through the use of the senses (Vealy & Greenleaf, 2006). It is a mental training technique that teaches the mind to respond as programmed. You can use imagery before, during and after exercise in any of the following ways: (1) to prepare yourself to get ready for exercise; (2) help you focus on exercising properly; (3) to enjoy exercising; (3) to accomplish challenging exercise goals that will improve your performance and level of fitness; (5) to feel your body become energized; (6) to overcome fatigue and persevere through your workout in order to achieve new performance levels (e.g., finishing that 10K race, getting that extra set in, stretching longer and further than you ever have before) and (7) to evaluate the success of your workout and correct any mistakes made so future workouts can become more efficient. For example, imagine if you took a few minutes out of your busy day to image how great you would feel later in the day after a workout. You begin to feel invigorated as you see yourself getting a good workout and think about the new performance levels that you have reached (e.g., reaching a new tension point, achieving a new level on the exercise bike, going for your longest run, getting in that extra rep on the chest press). Before you know it, you will start to feel better about yourself and look forward to finishing up school or work so you can get to the gym to exercise.

Using imagery effectively with exercise takes a little practice. In fact, there are three skills involved in imagery that you need to be aware of and eventually master in order to reap the benefits of imaging: Vividness, which is the clarity or clearness of the image; (2) Controllability, which is the ability to hold a desired image in your mind without being distracted and (3) Sensory Awareness which is the ability to utilize the senses to create a realistic sensory experience.

So take a few minutes and image your next workout. Imagine that you are exercising in a place that is aesthetically pleasing and enjoyable. Imagine the exercises that you plan to do, and imagine achieving your desired exercise goals. Imagine feeling energized all throughout the workout and being in a positive mood. By using imagery, you will learn to create positive experiences while exercising which will inevitably enhance your motivation and commitment to make exercise a major focal point in your life. Here are some suggestions for how to use imagery prior to, during and after exercise.

Using Imagery Before Exercise

Select a time anywhere between a few minutes and a few hours before your planned workout and image that you are going to have your best workout ever. See yourself improving your performance by exercising longer and challenging yourself to reach new levels of fitness. Envision an environment where you like to exercise (e.g., your local gym or exercise facility; at home, park bench, workplace, exercise class). Hear the sounds of your favorite music. Feel how your body becomes invigorated with each rep, set, and minute that you exercise.

Using Imagery During Exercise

While exercising, you can use imagery to create experiences that help you enjoy your workouts, improve performance and increase your motivation to continue. For example, you can image running on the beach while on a treadmill. You can image yourself looking and feeling great after performing a new exercise or getting in a few extra reps. You can image yourself stretching to a new tension point and feeling more flexible than ever. By creating an image of what you want to accomplish and using your senses to make it seem real, you are using your mind to prepare your body to achieve new performance levels.

Using Imagery After Exercise

After finishing your workout, you can use imagery as part of your cool-down period. You can imagine the tension caused from exercise overload disappearing and being replaced with a huge sense of accomplishment. You can imagine feeling energized as you think about how much better you feel after your workout than before you started. You can imagine hearing people compliment you on how good you look and you imagine seeing and feeling like you are in the best shape of your life, both mentally as well as physically.

How Committed Are You to Use Cognitive Strategies When You Exercise

Table 11.3 is a scale for you to use to determine how committed you are to use one of more of the four cognitive strategies presented in this chapter (association, dissociation, positive self-talk and imagery) with exercise.

Table 11.3
Determining Your Level of Commitment to use Cognitive Strategies During Exercise

	1 not committed	2	3	4	5	6	7	8	9 extremely committed
Association	1 not committed	2	3	4	5	6	7	8	9 extremely committed
Dissociation	1 not committed	2	3	4	5	6	7	8	9 extremely committed
Positive-Self Talk	1 not committed	2	3	4	5	6	7	8	9 extremely committed
Imagery	1 not committed	2	3	4	5	6	7	8	9 extremely committed

If for any reason you are not "extremely committed" to using any or all of the cognitive strategies during exercise, take a few moments to identify what is stopping you. Then proceed to the next section with an open mind and by the time you are finished you will truly embrace the value of knowing how and what to think about during exercise.

Using Cognitive Strategies During Exercise

A goal of this chapter is to show you how valuable cognitive strategies can be to increase your performance, enjoyment, motivation, and commitment to exercise. Whether it is using ***association*** to make sure you exercise safely and concentrate on incorporating proper technique; ***dissociation*** to take your mind off the demands of exercise and direct it towards pleasing thoughts); ***positive self-talk*** to take control of your thoughts and internalize the benefits that you are getting from exercise; or ***imagery*** to create an experience that prepares you to exercise, helps you during exercise, or allows you to evaluate your workouts positively after exercise, cognitive strategies are an excellent way to program your thoughts to work for you with exercise. You can determine which one(s) are for you as you practice each of these strategies in your lab assignments. Enjoy and think positively!

REVIEW QUESTIONS

1. Define cognitive strategies and explain how they can be used during exercise.

2. What is the difference between associating and dissociating during exercise?

3. Explain how and when you should associate during CRE activity?

4. Explain how and when you should dissociate during CRE activity?

5. Explain how and when you should associate during muscular fitness activity?

6. Explain how and when you should dissociate during muscular fitness activity?

7. Explain how and when you should associate during flexibility activity?

8. Explain how and when you should dissociate during flexibility activity?

9. What is positive self-talk and explain how you can use positive self-talk to increase the quality of your exercise experience.

10. Define imagery and list and explain three types of imagery skills.

11. Explain how you can incorporate imagery into your exercise program.

LAB ASSIGNMENT 11.1

Your assignment is to determine the effectiveness of using cognitive strategies on exercise performance, enjoyment, motivation, and commitment. Read the instructions below, answer the questions and have some fun!

Questions 1-3 should be answered before you begin exercising for the week.

1. Over the next two weeks, select 1 or more exercise(s) for each component of health-related fitness that you will do at least two times per week. In the column below, list the exercise(s) that you plan to use to improve your health-related fitness over the next two weeks.

CRE				
MF				
Flexibility				

2. Prior to using your cognitive strategies, rank your overall level of enjoyment, motivation, and commitment to exercise in each area of health-related fitness from 1 (extremely low) to 9 (extremely high).

Enjoyment

CRE	1	2	3	4	5	6	7	8	9
MF	1	2	3	4	5	6	7	8	9
Flexibility	1	2	3	4	5	6	7	8	9

Motivation

CRE	1	2	3	4	5	6	7	8	9
MF	1	2	3	4	5	6	7	8	9
Flexibility	1	2	3	4	5	6	7	8	9

Commitment

CRE	1	2	3	4	5	6	7	8	9
MF	1	2	3	4	5	6	7	8	9
Flexibility	1	2	3	4	5	6	7	8	9

3. Over the next two weeks, select 1 associative and 1 dissociative strategy that you will use during your exercise workouts. List the strategies and explain why you selected each?

	Associative Strategy	Disassociative Strategy
CRE	1.	1.
MF	1.	1.
Flexibility	1.	1.

Questions 4-11 should be answered after you have completed your two weeks of exercising.

4. Rank your overall level of enjoyment, motivation, and commitment to exercise in each area of health-related fitness from 1 (extremely low) to 9 (extremely high).

Enjoyment

CRE	1	2	3	4	5	6	7	8	9
MF	1	2	3	4	5	6	7	8	9
Flexibility	1	2	3	4	5	6	7	8	9

Motivation

CRE	1	2	3	4	5	6	7	8	9
MF	1	2	3	4	5	6	7	8	9
Flexibility	1	2	3	4	5	6	7	8	9

Commitment

CRE	1	2	3	4	5	6	7	8	9
MF	1	2	3	4	5	6	7	8	9
Flexibility	1	2	3	4	5	6	7	8	9

5. Circle the cognitive strategy you enjoyed the most for CRE, MF, and Flexibility and explain why you like it more than the other strategy?

CRE	Association	Dissociation
MF	Association	Dissociation
Flexibility	Association	Dissociation

6. Is there a strategy that you disliked? If so, for which exercise and explain why?

7. Which strategy increased your motivation to work on improving your CRE, MF, and Flexibility? Circle all that apply.

    Association   Dissociation   Both   Neither

8. Which strategy increased your level of commitment to work on improving your CRE, MF, and/or flexibility? Circle all that apply.

    Association   Dissociation   Both   Neither

9. Which strategy improved your performance more in your CRE, MF, and flexibility workouts? Circle all that apply.

CRE	Association	Dissociation	Both	Neither
MF	Association	Dissociation	Both	Neither
Flexibility	Association	Dissociation	Both	Neither

10. Discuss the overall success you had in implementing association and dissociation into your exercises.

11. Do you plan on using association and/or dissociation as part of your exercise program in the future? Please explain.

Association/Dissociation	CRE Exercises	YES	NO
Association/Dissociation	Muscular Fitness Exercises	YES	NO
Association/Dissociation	Flexibility Exercises	YES	NO

LAB ASSIGNMENT 11.2

Using Positive Self Talk to Increase Your Motivation to Exercise

1. Identify any components of health-related fitness that you have negative thoughts about and lack motivation to work on even though you know it will improve your health-related fitness.

2. Using the "Positive Self-Talk Sheet" in Appendix 11A list your negative thoughts in Column B.

3. Explain why you lack motivation to improve your fitness in these area(s).

4. Over the next week, you are invited to use positive self-talk with the areas of health-related fitness that you have negative thoughts about and listed in question 1. Please follow these guidelines.

a. Convert the negative statements that you listed in Column B into positive words or cues and list them in Column C. Make a few copies of your positive statements and put them in areas that you frequent and can remind you to be positive (e.g., exercise bag; cell phone; screen saver; car; appointment book, workout cards, desk, wall).

5. For the next week, plan to use these positive statements in your workouts. In fact, you can even set a SMAART to use a certain amount of positive statements in your workouts.

6. When the week is up, answer the following:

a. I enjoyed using positive self-talk while exercising

1	2	3	4	5	6	7	8	9
not at all				somewhat			very much	

b. Positive self-talk motivated me to want to exercise more

1	2	3	4	5	6	7	8	9
not at all				somewhat			very much	

c. Positive self-talk increased my commitment to make exercise a part of my life.

1	2	3	4	5	6	7	8	9
not at all				somewhat			very much	

d. Positive self-talk enhanced my exercise performance

1	2	3	4	5	6	7	8	9
not at all				somewhat			very much	

LAB ASSIGNMENT 11.3

Using Imagery to Enhance Your Exercise Experiences

Answer questions 1-3 before you use imagery with your exercise(s).

1. Take a few minutes and think about what you would like to image either before, during, or after you exercise.

2. Write down your imagery scenario and read it over a few times so you can experience the positive feelings and emotions that you would want to receive from exercising.

3. For the next week, select a time when you will use imagery either before, during, or after your exercises and fill in the following:

   a. I will use imagery   before   during   after   I exercise.

Questions 4-8 should be answered after you have completed imagery and have exercised.

4. I used imagery   before my exercise   during my exercise   after my exercise

5. Evaluate your success incorporating the three Imagery elements.

Vividness	1	2	3	4	5	6	7	8	9
	poor				average				excellent

Controllability	1	2	3	4	5	6	7	8	9
	poor				average				excellent

Sensory Awareness	1	2	3	4	5	6	7	8	9
	poor				average				excellent

6. Explain any problems you had with imagery.

7. Circle the number that best describes your experience using imagery with your exercises.

   a. I enjoyed using imagery with exercise

1	2	3	4	5	6	7	8	9
not at all				somewhat			very much	

   b. Imagery motivated me to want to exercise more

1	2	3	4	5	6	7	8	9
not at all				somewhat			very much	

   c. Imagery increased my commitment to make exercise a part of my life.

1	2	3	4	5	6	7	8	9
not at all				somewhat			very much	

    d. Imagery increased my exercise performance

       1   2   3   4   5   6   7   8   9
   not at all   somewhat   very much

    e. I will make imagery part of my exercise routine.

       1   2   3   4   5   6   7   8   9
  definitely not   maybe   definitely so

8. Which of the four cognitive strategies did you enjoy most and least and explain why?

9. Six months from now, which cognitive strategies can you see yourself using with your exercise? Circle all that apply and explain your answer..

    Association   Dissociation   Positive Self-Talk   Imagery

10. Which of the cognitive strategies would you recommend to a friend and why?

REFERENCES AND RECOMMENDED READINGS

Couture, R.T., Jerome, W., & Tihanyi, J. (1999). Can associative and dissociative strategies affect swimming performance of recreational swimmers? *The Sport Psychologist, 13,* 334-343.

Martin, J., Dubbert, P.M., Katell, A.D., Thompson, J.K., Raczynski, J.R., Lake, M.,Smith, P.O. Webster, J.S., Sikora, T., & Cohen, R.E. (1984). The behavioral control of exercise in sedentary adults: Studies 1 through 6. *Journal of Consulting and ClinicalPsychology, 52, 795-811.*

Masters, K.S. & Olges, B.M. (1998a). Associative and dissociative cognitive strategies in exercise and running: 20 years later, what do we know. *The Sport Psychologist, 12,* 253-270.

Mikes, J. (1987). Basketball fundamentals. A complete mental training guide. Champaign, Il: Leisure Press.

Morgan, W.P., & Pollack, M.L. (1977). Psychological characterization of the elite distance runner. *Annals of the New York Academy of Sciences, 301,* 382-403.

Nietfeld, J.L. (2003). An examination of metacognitive strategy use and monitoring skills by competitive middle distance runners. *Journal of Applied Sport Psychology,* **15,** 307-320.

Scott, M.L., Scott, D., Bedic, S.P., & Dowd, J. (1999).The effect of associative and dissociative strategies on rowing ergometer performance. *The Sport Psychologist, 13,* 57-68.

Vealy, R.S., & Greenleaf, C.A. (2006). Seeing is believing: Understanding and using imagery in sport. In J. M. Williams, Applied sport psychology: Personal growth to peak performance, 5th edition, pp 306-307.

Weinberg, R.S., & D. Gould. (2003). Exercise behavior and adherence. In Weinberg, R.S. & Gould, D. *Foundations of Sport and Exercise Psychology*, 3rd edition, pp 418-419. Human Kinetics: Champaign, IL.

Weinberg, R.S. & Gould, D. (2003). Self-talk. In Weinberg, R.S. & Gould, D. *Foundations of sport and exercise psychology*, 3rd edition, pp 364-367. Human Kinetics: Champaign, IL.

APPENDIX 11A
USING POSITIVE SELF-TALK DURING EXERCISE

Column A Exercises	Column B Negative Statements that you've used to minimize or prevent participation of these exercises	Column C Positive Statements using Mike's 6 rules for Self-Talk

In Column A, list different exercises that represent the following: (a) exercises that you do that you do not enjoy; (b) exercises that you have never done, but you want to start doing and (c) exercises that you did in the past and stopped doing them. In Column B, list the negative statements associated with these exercises. For each negative statement that you have used in Column B, create a positive statement using Mikes' 6 rules for self-talk and list them in Column C.

Chapter 12

Managing Your Stress

OVERVIEW

In this chapter you will:

- Learn what stress is
- Identify stressors in your life
- Discover how to take control of your stress
- Incorporate stress management techniques into your daily life
- Determine how exercise transforms negative stress into positive stress

At some point in our lives, we have all experienced a great deal of stress. According to the Anxiety and Depression Association of America (ADAA, 2017), seven out of ten adults in the United States say they experience stress or anxiety daily, and most say it interferes at least moderately with their lives. The fact is that many of us are surrounded by stress on a daily basis as we strive to achieve countless challenges including: (1) doing well in school or work; (2) taking care of our finances; (3) managing our time effectively; (4) building positive relationships; (5) fulfilling family obligations and (6) taking better care of ourselves.

Approximately two-thirds of adults experience large amounts of stress at least one day a week and it is estimated that it costs the United States government and businesses between 30 and 44 billion dollars annually for the treatment and consequences of stress and stress-related illness, (health care costs; worker absenteeism; reduction in job productivity) (International Labour Organization, 2000). The simple fact is that stress is everywhere (Blonna, 2012). Whether in school (adjusting to a new living environment, dealing with academic pressure, meeting new people), at home (balancing relationship demands, family and financial responsibilities), at work (succeeding at work, getting along with peers, handling the pressure of job responsibilities), playing sports (pressure to win; dealing with losing) or exercising (uncertainty of using equipment properly, being uncomfortable around others, not seeing results, feeling guilty if you miss a workout), you will find stress. And if you don't find stress, then stress with find you.

According to Stress Statistics, there are several top causes of stress in the United States that impact the lives of millions of people both physically and mentally. See Tables 12.1 to 12.5 for a list of causes of stress (Table 12.1), the statistics on stress (Table 12.2), the impact that stress has on people lives (Table 12.3), physical (Table 12.4) and psychological symptoms of stress (Table 12.5).

Table 12.1
List of Causes of Stress

	Top Causes of Stress in the United States	Factors
1	Job Pressure	Co-Worker Tension, bosses, Work Overload
2	Money	Loss of Job, Reduced Retirement, Medical Expenses
3	Health	Health Crisis, Terminal or Chronic Illness
4	Relationships	Divorce, Death of Spouse, Arguments with Friends, Loneliness
5	Poor Nutrition	Inadequate Nutrition, Caffeine, Processed Foods, Refined Sugars
6	Media Overload	Television, Radio, Internet, E-mail, Cellphone, Social Networking
7	Sleep Deprivation	Inability to release adrenaline and other stress hormones

Table 12.2
Stress Statistics

	Data	People in the United States
1	77%	regularly experience physical symptoms caused by stress
2	73%	regularly experience psychological symptoms caused by stress
3	33%	feel they are living with extreme stress
4	48%	feel their stress has increased over the past 5 years
5	76%	cited work and money as the leading causes of their stress
6	48%	reported lying awake at night due to stress

Table 12.3
Stress Impact Statistics

	Data	People in the United States
1	48%	stated that stress has a negative impact on their personal and professional life
2	31%	employed adults say they have difficulty managing work and family responsibilities
3	35%	cited jobs interfering with their family or personal time as a significant source of their stress
4	54%	said stress has caused them to fight with people close to them
5	26%	reported being alienated from a friend or family member because of stress
6	30%	say there are "always: or "often" under stress at work.

Table 12.4
Physical Symptoms of Stress

	Data	Physical Symptoms
1	51%	Fatigue
2	44%	Headache
3	34%	Upset Stomach
4	30%	Muscle Tension
5	23%	Change in Appetite
6	17%	Teeth Grinding
7	15%	Change in Sex Drive
8	13%	Feeling Dizzy

Table 12.5
Psychological Symptoms of Stress

	Data	People in the United States
1	50%	Irritability or Anger
2	45%	Feeling Nervous
3	45%	Lack of Energy
4	35%	Feeling as Though You Could Cry

Recently, the World Health organization has labeled "Stress" as "The Health Epidemic of the 21st Century and it is estimated to cost American businesses up to $300 billion per year due to stress and stress-related illness resulting in greater worker absenteeism, decreased job productivity and increased medial expenses. Now that you know the statistics and recognize the significant role that stress plans in our life, the question becomes what will you do about it?

In this chapter you will learn what stress is and how to deal with it effectively in your lives. In addition, you will learn a variety of coping strategies designed to transform negative stress (distress) into positive stress (eustress). Finally, you will learn how to take control of your stress and empower yourself to live your life the way you choose to rather than have to.

WHAT IS STRESS?

Over the years, there has been a considerable amount of work done in the area of stress and stress and management. Consequently, a number of popular definitions are currently being used to define and understand what stress is. For example, renowned researcher Robert Lazarus defined stress as a state of anxiety produced when events and responsibilities exceed one's coping abilities (Lazuras & DeLongis, 1983). McGrath (1970) defined stress as a substantial imbalance between psychological and/or physical demand and response capability, under where failure to meet that demand has important consequences. The American Psychological Association defines stress as any uncomfortable emotional experience accompanied by predictable, biochemical, physiological and behavioral changes (www.reference.com/world-view/psychological-definition-stress). Perhaps, the most popular definition of stress comes from Hans Selye, one of the leading authorities on stress who defined stress as a nonspecific response of the body to any demand placed upon it (Selye, 1976). In essence, any time the body reacts to a demand (e.g., exercise overload, job promotion, family argument) you are under stress. One final way to define stress is to view it as the result of imbalance between life's demands and one's ability to handle these demands. For example, when you never seem to have enough time to do what you want to do or when your mind is racing with ideas and you just cannot seem to get your thoughts straight there is an imbalance between life's demands and your ability to handle them thus creating stress.

What Causes Stress?

Any fact or situation, event or circumstance, feedback or stimulus that is perceived to be a threat is known as a stressor or that which causes or promotes stress. Stressors can be identified by time and how long they last. For example, acute stressors are often the result of a rapid-onset of stress which pops up unexpectedly (e.g., hearing a loud noise late at night while you were sleeping) and then goes away. Chronic stressors are long lasting and usually unassociated with an immediate warning. This causes physiological arousal to last for extended periods of time (days, weeks, months, years). For example, Joyce is a woman who worries on a daily basis regardless of any new events occurring in her life. She worries about getting her children off to school on time, making sure the house is clean, getting to work on time and being productive, making dinner that her family likes, helping her husband with his career and spending quality time with her family. Even though she has a set routine and successfully completes it all, it does not stop Joyce from feeling stressed on a daily basis. Consequently, Joyce's life appears to be one big chronic stress.

Sources of Stressors

Stressors can come from a variety of sources that people encounter in their lives and they include:

- *physical stressors*—happen when the body is overloaded resulting in tension, discomfort or pain in one or more parts of the body (e.g., muscles, joints, etc);
- *psychological stressors*—occur when the mind is preoccupied with thoughts of worry, nervousness, apprehension or there is a threat to one's self-esteem;
- *social stressors*—are when people feel uncomfortable in crowds and/or have difficulty being around others;

- *environmental stressors*—are related to air pollution, noise, weather and temperature that are known to affect one's mood, attitude, and the amount of stress perceived on a daily basis;

- *biochemical stressors*—are related to the changes that the body undergoes resulting from air pollution, temperature, humidity, nutrition, drugs, and alcohol;

- *nutritional stressors*—deal with your eating patterns; when you eat poorly (e.g., overeat, skip meals, binge eat, consume lots of processed foods) you may become nutrient deficient causing the body to overwork itself and function inefficiently;

- *academic stressors*—can result from having difficulty in school (e.g., not enjoying classes, poor communication with instructors and administrators, difficulty understanding coursework; can't find a major of interest; being overloaded with exams, etc);

- *philosophical stressors*—occur when you have a lack of purpose or direction in life (e.g. not knowing what you want out of life, uncertainty about what to major in college, being in the wrong job or career or questioning whether you are going in the right direction);

STRESS AND THE STRESS PROCESS

After being confronted with stress, people exhibit a certain behavioral pattern known as stress reactivity. (See Table 12.6 for a list of common reactions people have when confronted by stressors). Over the years, there have been several explanations for how people react when confronted by stressors. This section introduces two different explanations for how people react to stress: (1) fight or flight and (2) general adaptation syndrome (GAS).

Table 12.6
Reactions to Stress

1. Elevated heart rate	8. Shortness of breath
2. Rapid breathing	9. Fatigue
3. Diarrhea	10. Headaches
4. Constipation	11. Dizziness
5. Dry mouth	12. Sleep disturbances
6. Low back pain	13. Memory problems
7. Irritability and moodiness	14. Lack of concentration

Fight or Flight

Walter Cannon was a Harvard University physiologist who in the early 1900's was the first to explain how people react to stress as the fight-or-flight response. According to Cannon, when people are faced with stress, they have two choices: (1) stand up and confront the stress = "fight it" or (2) run away from it = "flight" (Cannon, 1922). Here's an example of the fight or flight response.

Adam has been working for his boss Janet for the past four years and he is upset with her for not getting the promotion he was promised. Each time he sees her, Adam wants to convey his feelings (fight) to Janet only to be stopped by his fear of upsetting his boss and possibly losing his job so he keeps his emotions to himself (flight). He is concerned, however, that if he does not speak with Janet (Flight), his anger will get the best of him and cause him to overreact and lose focus at a job that he loves so much. Consequently, Adam has kept his emotions inside of himself (flight) leaving him with a very important choice: (1) speak with Janet and let her know how he feels (fight) or (2) avoid talking with her about his upset and keep it inside (flight). After careful consideration, Adam decides to talk to Janet, recognizing that the only way he could truly get rid of his stress was to have a conversation with Janet and let her know about how he felt about not getting promoted. While Adam may not have control over Janet's final decision, he does have a choice in the way he chooses to deal with the stress that he is confronted with in the form of flight or fight. By speaking with Janet, Adam has created an opportunity to take control of his stress by expressing his thoughts, feelings and emotions.

Does this ring a bell for you? Are you confronted with stress in your life that has you thinking fight or flight? Has it worked for you? If not, maybe you should consider the opposite approach. In other words, if you have been doing a lot of fighting then maybe you are better off taking a few steps back and just leave it be. Clearly, the fighting hasn't worked so maybe the flight will. Conversely, have you been avoiding someone or something because you are perceiving a significant amount of stress and fearing a conversation may make it worse? Maybe it's time to confront this stress by expressing yourself. Tell this significant other what's on your mind. Go talk with your boss, friends, teacher or significant other and simply let them know what's on your mind since keeping it inside this long has been ineffective.

It is important to note that neither "flight or fight" is necessarily any better or worse than the other. It all depends on the situation. Sometimes, you may be better off standing your ground and taking action (fight) while other times you might be better off looking the other way (flight) and avoiding the possibility of confrontation. It really depends on you, the stressors you are dealing with and the situation that you are in.

It is important to note that neither "flight or "fight" is necessarily any better or worse than the other. In some instances, you may be better off standing your ground and take action (fight) while other times you may be better off looking the other way (fight) and not letting stress get the best of you by acting inappropriately. It really depends on you, the stressors you are dealing with and the situation(s) that you are in.

GENERAL ADAPTATION SYNDROME (GAS)

Developed by Selye, GAS is a three-stage process that explains how people react to stress: (1) alarm; (2) resistance; (3) exhaustion (Selye, 1974).

Alarm Phase—As you perceive a stressor(s), your body's balance becomes disturbed and prepares itself for sudden action. For example, you are sleeping in your bed late at night and you hear a loud noise. Immediately, your senses become sharpened, resulting in several physiological changes (e.g., heart starts to beat faster; muscles begin to tighten; respiration, blood pressure and perspiration increases).

Resistance Phase—After you have become aware of the stressors(s) that have confronted you, your body attempts to adjust back to its' normal physiological balance called homeostasis. Your heart rate, respiration, blood pressure, perspiration and muscular tension all begin to decrease as you prepare to make decisions about how to handle your stress (e.g., turn the alarm off). However, if stress continues and you cannot adapt to it, you will enter the third and final phase.

Exhaustion Phase—Your endocrine system cannot produce a sufficient amount of hormones to counter the chronic stressors you are dealing with. If this continues over long periods of time (weeks, months or even years), it can affect your heart, blood pressure, stomach, muscles and joints causing headaches, fatigue, dizziness, cramping, and other more serious debilitating conditions (e.g., heart disease).

Here is an example of how GAS works. Let's use Stephanie, a young elementary school teacher studying for her MS degree. She comes home from a long day of teaching at school and she decides she wants to catch up on some well-needed sleep. As she prepares to take her nap, she suddenly remembers that she has an important paper due tomorrow that she has not started yet. Immediately, her bodily functions begin to change as she starts to experience an increase in heart rate and tightness in her muscles (alarm phase). In order to counter these feelings, Stephanie decides to sit down for an hour and start writing her paper. Upon doing so, Stephanie has redirected her focus from feeling stressed about forgetting her paper to getting it done (resistance phase). Consequently, she has successfully resisted her stress and now she feels better. However, if at any point Stephanie thinks she will never finish her paper on time or if she allows herself to get upset about leaving her schoolwork for the last minute, her stress will automatically increase and cause possible exhaustion, especially if this type of behavior lingers on.

TAKING RESPONSIBILITY AND CONTROL OF YOUR STRESS

In life, there are many things that can cause you stress. For example, losing your job, failing an exam, mourning the loss of a loved one or having a fight with a significant other can certainly create stress for you. However, what determines whether your stress goes away or lingers on in your life is how you choose to deal with it. Will you take responsibility for your stress and gain control over it or will you attempt to push it away and blame others, find excuses, or pretend everything is ok when you know it is not? (See Table 12.7 for a list of perceived causes of stress).

Table 12.7
Perceived Causes of Stress

Health	Family	School	Work	Friends	Finances
Acute or chronic conditions	Parents	Teachers	Bosses	Relationships	Money
Level of Fitness	Siblings	Classmates	Co-workers	Trust or Lack there-of	Salary
	Other family members	Courses	Salary		Bills
		Homework	Benefits		
			Responsibilities		

All too often, people look to blame others for their stressors and neglect to take full responsibility for their actions or interpretations. Phrases like: "It's your fault that I... If only you would have... You make me so mad... It's not fair that you got... I did it because you... are prime examples of how we attempt to redirect our stress by justifying its causes and blaming others while making up reasons for our actions. If only it was that easy. Just blame someone else every time things do not go your way and you get upset. The problem is that when you do that, you wind up holding on to your stress. In fact, it is rather common for people to experience high levels of stress simply by thinking about someone whom they have had disagreements with, became upset with or argued with in the past (even when these people are not around you).

Unfortunately, blaming others for your stress or justifying how things are unfair when situations or opportunities do not go your way is not going to take the stress away. In fact, your stress level will only increase. For example, take Brady and Keisha, a happily married couple who get into an argument resulting in each of them getting very angry and barking profanities at each other. Their choices are to take responsibility for what they said and/or did or blame the other for their stress-provoking actions. Doing the former will most likely lead to a reduction and possible elimination of stress because they both recognized that their causes of stress came from themselves and not the other, thus giving them the freedom to choose how to handle their stress.

Conversely, blaming each other for your own stress and neglecting to take full responsibility for your actions will only result in your stress increasing because your perceived stressors (what you think is causing your stress) is not within your control. So while Brady cannot control what Keisha said and vice versa, each can control the way they interpret what was said. They can choose to react in rage or anger or apologize for the other being upset. They can choose to blame the other for their stress or walk away from the situation before losing control. Finally, they can stop talking to each other and keep the stress inside or they can let each other know that they were upset with what was said to them.

To put it simply, if you cannot control your stressor, then do not waste time thinking about it. Taking control of your stress means that you perceive yourself to be the cause of your stress response and once you recognize that the way you handle your stress is 100% within your control, then you are on your way towards living a healthier, stress-free lifestyle (most of the time). Below is a list of six common, potentially stressful situations that identify what you are and are not in control of in order to reduce your stress.

1. *Health*—Over the past few months you have noticed that you haven't been feeling well. You started a new job, your sleep is erratic, your healthy eating habits have diminished rapidly and you haven't exercised in several months. While you may not be in control of the hours you put in at work, you are certainly in control of what you choose to do with your time after work and on your days off. Will you start to go to sleep at a normal hour? Will you plan your meals again? How about going back to the gym one night after work and one day on the weekend?

2. *Relationships*—You have an argument with a significant other and you are hurt by what was said to you. Although you cannot control what your significant other said, you can control the way you perceive what was said. Do you let it continue to bother you or do you look to get rid of your stress by speaking with him/her or interpreting what was said in a less stressful manner?

3. *School*—You feel stressed in one of your classes because of all the work that has to be done to get a good grade. Moreover, you are unhappy with one of the grades that you received. While you cannot control the amount of coursework given in the class, you can control how much time you study. Although you cannot control the grade that you received, you can choose whether to speak with your teacher about your grade and explain why you think you deserved a higher grade.

4. *Work*—Sometimes you may become stressed at work because you do not like the way your boss is treating you, the work that you do or the environment that you spend a significant amount of time in. What you cannot control is your boss' behavior. However, what you can control is how you interpret what your boss says. You can choose to accept the way your boss is and what he/she tells you regardless of the way it was expressed (i.e., yelling) or you can choose to speak with your boss and let him/her know what's on your mind and how you feel rather than keep it all inside of you. You can also choose to quit your job and find something else. In time, you will realize that sometimes when you take a proactive stand to get rid of your stressors by choosing to do something about it, rather than adopting a defeatist attitude that there is

nothing you can do, the stress that appears to surround you begins to disappear and you become empowered in your life.

5. *Finances*—You may be stressed because you do not have enough money and you may even be faced with financial debt (student loans, rent, mortgage, taxes, car payments). It is important to note that you are the one who controls how much money you make as well as how much money you spend. Granted, times are tough for many people. Presently, the cost of living has exceeded the annual raises that people are getting in many popular professions (e.g., teaching) resulting in what once may have been afford-able, now becoming too costly. Choosing to take control over your finances means that you will figure a way to earn more money and/or spend your money more efficiently.

6. *Time Management*—Do you ever think that there's not enough time in the day to accomplish all of the things that you want to do? How about investigating your time management skills? No matter how much you accomplish in any given day, there is always more to do the next day? Well, how much time do you create to procrastinate (e.g., watch television, play video games, talk or text on your cell phone, interact on social media)? There are 24 hours, 1440 minutes and 86,400 seconds in every day. While some days may indeed be busier than others, everyone has at least a few minutes each and every day to find the time to accomplish what they set out to do. In fact, when you believe that you would be doing more things that you want to (e.g., exercising, eating healthier) if you only had the "time" you are really making a choice to do other things with your time. Now imagine for a moment that you planned to take a few minutes out of your day to do something because you wanted to and not because you thought you had to. Your stress would decrease and you would probably accomplish more in that day that you usually do. In Lab 12.6 you will learn how to decrease your stress by managing your time more effectively.

So anytime you find yourself blaming others for your stress and resenting the fact that this is happening to you, take a step back and take control. Choose what you can do to get rid of your stress and do it. And remember, if the stressor is out of your control and there is nothing you can do to get rid of it then let go of it and move on.

REDUCING YOUR STRESS

There are many different stress management techniques designed to help people decrease their stress. This section provides five different stress management techniques (1) Progressive muscle relaxation; (2) Relaxation response; (3) Yogic Breathing; (4) Time Out and (5) Exercise. The key is to find the one(s) that work best for you.

Progressive Muscle Relaxation (PMR) was developed by Edmond Jacobson in the 1930's and it teaches you how to distinguish muscular tension from muscular relaxation by creating tension throughout the body and then relaxing. Over time, this process will allow you to become more sensitive to how your body feels when you become stressed, thus enabling you to relax your muscles before they become too tense. Unfortunately, many people often do not realize when they are under physical stress until they begin to experience extreme discomfort or pain (e.g., back aches after sitting arched behind your desk for hours at a time, muscle cramps after over-exercising or putting too much stress on your body, stomach aches due to overeating or eating poorly). PMR heightens your awareness to become more receptive to muscular tension before actually feeling pain by becoming more aware of the physiological messages received from your body (e.g., slight muscle aches, body discomfort). PMR can be done for short (a few minutes) or long (thirty minutes or more) periods of time as well as in a variety of locations (e.g., at your desk; in your car; on the bus or train; in the lunchroom, in your bed, at the gym, shower, standing, sitting. In fact, PMR can be done almost anywhere. Since PMR is a physical to mental technique, it is recommended for people who experience physical stress before mental stress. In other words, aches and pains come before thoughts about feeling stressed. Common symptoms that generally let you know that you are under physical stress include muscular tension, aches and pains, cramping, gastrointestinal problems, headaches, nausea. See Figure 12.1 to learn how PMR works.

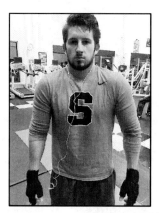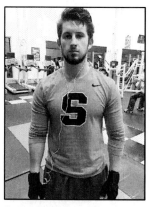

Progressive Muscle Relaxation

By manipulating tension in each part of your body and then exhaling that tension away, you should feel more relaxed. In addition to using PMR as a total body relaxation exercise, you can also you it when you are beginning to feel tension in a certain part of the body by simply inhaling when you recognize the tension you feel and then slowly exhaling it out (i.e., in your car; behind the desk; before a presentation or exam; job interview, etc.).

Here is how PMR works:
- Start off by inhaling a few times for 3-5 sections through your nose and then exhale for 3-5 through your mouth. This begins to get your focused on your breathing. Then do the following
- Inhale for 3-5 seconds and tighten the toes on your left foot.
- Exhale for 3-5 seconds and relax the toes on your left foot.

- Keep the toes on your left foot relaxed and inhale for 3-5 seconds and then exhale for 3-5 seconds.
- Repeat 1-2 times.

- Inhale for 3-5 seconds and tighten the toes on your right foot.
- Exhale for 3-5 seconds and relax the toes on your right foot.
- Keep the toes on your right foot relaxed and inhale for 3-5 seconds and then exhale for 3-5 seconds.
- Repeat 1-2 times.

- Inhale for 3-5 seconds and tighten your left ankle.
- Exhale for 3-5 seconds and relax your left ankle.
- Keep your left ankle completely relaxed and inhale for 3-5 seconds and then exhale for 3-5 seconds. Repeat 1-2 times.
- Inhale for 3-5 seconds and tighten your right ankle.
- Exhale for 3-5 seconds and relax your right ankle.
- Keep your right ankle completely relaxed and inhale for 3-5 seconds and then exhale for 3-5 seconds.
- Repeat 1-2 times.

- Inhale for 3-5 seconds and tighten your left calf.
- Exhale for 3-5 seconds and relax your left calf.
- Keep your left calf completely relaxed and inhale for 3-5 seconds and then exhale for 3-5 seconds.
- Repeat 1-2 times.

- Inhale for 3-5 seconds and tighten your right calf.
- Exhale for 3-5 seconds and relax your right calf.
- Keep your right calf completely relaxed and inhale for 3-5 seconds and then exhale for 3-5 seconds.
- Repeat 1-2 times.

- Inhale for 3-5 seconds and tighten your left hamstring.
- Exhale for 3-5 seconds and relax your left hamstring.
- Keep your left hamstring completely relaxed and inhale for 3-5 seconds and then exhale for 3-5 seconds.
- Repeat 1-2 times.

- Inhale for 3-5 seconds and tighten your right hamstring.
- Exhale for 3-5 seconds and relax your right hamstring.
- Keep your right hamstring completely relaxed and inhale for 3-5 seconds and then exhale for 3-5 seconds.
- Repeat 1-2 times.

- Inhale for 3-5 seconds and tighten your left quadricep.
- Exhale for 3-5 seconds and relax your left quadriceps.
- Keep your left quadricep completely relaxed and inhale for 3-5 seconds and then exhale for 3-5 seconds.
- Repeat 1-2 times.

- Inhale for 3-5 seconds and tighten your right quadriceps.
- Exhale for 3-5 seconds and relax your right quadriceps.

- Keep your right quadricep completely relaxed and inhale for 3-5 seconds and then exhale for 3-5 seconds.
- Repeat 1-2 times.

- Inhale for 3-5 seconds and expand your stomach up to the ceiling.
- Exhale for 3-5 seconds and relax your stomach.
- Keep your stomach completely relaxed and inhale for 3-5 seconds and then exhale for 3-5 seconds.
- Repeat 1-2 times.

- Inhale for 3-5 seconds and expand your chest up to the ceiling.
- Exhale for 3-5 seconds and relax your chest.
- Keep your chest completely relaxed and inhale for 3-5 seconds and then exhale for 3-5 seconds.
- Repeat 1-2 times.

- Inhale for 3-5 seconds as you raise your shoulders up to the sky.
- Exhale for 3-5 seconds and relax your shoulders.
- Keep your shoulders completely relaxed and inhale for 3-5 seconds and then exhale for 3-5 seconds.
- Repeat 1-2 times.

- Inhale for 3-5 seconds and turn your neck as far to the left as you can.
- Exhale for 3-5 seconds and bring your neck back to center.
- Keep your neck completely relaxed and inhale for 3-5 seconds and then exhale for 3-5 seconds.
- Repeat 1-2 times.

- Inhale for 3-5 seconds and turn your neck as far to the right as you can.
- Exhale for 3-5 seconds and bring your neck back to center.
- Keep your neck completely relaxed and inhale for 3-5 seconds and then exhale for 3-5 seconds.
- Repeat 1-2 times.

- Inhale for 3-5 seconds and bring your chin to to your chest.
- Exhale for 3-5 seconds and allow your chin to return to center, facing straight ahead.
- Keep your chin completely relaxed and inhale for 3-5 seconds and then exhale for 3-5 seconds.
- Repeat 1-2 times.

- Inhale for 3-5 seconds and tilt your head all the way back.
- Exhale for 3-5 seconds and allow you head to return back to return to it's normal resting place facing forward.
- Keep your head completely relaxed and inhale for 3-5 seconds and exhale for 3-5 seconds.
- Repeat 1-2 times.

- Inhale for 3-5 seconds and you smile as wide as you can.
- Exhale for 3-5 seconds and let your face relax.
- Keep your face relaxed and inhale for 3-5 seconds and exhale for 3-5 seconds.
- Repeat 1-2 times.

- Inhale for 3-5 seconds and raise your eyebrows to the top of your head.
- Exhale for 3-5 seconds and allow your eyebrows to descend back to it's normal resting place.
- Keep your eyebrows completely relaxed and inhale for 3-5 seconds and then exhale for 3-5 seconds.
- Repeat 1-2 times.

- Inhale for 5 seconds and make a tight fist with your left hand.
- Exhale for 5 seconds and slowly relax and extend each finger on your left hand one at a time starting with your thumb-index finger-middle finger-ring finger-pinky.
- Keep your left hand completely relaxed with fingers softly extended and inhale for 5 seconds and then exhale for 5 seconds.
- Repeat 1-2 times.

- Inhale for 5 seconds and make a tight fist with your right hand.
- Exhale for 5 seconds and slowly relax and extend each finger on your right hand one at a time starting with your thumb-index finger-middle finger-ring finger-pinky.
- Keep your right hand completely relaxed with fingers softly extended and inhale for 5 seconds and then exhale for 5 seconds.
- Repeat 1-2 times.

- Put your palms together and start to rub your hands slowly and then faster and faster until you feel your palms warming up. Then place your palms over your eyelids. The warm sensation you are feeling represents a transformation from physical stress to total relaxation.
- Repeat 1-2 times.

Figure 12.1—Progressive Muscle Relaxation

Relaxation Response (RR)—was developed by Herbert Benson (1975) and emphasizes a state of deep rest that includes the following four components:

1. a quiet environment—select a place that is free from noise or distractions that allows you to focus on yourself without being interrupted;

2. a passive attitude—allow your thoughts to enter and exit your mind without analyzing, evaluating, criticizing or questioning; avoid over-thinking; in time, these thoughts will learn to disappear just as quickly as they appear;

3. a comfortable position—select a position that you feel comfortable and can stay in for at least 20 minutes without having to move around too much; the key is to feel comfortable, but not so comfortable that you will fall asleep;

4. a mantra—choose a word that you can repeat over and over again (either verbally or nonverbally) that creates a feeling of relaxation; For example, say you pick the word "relax" and begin to repeat "relax" to yourself. As time goes by, the word "relax" will enter your mind and push out thoughts that create stress for you (e.g., I have so much to do today; I am so tired). Once your mantra has kicked out your unwanted "stress provoking" thoughts, you are now free to allow you mind to wander freely and explore places that create an immediate sense of freedom, tranquility and total mind-body relaxation.

Unlike PMR which focuses on doing something physical in order to feel physically and then mentally relaxed, RR is more of mental approach designed for individuals who are experiencing mental stress (i.e. anxiety, worry, overthinking) before physical stress. For example, Link is someone who is constantly on the go thinking about all the things he has to accomplish each and every day. No matter how much work he gets done in a day, it never seems like it's enough and there's always more to do. Even when he is physically drained, his mind is always working, non-stop, often thinking to excess about what has to be done next, evaluating how the previous task was done, if it could have been done better, etc. What Link needs to do is take control of his thoughts and RR is one way to do this. For instance, Link could begin by sitting in his car before he leaves for work or even at his office. Both places are quiet and can be used to sit in a comfortable position. Next, Link can close his eyes and allow his thoughts to enter and exit his mind as he begins to use his mantra. In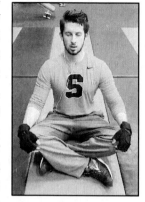
time, Link can even start using his mantra in situations where he is experiencing sudden and/or significant amounts of mental stress (e.g., in traffic, writing a paper or studying during finals week, deadline at work, job interview). All he has to do is acknowledge the mental stress that he is feeling and then start reciting the mantra to allow himself to kick out the stressful thoughts and replace it with relaxing thoughts. See Figure 12.2 to familiarize yourself with Relaxation Response.

Yogic Breathing—involves manipulating your breathing pattern so that you eventually learn how to control your breathing response; Yogic Breathing works on a 1:4:2 count and starts with inhaling for 4 seconds followed by holding your breath for 16 seconds and then exhaling for 8 seconds. Typically, when someone is stressed their breathing pattern becomes labored resulting in rapid inhaling and exhaling leading to possible shortness of breath. Through yogic breathing, you will become more sensitive to your normal breathing pattern and

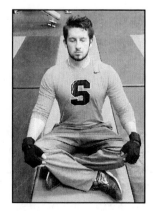 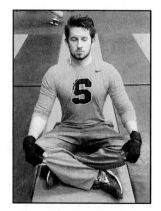 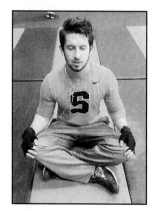

Figure 12.3. Yogic Breathing
Inhalation — Holding Breath — Exhalation

in times of stress, your awareness of your breathing will be heightened, thus helping you to concentrate and eventually control your breathing pattern. This will inevitably take your mind off of your stressors and onto regulating your breathing which will decrease your stress and make you feel more relaxed.

Time Out—In times where you recognize that you are under high levels of stress that just won't go away, an effective strategy for you to employ is to remove yourself from that stressful environment and take a "time out." For example, in sport, when a coach sees his team playing poorly and not performing up to their potential, he/she calls a time out to stop things from getting worse. In your case, you are calling a time out to stop your stress from increasing. Simply remove yourself from your stressful situation and go someplace else. By walking away. you are stopping yourself from fighting a losing battle and giving yourself an opportunity to redirect your thoughts, channel your energy and empower yourself towards overcoming your stressors and feeling better.

Exercise—Last, but certainly not least is exercise. Over the years, research has found exercise to be a successful method for reducing stress across a variety of populations (e.g., college students, fit & unfit individuals, athletes & non-athletes, spinal cord injury patients, mental disorders, Berger & Owen, 1988; Berger, Friedman & Eaton, 1988, Crews & Landers, 1987, Latimer et al., 2004). According to the Mayo Clinic, virtually any form of exercise from yoga to aerobics can act as a stress reliever. Regardless of whether you are an athlete or you are out of shape, a little exercise can go a long way toward stress management. (Mayo Clinic, 2015). Here are a few explanations of how exercise helps to reduce stress:

1. As you exercise, you begin to place more than the usual amount of physical stress on the body (overload) which can redirect you from distress (negative stress) to eustress (positive stress) and invigorate your body and mind and make you feel better.

2. During exercise, the body releases endorphins which are a morphine-like substance that act as natural painkillers, creating a euphoric like state of well-being that makes you feel good.

3. Exercise is like meditation in motion (Mayo Clinic, 2015). It can create a distraction from daily stressors by forcing you to associate (at least some of the time) on important exercise information (heart rate, breathing pattern, muscular tension, proper form, pace, equipment, environment) as well as dissociate by listening to music, watching television or interacting on your cell phone. After just a few minutes of exercise (swimming a few laps in the pool, jogging a few minutes on the treadmill, doing of few reps lifting weights), you will often find that your focus on the stress that confronted you before exercise has now been replaced with more empowering thoughts like how good your body feels or how happy you are. As time goes on and you continue to engage in exercise and/or sport-related activities, you may discover that the mere thought of these activities can create a sense of energy and optimism which can help you remain calm and clear in

everything you do (i.e. I need to go for a run; I want to go to the gym and lift; I can't wait to do Yoga later).

4. Exercise is vital for maintaining mental fitness and studies have shown that exercise is very effective at reducing fatigue, improving alertness and concentration, and enhancing overall cognitive function (ADAA, 2017). So the next time you think you can't concentrate because you are under distress, go exercise so you can deplete your stress and enhance your energy and ability to concentrate.

5. Exercise improves your mood. I'm sure you've noticed that no matter how you feel before you exercise, you always feel better after you exercise. That, by itself, should be more than enough to get you to exercise when you feel stressed out. In fact, research has consistently demonstrated that exercise enhances positive mood states (e.g., happiness, vigor) and decreases negative mood states (e.g., anger, anxiety, depression).

6. Once you begin to see and feel improvements from exercise your self-esteem may increase (especially if you are exercising with SMAART goals) and you will begin to look at exercise as something positive and worthwhile, especially under times of stress. Consequently, when you think and feel stressed, you will immediately resort to exercise to reduce your stress and feel better.

7. Exercise increases your overall health and your sense of well-being, which puts more pep in your step every day which will decrease your stress. All of these exercise benefits can ease your stress levels and give you a sense of command over your body and your life (Mayo Clinic, 2015).

In conclusion, stress is something that is part of everyone's daily life. However, the amount of stress you encounter on a daily basis and the way you choose to handle your stress is totally up to you. Learning how to take responsibility for your stressors and control the way you react to them is a formidable way to live. So, the next time you are under stress, I invite you to ask yourself, "Who's in control of my stress?" Then, powerfully look in the mirror and respond, "I am." Finally, choose any of the stress managements techniques presented in this chapter and use them when you feel stressed and/or if you simply want to energize and empower yourself. Most important, be proud of yourself for the choices that you have made and all that you have accomplished.

REVIEW QUESTIONS

1. Identify one stressful situation that occurred in your life this week and answer the following: Stress occurred in my life when _____ ....

2. List three to five sources of stress and describe how each exists in your life.

3. Define the "Fight vs. Flight" response and give an example of how you have used each in your life.

4. What is the General Adaptation Syndrome?

5. If you are not in control of your stress, discuss why you are choosing to be this way and how does it make you feel? So, what will you do about that?

6. Identify a situation in your life where you have not taken control of the stress in your life. What were the results? What could you have done differently to decrease your stress better than what you did?

7. What will you do this week to take control of the stress that you are presently experiencing in your life?

8. List at least three different stress management techniques and explain how to use each.

9. Can you see yourself seeking success on a daily basis? If so, explain what you need to focus on to achieve success today, tomorrow and the rest of this week? If you cannot see yourself seeking success on a daily basis then write down what is stopping you from success and what you plan to do to overcome this barrier.

LAB ASSIGNMENT 12.1
TAKING CONTROL OF YOUR STRESS

Answer the following:

1. Identify one stressful situation that occurred in your life this week and answer the following: Stress occurred in my life when _____

   _____

   _____

2. Explain the causes(s) of your stress?

3. Are you in control of the stress that occurred in your life the last week?

   YES   NO   NOT SURE

4. If you are in control of your stress, what do you do to stay in control?

5. If you are not in control of your stress, discuss why you are choosing to be this way and how does this make you feel? So what will you do about that?

LAB ASSIGNMENT 12.2
TRANSFORMING STRESS INTO SUCCESS

1. Identify one successful and one unsuccessful experience that occurred in your life.
   Successful experience _____

   _____

   _____

   Unsuccessful experience _____

   _____

   _____

2. Explain the differences in your perceptions and behaviors for each experience.

3. For your successful experience—List three strengths that helped you to achieve success

4. For your unsuccessful experience—List three barriers that stopped you from being more successful.

5. Is it within your control to live a successful life? If so explain how and if not, explain what is presently stopping you.

6. Over the next week, your assignment is to create one successful experience that you want to happen. What strengths will you utilize to create success? What strategies will you incorporate in the event you get stopped?

7. In order for me to succeed this week, I will _____

   _____

   _____

   and I will not _____

   _____

   _____

After the week is up, answer the following:

8. Were you successful? Explain why or why not.

9. How did this experience affect the level of stress in your life (e.g., increase, decrease, stayed the same).

10. Can you see yourself seeking success on a daily basis? If so, explain what you will need to focus on in order to achieve success today, tomorrow and the rest of this week. If you cannot see yourself seeking success on a daily basis, then write down what is stopping you from success and what you plan to do to overcome this barrier.

LAB ASSIGNMENT 12.3
PROGRESSIVE MUSCLE RELAXATION

Over the next two weeks, practice each of these five stress management techniques listed below and answer the following:

1. Define each of these stress management techniques.
    A. Progressive Muscle Relaxation
    B. Relaxation Response
    C. Yogic Breathing
    D. Time Out
    E. Exercise

2. Draw a line from the words in Column A that match with the words in Column B

Jacobson	Endorphins
Benson	1:4:2
Mantra	Walk Away from Stress
Time Out	Progressive Muscle Relaxation
Exercise	Word to repeat
Yogic Breathing	Relaxation Response

3. Please rate your level of enjoyment for each of the 5 stress managements techniques that you have used over the past two weeks from 1 (least enjoyed) to 5 (most enjoyed).
    Progressive Muscle Relaxation

    Relaxation Response

    Yogic Breathing

    Time Out

    Exercise

4. What were your thoughts prior to and after practicing each technique?

5. Which of the stress management techniques that you practiced over the past two weeks can you see yourself using on a weekly basis and why?

LAB ASSIGNMENT 12.4
RELAXATION RESPONSE

Over the next week, select a day and time that you are committed to practicing Relaxation Response (RR) and jot it down in the space below.

I will practice PMR on _____, the _____ day of _____ at _____ AM/PM at _____ (name of place).

Once you have completed RR answer the following questions:

1. Who invented relaxation response (RR)?
2. Define the four components of RR?
3. What is the mantra that you used and did it work to take your mind off of your stress?
4. What did you like about RR?
5. How did RR affect your level of stress?
6. Can you see yourself using RR to reduce your stress on a weekly basis?
7. If yes, list two different times and places that you will consider incorporating RR into your life?
8. If no, explain what you disliked about RR?

LAB ASSIGNMENT 12.5
YOGIC BREATHING

Over the next week, select a day and time that you are committed to practicing Yogie Breathing and jot it down in the space below.

I will practice PMR on _____, the _____ day of _____ at _____ AM/PM at _____ (name of place).

Once you have completed yogic breathing, answer the following questions.

1. Define the proper breathing pattern for Yogic Breathing.
2. What did you like about Yogic Breathing?
3. How did Yogic Breathing affect your level of stress?
4. Can you see yourself using Yogic Breathing to reduce your stress on a weekly basis?
5. If yes, list two different times and places that you will consider incorporating Yogic Breathing into your life?
6. If no, explain what you disliked about Yogic Breathing?

LAB ASSIGNMENT 12.6
TAKING CONTROL OF YOUR TIME

The purpose of this assignment is for you to learn how to take control of your time and manage it successfully.

1. Over the next 24 hours, your time will be broken down into one-hour increments where you should record everything that you do in the column marked "Activity." Then in the column marked "Level of Stress Experienced", rank the stress that you have experienced from 1 (low) to 5 (moderate) to 9 (high) during that time period. In the third column, marked "How do you feel at this time?" record the thoughts that you are experiencing (e.g., happy, angry, energetic, sad, satisfied, etc) during this time period. If one day is not enough time for you to determine how you manage your time, you can repeat this exercise for as many consecutive days as you think you need to get a handle on your time management skills.

	Activity	Level of Stress Experienced	How do you feel at this time?
7 AM			
8 AM			
9 AM			
10 AM			
11 AM			
12 AM			
1 PM			
2 PM			
3 PM			
4 PM			
5 PM			
6 PM			
7 PM			
8 PM			
9 PM			
10 PM			
11 PM			
12 AM			
1 AM			
2 AM			

3 AM			
4 AM			
5 AM			
6 AM			

After completing the recording of your activities, answer the following.

2. What have you noticed about what you do with your time?

3. Explain how your time management skills play a role in the level of stress that you experience.

4. For the next week, organize yourself in the following manner. List all of the things you must do or get accomplished in the next day under Priority Column A. Then list all of the things that you would like to get accomplished, but can wait at least one day, but not more than three days under Priority Column B. Finally, in Priority Column C include all the things that you would like to accomplish, but can wait at least five or more days.

	Priority Column A Must Accomplish Today	Priority Column B Must Accomplish in Next 2-3 Days	Priority Column C Can Wait until Next Week
1.			
2.			
3.			
4.			
5.			
6.			
7.			
8.			

After the week is over, answer the following questions:

5. Place a check mark next to all of the items that you have listed and completed from your priority list in Q4.

6. Did you complete everything from your Priority A List?   YES   NO
Explain why or why not?

7. If you answered "YES," explain how your stress has been affected by your accomplishments? If you answered "NO" explain what stopped you from accomplishing all of the items on Priority Lists A and B?

8. Explain how this exercise (writing down and ranking your list of priorities by importance) has helped you decrease your level of stress.

9. What do you have planned for next week?

10. What strategies will you incorporate to accomplish your agenda items on priority lists A and B.

LAB ASSIGNMENT 12.7
EXERCISE YOUR STRESS AWAY

1. Over the next week, select two days that will exercise and two days that you will not and jot down your schedule for each in the spaces listed below.

   Exercise Day 1 Time _____ Place _____ Activity _____

   Exercise Day 2 Time _____ Place _____ Activity _____

   No exercise   Date 1 _____   Date 2 _____

2. Prior to exercising answer the following:

   A. My mood is

       1   2   3   4   5   6   7   8   9

     Bad   Excellent

   B. My level of stress is

       1   2   3   4   5   6   7   8   9

     Low   High

   C. I am looking forward to exercising today

       1   2   3   4   5   6   7   8   9

     Not at All   Very Much

3. Write down the following as it pertains to your exercise workout:

   Activities you plan to do   _____

   Time Committed to Exercising _____

   Place of Exercise _____

4. After completing your exercise answer the following:

   A. As a result of exercising my level of stress has

       INCREASED   DECREASED   REMAINED THE SAME

B. My mood is

BETTER   WORSE   THE SAME

C. I have MORE LESS the SAME amount of energy now than before I started exercising

5. Explain the effect that exercise had on your level of stress.

6. Answer the following questions on the days that you did not exercise:

A. My mood is

1	2	3	4	5	6	7	8	9
Bad								Excellent

B. My level of stress is

1	2	3	4	5	6	7	8	9
Low								High

C. I am looking forward to exercising today

1	2	3	4	5	6	7	8	9
Not at All								Very Much

7. What have you noticed about your level of stress on the days that you exercised vs. the days that you did not?

8. Do you plan to incorporate exercise into your life as a way to manage your stress? If so, explain when? If not, explain what is stopping you and what you plan to do to overcome your barriers?

LAB ASSIGNMENT 12.8

Now that you have practiced each of the five stress management techniques introduced in labs 10.3-10.7 let's see which ones are really for you.

1. Please rank the order of enjoyment for each of the five stress management techniques that you have been practicing for the past few weeks from 1 (did not enjoy) to 5 (enjoyed the most):

Progressive Muscle Relaxation   _____

Managing My Time Successfully   _____

Relaxation Response   _____

Exercise My Stress Away   _____

Yogic Breathing   _____

2. Explain what you liked and/or disliked about each.

   Progressive Muscle Relaxation _____

   Relaxation Response _____

   Yogic Breathing _____

   Managing Time _____

   Exercise _____

3. What were your thoughts prior to and after practicing each technique?

4. Did you have any difficulties practicing any of these techniques? If so, list each.

5. Which of these techniques allowed you to feel 100% in control of your stress?

6. Five years from now, which techniques do you see as part of your lifestyle behavior and why?

REFERENCES AND RECOMMENDED READINGS

Anxiety and Depression Association of America (2017). Physical activity reduces stress. https://adaa.org/understanding-anxiety/related-illnesses/other-related-conditions/stress/physical-activity-reduces-stress.

Benson, H. (1975). The relaxation response. New York: Avon Books

Berger, B.G., & Owen, D.R. (1988). Stress reduction and mood enhancement in four exercise modes: Swimming, body conditioning, Hatha yoga, and fencing. *Research Quarterly for Exercise and Sport, 59,* 148-159.

Berger, B., Friedman, E., & Eaton, M. (1988). Comparison of jogging, the Relaxation Response, and group interaction for stress reduction. *Journal of Sport & Exercise Psychology, 10,* 431-447.

Blonna, R. (2012). *Coping with stress in a changing world,* fifth edition. McGraw-Hill, New York, NY.

Cannon, W. (1922). The wisdom of the body. New York: W.W. Norton.

Crews, D.J., & Landers, D.M. (1987). A meta-analytic review of aerobic fitness and reactivity to Psychosocial stressors. *Medicine and Science in Sports and Exercise, 19,* 114-120.

International Labour Organization (2000). Press release Index: ILO report examines mental health in the workplace, in Finland, Germany, Poland, United Kingdom, United States, Costs of workplace stress are rising with depression increasingly common. October, 2000.

Jacobson, E. (1938). Progressive relaxation. 2nd edition. Chicago: University of Chicago Press.

Latimer, A.E., Martin Ginis, K.A., Hicks, A.L., & McCartney, N. (2004). An examination of the mechanisms of exercise-induced change in psychological well-being among people with spinal cord injury. *Journal of Rehabilitation Research & Development, 41*, 643-652.

Lazuras, R., & DeLongis, A. (1983). Psychological stress and coping in aging. *American Psychologist*, 38, 245-254.

Lox, C.L., Martin Ginis, K.A., & Petruzzello, S.J. (2006). The psychology of exercise: Integrating theory and practice, 2nd ed. pp 269-292, 346. Holcomb Hathaway: Scottsdale, AZ.

Mayo Clinic Staff (2015). *Exercise and stress: Get moving to manage stress.* www.mayoclinic.org. April 16, 2015

McGrath, J.E. (1970). Major methodological issues. In J.E. McGrath (Ed.), Social and psychological factors in stress (pp. 20). New York: Holt, Renehart, & Winston.

Selye, H. (1976). *The stress of life.* McGraw-Hill, New York.

Selye, H. (1974). *Stress without distress.* Lippincott, New York.

Smith, N. (2012). Employees reveal how stress affects their jobs. Business News Daily, March 28, 2012. www.businessnewsdaily.com/2267-workplace-stress-health-epidemic-preventable-employee-assistance-programs-html

Statistical Brain Research Institute (2017). American Institute of Stress, NY. www.statisticbrain.com/stress-statistics, May 128, 2017.

www.reference.com/world-view/psychological-definition-stress.

www.reference.com/health/operational-definition-stress.

Chapter 13

It's Time to Stop Smoking

OBJECTIVES

After reading this chapter, you will be able to:

- become familiar with the prevalence of smoking in adult and adolescent populations in the United States
- understand the factors associated with youth tobacco use
- recognize the harmful effects of smoking tobacco by learning the correlation between smoking and illness and disease
- discover the costs of smoking
- learn how to stop smoking

MY STORY

As I reflect back to the period of time I grew up in the 1970's, I recall a world surrounded by smoke. You see, I grew up in a family of smokers. In fact, it is hard pressed for me to remember many adults in my immediate world that didn't smoke at one time or another in their lives. Going as far back as I can remember, my grandfather was a smoker. So were my mom and dad (although Dad smoked cigars). Most of my aunts and uncles were smokers as were many of my parents' friends, too. I can even recall teachers at my elementary school lightening up once classes were dismissed as they walked to their cars.

The majority of my elders were born in the 1920s, 1930s and 1940s and during their teenage years smoking was advertised as a "relaxant," "stylish," "the thing to do." All it took was for one person to light up and smoke a cigarette and before you knew it, the entire room was filled with smoke. Back then, little if any information was published about the harmful effects of smoking and the damage it caused to one's health. In fact, it was quite the opposite. Tobacco companies created a wealth of advertisements and catchy slogans all designed to attract people to smoking. Table 13.1 includes a list of 15 of the most popular tobacco companies and their slogans for smoking.

I guess, at that time, it was less about whether one should start smoking and more about which brand of cigarette best fit the individual smoker or smoker to be. Tobacco companies used a powerful ploy to attract customers to smoke their cigarettes by targeting specific audiences and advertising their brand during popular TV shows like the *Flintstones* and *The Beverly Hillbillies* because they were watched by many children and teens (Pollay, 1964). Celebrities like Bob Hope, Bing Crosby, Frank Sinatra, Spencer Tracy, Lucille Ball, Desi Arnaz, Barbara Stanwyck, Ed Sullivan and Laurel & Hardy were hired during the highlight of

Table 13.1
List of the Most Popular Tobacco Companies and Their slogans

	Company	Slogan
1.	Virginia Slims Women's Cigarettes	It's A Woman's Thing. You've come a long way, baby
2.	Marlboro Cigarettes	You've got a lot to like with a Marlboro Come to Marlboro Country Come where the flavor is
3.	Strand Cigarettes	You're never alone with a Strand
4.	Doral Cigarettes	Taste Me! Taste Me! Come and Taste Me!
5.	Winfield Cigarettes	Anyhow…Have a Winfield
6.	Chesterfield Cigarettes	Chesterfield. Blow some my way.
7.	Camel Cigarettes	Slow down. Pleasure Up. It's your taste. Where a man belongs. More Doctors smoke Camels than any other cigarette For digestion sake-Smoke Camels I'd walk a mile for a Camel
8.	Carlton Cigarettes	If you smoke, please smoke Carlton
9.	Pall Mall Brand	Wherever particular people congregate
10.	L&M Brand	Just what the doctor ordered
11.	Kool Menthol Cigarette Brand	Kool. The House of Menthol Mild, but not too light (for Kool mild). Lady be cool Enjoy a cooler side of mild Come all the way to Kool
12.	Winston Brand	Winston tastes good like a cigarette should.
13.	Peter Stuyvesant Dutch Cigarette Brand	The international passport to smoking pleasure Peter Stuyvesant. So much to enjoy
14	Consulate Brand	Cool as a mountain stream Menthol fresh, cool clean, consulate Cool, Fresh, Consulate
15	Eve Cigarette Brand	Farewell to the Ugly Cigarette

their careers to advertise cigarette brands both in commercials and in movies. Models were put on the covers of magazines and professional athletes like Hank Aaron, Willie Mays, Joe Lewis, Jesse Owens, Joe DiMaggio, Paul Hornung and Frank Gifford were often photographed with a cigarette or a cigar in their hand, all designed to make smoking look more appealing. Even today, one of the expressions for success in Major League Baseball after a team wins the World Series is to celebrate by smoking a cigar. Disheartening as it is, by the time many people who began smoking during that era knew smoking was harmful to their health, it was too late. They were hooked for the rest of their lives.

As I reflect back to the early 1980's, what hit me the hardest was seeing my mom live with emphysema in her mid 40's. She would come home from work and walk up the stoop into our house and then she would have to sit down for several minutes to catch her breath. By the time she realized that smoking was bad for her it was, indeed, too late. Five years later, she died from complications due to her battle with emphysema.

From that time on, I knew I could never be a smoker, not that I ever thought I would anyway. To me, it was just senseless how people could focus on the temporary satisfaction of smoking and neglect the long-term ill effects. Having witnessed my mom as well as several other significant members of my family die from smoking-related illness, I am committed to educating the population in any way I can on the dangers of smoking and introducing viable strategies to stop smoking once you start and/or get hooked.

PREVALENCE OF SMOKING IN THE U.S.

Adult Smoking

On January 11, 1964, Dr. Luther L. Terry, Surgeon General of the United States, released Smoking and Health: Report of the Advisory Committee of the Surgeon General of the Public Health Service – the first federal government report on Smoking and Health, linking smoking and specific diseases. 2014 marked the 50th anniversary of this landmark report which is now called The Surgeon General's Report. Here is a summary of the Surgeon General's findings regarding the health consequences of smoking over the past 50 years 1964-2014 (USDHHS, 2014).

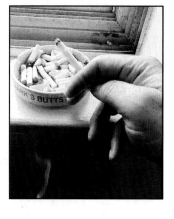

- More than 20 million Americans have died because of smoking since the first Surgeon General's Report was published.

- 2.5 million of these deaths have been among nonsmokers who died from diseases caused by exposure to second-hand smoke.

- More than 16 million Americans suffer from a disease caused by smoking.

- Nearly half a million Americans die prematurely from smoking and 42,000 deaths are caused by second-hand smoke exposure each year.

- Compared to nonsmokers, smokers suffer more health problems and disability due to their smoking and ultimately lose more than a decade of life.

- For every person who dies because of smoking, at least 30 people live with a serious smoking-related illness.

- More than 100,000 babies have died from Sudden Infant Death Syndrome, complications from prematurity, low birth weight, and other pregnancy problems resulting from parental smoking.

- Smoking rates among adults and teens are less than half of what they were in 1964, however, 42 million American adults and about 3 million middle and high school students continue to smoke.

- If current rates continue, 5.6 million Americans younger than 18 years of age who are alive today are projected to die prematurely from smoking-related disease.

In addition to the work by the Surgeon General, many other organizations including the Center for Disease Control and Prevention (CDC), United States Department of Health and Human Services (USDHHS) and the World Health Organization (WHO) have worked diligently conducting research and educating the world on the dangers of smoking. Below is a summary of their findings over the past 10 years.

- An estimated 45.3 to 55.8 million people, or approximately 19.3% to 23.8% of adults (aged 18 years or older) in the United States smoke cigarettes.

- As of 2013, there were also 12.4 million cigar smokers, 8.8 million smokeless tobacco users and 2.3 million people who smoke tobacco in pipes.

- Cigarette smoking has now become the leading cause of preventable death in the United States accounting for approximately one in five deaths annually or 1300 deaths every day.

In the United States, smoking causes early deaths of about 443,000 people per year (USDHHS, 2014). In addition, it is estimated that adult male smokers lost an average of 13.2 years of life and female smokers lost 14.5 years of life because of smoking. Moreover, compared to nonsmokers, smokers were found to suffer more health problems and disability resulting in a decrease in their quality of life due to the limitation of daily activities often caused by difficulties in breathing, thus making it hard to work, play or simply move around.

The simple fact is that more deaths are caused by tobacco use than by all deaths from human immunodeficiency virus (HIV), illegal drug use, alcohol use, motor vehicle injuries, suicides, and murders, combined (CDC, 2004; Mokdad, Marks, Stroup & Gerberding, 2004). Across the globe, tobacco use causes nearly 6 million deaths per year, and current trends show that tobacco use will cause more than 8 million deaths annually by 2030 (WHO, 2011).

Youth and Adolescent Smoking

Unfortunately, the prevalence of smoking is not limited to adults alone. Each day in the U.S., 3,200 youth ages 18 years or younger smoke their first cigarette and an additional 2,100 youth and young adults who have been occasional smokers become daily cigarette smokers (USDHHS, 2012). According to the USDHHS, tobacco use is started and established primarily during adolescence with nearly 9 out of 10 cigarette smokers first starting by age 18. Moreover, the Surgeon General has reported that one out of four high school seniors and one in three young adults will become regular cigarette smokers.

Cigarette Smoking Is Declining Among Youth in the U.S.

It is important to note that from 2011 to 2015, cigarette smoking has declined among middle and high school students. In 2011, the CDC revealed that approximately 4.3% of middle school students smoke cigarettes and 7.1% used some form of tobacco. This number has decreased to 2.3% in 2015. In high school, the rate of cigarette smoking decreased from to 15.8% in 2011 to 9.3% in 2015, however the use of electronic cigarettes increased slightly in both middle school (5.3% up 0.6%) and high school (14.5% in 2011 to 16.0 in 2015) (CDC, 2016).

While it is optimistic to think that smoking will continue to decrease among our youth and adolescent populations, the prevalence of smokers in this population is still quite alarming. (See Table 13.2 Tobacco Use Among High School Students in 2015 and Table 13.3 Tobacco Use Among Middle School Students in 2015). The startling fact remains that nearly 1.5 million youth smoke each day in the United States (USDHHS, 2012). Ironically, while only 5 percent of high school smokers said that they would definitely be smoking five years later, close to 75 percent were still smoking 7 to 9 years later. Eventually, this will lead to approximately 20% of our youth becoming daily smokers throughout their adult lives. That equates to over 40 million people and that is simply too much.

Table 13.2
Tobacco Use among High School Students in 2015

Tobacco Product	Overall	Females	Males
Any Tobacco Product	25.3%	20.3%	30.0%
Electronic Cigarettes	16.0%	12.8%	19.0%
Cigarettes	9.3%	7.7%	10.7%
Cigars	8.6%	5.6%	11.5%
Hookas	7.2%	6.9%	7.4%
Smokeless Tobacco	6.0%	1.8%	10.0%
Pipes	1.0%	0.7%	1.4%
Bidis	0.6%	0.4%	0.9%

Table 13.3
Tobacco Use among Middle School Students in 2015

Tobacco Product	Overall	Females	Males
Any Tobacco Product	7.4%	6.4%	8.3%
Electronic Cigarettes	5.3%	4.8%	5.9%
Cigarettes	2.3%	2.2%	2.3%
Cigars	2.0%	2.0%	1.9%
Hookas	1.8%	1.1%	----
Smokeless Tobacco	1.6%	1.4%	1.8%
Pipes	0.4%	----	----
Bidis	0.2%	----	----

Factors Associated with Youth Tobacco Use

While smoking has decreased over the past few years, the evidence remains that too many young people smoke today, get sick and die well before they should. The big question is why do young people start and continue to smoke despite the fact that they know it is harmful to their health? Research has discovered a variety of factors attracting our youth population to smoking and they include:

Social and Physical Environments

1. Mass media shows tobacco use as a normal activity who can promote smoking among young people. There is a pervasive presence of tobacco product marketing, advertisements in magazines, youth-generated posts on social networking sites, images of smoking in the movies that conveys a message that makes smoking use attractive to youth and young adults.

2. Youth are more likely to use tobacco if they see tobacco use is acceptable or normal among their peers. There's a feeling of comfort around friends that smoke. Smoking can create an acceptance into a group especially when the majority of people around you do not smoke;

3. High school athletes are more likely to use smokeless tobacco than their peers who are non-athletes (CDC, Morbidity and Mortality Weekly Report, 2015).

4. If parents smoke then there is a higher probability that their children may smoke.

Biological and Genetic Factors

1. Youth may be more sensitive to nicotine and once they start using tobacco they may become dependent on nicotine sooner than adults.

2. If the mother smoked during pregnancy it may increase the likelihood that her offspring will become regular smokers.

Mental Health Factors

1. There are expectations of positive outcomes from smoking, such as coping with stress, calming oneself down and controlling weight.
2. There is a strong relationship between youth smoking and depression, anxiety, and stress (USDHHS, 1994).

Other Factors to Recognize

1. There is a positive correlation between lower socioeconomic status, including lower income or education and smoking.
2. Adolescents and youth who lack the skills to resist the influence of tobacco use are more likely to start smoking and become addicted.
3. When there is a lack of support or involvement in life from parents, it can increase smoking rates in children, youth and adolescents.
4. When accessibility, availability, and price are within reach, then smoking is increased.
5. When academic achievement is low, smoking rates can increase.
6. When youth have a low self-image or self-esteem, they may be more susceptible to smoking.
7. When there is a greater frequency of exposure to tobacco advertising, smoking can be interpreted as something positive or rewarding in which to participate.
8. The act of smoking is perceived as enjoyable because many tobacco products are flavored and designed to attract the taste buds of youth and young adults.
9. Smoking becomes something to do when one gets bored.

It has also been discovered that young adults who have fewer pro-social bonds to conventional institutions, such as school, organized sports and places of worship are also more likely to use tobacco (Choi et al., 2002, Metzger et al., 2011). This is evidenced by the compelling associations between low academic achievement and smoking onset and use among adolescents (Dewey, 1999, Tucker et al., 2008). Even exposure to smoking by actors in movies increases the likelihood that a young person will begin to smoke (Sargent et al, 2001, 2005, Thrasher et al., 2008).

Here are some common experiences from teens who smoke.
1. They tried their first cigarette in sixth or seventh grade.
2. They often do not perform well in school.
3. They feel like they are not a part of the school.
4. They become isolated from other students.

5. They can't perform as well at sports events.

6. They feel like they have little hope of going to college.

7. They feel like they need a job to support their smoking habit.

8. They are reported to school officials for skipping classes.

9. They start using other illegal substances.

10. They begin experimenting with alcohol and other drugs.

11. They experience pressure from home and school and use tobacco as a form of relief.

12. Teen smokers enjoy trying to hide their smoking.

13. School has become more fun for some tobacco users.

The Influence of Peers

These above-mentioned types of behaviors get attention because the initiation of smoking is influenced by having a friend, particularly a best friend, who smokes. The health risk factors of smoking do not apply because those who are young often think that they are invincible. In addition, the perceived immediate benefits to smoke far outweigh the costs both in the immediate short-term and in the long-term future. Conversely, if the teen becomes a member of a pro-social group, such as those participating in sports, cheerleading, or any club that promotes healthy living, the likelihood that the teen will attempt to stop smoking improves.

If smoking continues at the current rate among youth in the United States, 5.6 million of today's Americans younger than 18 will die early from a smoking-related illness. That's approximately 1 of every 13 Americans aged 17 years or younger who are alive today (USDHHS, 2014). Among those who persist in smoking, one will die about 13 years earlier than his or her nonsmoking peers. Ironically, it has also been reported that if young people can remain free of tobacco use until the age of 18, most will never start to smoke.

How To Reduce Youth Tobacco Use

In order to reduce and prevent youth tobacco use, national, state and local programs have worked together to implement the following:

1. Increasing the cost of tobacco products making it harder for teenagers to afford to buy cigarettes (King, B.A., Jama, A.O., Marynak, K.L., Promoff, G.R., 2015).

2. Prohibiting smoking in indoor areas of worksites and public places (CDC, 2014).

3. Raising the minimum age of sale for tobacco products to 21 years.

4. TV and radio commercials, posters, and other media messages targeted toward youth to counter tobacco product advertisements.

5. Community programs and school and college policies and interventions that encourage tobacco-free environments and lifestyles.

6. Mass media campaigns that reduce tobacco advertising, promotions, and availability of tobacco products.

7. The truth on the effects of nicotine that are in tobacco products are listed on the products.

CONCLUSIONS ABOUT THE PREVALENCE OF YOUTH AND ADULT SMOKING

1. Cigarette smoking by youth and young adults has immediate adverse health consequences, including addiction, and accelerates the development of chronic diseases across the lifespan.

2. Prevention efforts must focus on both adolescents and young adults because among young adults who become daily smokers, nearly all first use of cigarettes occurs by age 18 (88%), with 99% of first use by 26 years of age.

3. Advertising and promotional activities by tobacco companies have been shown to cause the onset and continuation of smoking among adolescent and young adults.

4. To reduce the use of smoking and tobacco there has been a coordinated, multicomponent intervention that has combined mass media campaigns, tax increases in tobacco products, school-based policies and programs, and statewide or community-wide changes in smoke free policies and norms.

THE HARMFUL EFFECTS OF SMOKING TOBACCO

Did you know that there are more than 7000 chemicals and compounds in tobacco smoke with hundreds of these being toxic, and at least 69 cancer causing? Research has discovered that smoking harms nearly every organ of the body and can reduce one's health and cause many illnesses and diseases which often results in a shortened lifespan. From the moment you smoke, the poisonous chemicals in tobacco smoke quickly reach your lungs as you inhale. Once these toxicants enter the lungs they rapidly spread through your bloodstream and reach cells throughout the body causing immediate damage to tissues and cell structure and thus interfering with the body's normal processes.

A simplistic way to view this is to imagine that you burned a part of your body and it became inflamed. Rather than rest it and give it a chance to heal, you continue to let that same part of your body burn over and over again, preventing it from healing. It would stay, red, irritated, and inflamed and never be able to function properly again. Well, that's exactly what happens when you smoke. The organs in your body have a lining that is similar to your skin. Chemicals in tobacco smoke cause inflammation and damage to the lining and to the cells inside the lining. When you keep smoking, the body is forced to continuously overwork itself and eventually your immune system will break down and increase your risk of many illnesses and diseases.

The truth is that there are no physical reasons to start smoking. The body doesn't need tobacco the way it needs food, water, sleep, and exercise. Moreover, many of the chemicals in cigarettes, like nicotine and cyanide, are actually poisons that can kill in high enough doses. The consequences of this poisoning happen gradually and over the long term, smoking leads people to develop a variety of health problems. This section focuses on the harmful effects of smoking and the following smoke-related illnesses and diseases:

Smoking and Coronary Heart Disease and Stroke

Smoking and Respiratory Disease

Smoking and COPD—Emphysema and Chronic Bronchitis

Smoking and Cancer

Smoking and the Circulatory System

Smoking and Asthma

Smoking and Reproductive Health

The Effects of Secondhand Smoke

The Effects of Smoking on Your Body

Smoking and Death

Smoking and Coronary Heart Disease (CHD)

CHD is the leading cause of death in the United States and people who smoke significantly increase their chances of acquiring CHD by 2 to 4 times more than nonsmokers. About 20% of all deaths from heart disease in the U.S. are directly related to cigarette smoking (www. medicinenet.com/smoking_and_heart_disease/article.htm).

What happens to your cardiovascular (CV) system when you smoke?

Breathing tobacco smoke quickly affects blood chemistry and damages the delicate cells that line blood vessels throughout the body. These important cells help maintain blood flow. When they are damaged by the chemicals in tobacco smoke, they do not work properly. Over time, the cells of the blood vessels will thicken and the vessels will become narrower which will decrease normal blood flow in the body and increase both heart rate and blood pressure making your cardiovascular system work harder and harder just to produce normal, daily life functions (e.g., breathing, circulation; physical activity).

A simple way to understand how smoking negatively affects the cardiovascular system is to picture this—you are watering your lawn and about 50 feet behind you there is a brick on your hose causing a decrease in the water coming out of the nozzle. You can't see the brick because it is so far behind you, but you do see that the amount of water coming out of your hose is minimal. Logically, you squeeze the nozzle harder in order to increase the pressure to get more water out, but because the brick is on the hose the water remains at a standstill. The end result is more pressure is being used to get water out with less water actually coming out.

In essence, one's blood vessels are like your water hose. When the hose is blocked, water cannot flow through it which can cause an increase in pressure and possibly break the hose, the pipes and cause a flood. In your body, when the vessels become narrow there is a restriction of blood flow causing the heart and lungs to work harder and produce less (i.e., faster heart rate with less oxygen coming out). Over time, this can damage the cardiovascular system and cause a heart attack (USDHHS, 2004).

Heart disease includes several types of heart conditions with the most common in the United States called coronary heart disease, which is the narrowing of the blood vessels that carry blood to the heart (CDC, 2015). Signs and symptoms of heart disease due to smoking include:

Chest pain

Shortness of breath

Increase in Blood Pressure and Heart Rate

Increase in Blood Clotting

Damage to the cells that line the coronary arteries and other blood vessels

Arrhythmia—when the heart beats too fast, too slow or irregularly.

Smoking and Stroke

When people smoke it makes the blood in the body sticky and more likely to clot which can block blood flow to the heart and brain. A stroke occurs when the blood supply to the brain is blocked or when a blood vessel in the brain bursts, causing brain tissue to die (CDC, 2015). Research has discovered that smoking makes a significant independent contribution to the risk of stroke (Wolf et al., 1988). More specifically, heavy smokers (>40 cigarettes/day) have a relative risk of stroke that is twice that of light smokers (< 10 cigarettes/day) and 2-4 times greater than non-smokers (Wannamathee, Shaper, Whincup & Walker, 1995). Approximately 700,000 strokes occur annually with 20% being directly related to smoking (Shah & Cole, 2010). Once someone gets a stroke it can cause a variety of disabilities including paralysis, muscle weakness, difficulty speaking, memory loss or death.

Smoking and Respiratory Disease

Healthy lungs are like balloons. They expand when you inhale and compress when you exhale. When you smoke, the poisons in tobacco break down the lining of your lungs which will decrease the elasticity of the lungs so that they can no longer stretch and extend to exchange air flow. A common reaction when you first start smoking is a burning sensation in the lungs causing you to cough. This is your body's message to you! "Stop!" "I am being poisoned." "This is not good for me." While your body uses tiny brushes to sweep out the mucus and dirt in your lungs when you first begin to smoke, over time smoking will damage and destroy these brushes resulting in "smokers cough"—the bodies inability to clear out the lungs from smoke.

Smoking and COPD

As a result of smoking, one becomes more susceptible to acquiring several respiratory illnesses including chronic obstructive pulmonary disease (COPD). In 2011, COPD was the third leading cause of death in the United States with over 15 million Americans reporting that they have been diagnosed with COPD.

What is COPD?

COPD refers to a group of diseases that cause airflow blockage and breathing-related problems. It includes emphysema, chronic bronchitis, and in some cases asthma (CDC, 2015). Symptoms of COPD include: shortness of breath, wheezing, chronic coughing with mucus, tightness in the chest and fatigue.

Emphysema

Emphysema is a form of chronic (long-term) lung disease that causes difficulty in breathing due to a limitation in blowing air out. Emphysema causes the walls between the air sacs in the lungs to lose their ability to stretch and shrink back. The air sacs become weaker and wider, and air gets trapped in the lungs. In short, with emphysema, lung tissue is destroyed, making it difficult for the body to acquire enough oxygen.

A simple way to understand Emphysema is to picture this—imagine for a moment that your bicycle has a flat tire with microscopic holes in it that are unrecognizable to the human eye. You take out your old air pump and begin to vigorously squeeze it to push air into your tire. Even though air is getting pushed into the tire, the holes are preventing the air from staying in and being transported to where it is needed. Over time, fatigue sets in and your pumping slowly fades due to the hard work and effort that you expended to no avail. Despite your hard work, your tire remains flat.

While there are multiple causes of emphysema, smoking is by far the most common cause (www.webmd.com/lung/copd/what-is-emphysema). Unfortunately, there is no cure for emphysema. The body simply cannot manufacture enough air for people with emphysema to breathe on their own and so they will eventually die from a lack of air. However, quitting smoking will reduce the speed at which the disease gets worse which can certainly expand one's lifespan.

Bronchitis

Bronchitis is the swelling of the lining of the bronchial tubes. When the bronchioles are swollen, they become narrower, and less air flows to and from the lungs. Chronic inflammation of the bronchioles can cause mucus to build up in the lungs making it harder to breathe. Over time, the lining of the bronchial tubes thickens and airways eventually become scarred, again making in more difficult to breathe. There are three different types of bronchitis, all with similar symptoms, yet caused by very different circumstances and they are: (1) acute bronchitis, (2) asthmatic bronchitis and (3) chronic bronchitis. Below is a brief description of each.

Acute Bronchitis—affects about 10 million people per year and occurs before the age of 5.

Asthmatic Bronchitis—seen in people with continual asthma.

Chronic Bronchitis—affects about 9 million people each year and is most common with people who smoke and/or are over 45 years of age.

Symptoms of Bronchitis

- Persistent cough that feels like a cold
- Mucus build up
- Fatigue
- Wheezing
- Chest Pain
- Difficulty Breathing

For those people with chronic bronchitis, the coughing and mucus buildup can last for several months and include tightness, chest discomfort, headaches, running nose and impaired voice (Gilligan, 2015).

What Causes COPD?

According to the CDC, COPD is caused by smoking with smokers 12 to 13 times more likely to die from COPD than nonsmokers. A key factor in the development and progression of COPD is tobacco smoke (CDC, 2005). When someone has COPD, there is less air that flows through their airways (the tubes that carry air in and out of the lungs) due to one or more of the following:

- The walls between the air sacs are destroyed.

- The airways and tiny air sacs in the lungs lose their ability to stretch & shrink back thus decreasing the amount of air that can go in and out of the lungs.

- The walls of the airways become thick and inflamed (irritated and swollen).

- The airways develop more mucus than usual, which can cause clogging and block air flow. (National Heart, Lung, and Blood Institute, 2015).

- In the early stages of COPD, there may not be any symptoms, or there may be only mild symptoms such as:

   A nagging cough (often called "smoker's cough)
   Shortness of breath, especially during physical activity
   Wheezing (a whistling sound when you breathe)
   Tightness in the chest

- As the disease gets worse, symptoms may include:

   Having trouble breathing or catching your breath
   Difficulty speaking
   Blue or gray lips and/or fingernails (a sign of low oxygen levels in your blood)

Trouble with mental alertness
A rapid heartbeat
Swelling in the feet and ankles
Weight loss
(National Heart, Lung, and Blood Institute, 2015).

The severity of COPD symptoms is dependent on how damaged your lungs are. The more you continue to smoke, the greater and faster the damage will occur. Among the 15 million Americans with COPD, 39% continue to smoke and approximately 8 out of 10 COPD-related deaths is due to smoking (CDC, 2011).

How Can COPD be Prevented?

Clearly, the best and most effective way to prevent COPD is to never start smoking, and if you do smoke then quit. In addition, stay away from secondhand smoke.

How is COPD Treated?

For those people who have been diagnosed and are living with COPD, the National Heart, Lung, and Blood Institute has recommended the following strategies to treat COPD:

1. To avoid shortness of breath while eating, follow a special meal plan with smaller, more frequent meals
2. Rest before eating
3. Taking vitamins and nutritional supplements

To improve the health and well-being:

1. Exercise
2. Nutritional counseling
3. Education on lung disease and how to manage it
4. Energy-conserving techniques
5. Breathing strategies
6. Psychological counseling and/or group support

According to the American Lung Association, there are several different categories of treatments for people with COPD based on the severity of their condition and they include: (1) pulmonary rehabilitation; (2) medications; (3) supplemental oxygen; (4) surgery; (5) clinical trials; and (6) complimentary therapies;

1. ***Pulmonary Rehabilitation*** is a program of education and exercise classes that teach people with COPD about their lungs and their illness and how to exercise and be more active with less shortness of breath. Classes often take place in a group setting in order to give each individual an opportunity to meet others with the same condition so they

can provide and receive necessary social support and encouragement, feel better and learn how to manage their own COPD (www.lung.org). According to the American Lung Association, people with COPD who participate in Pulmonary Rehabilitation will become stronger and get into better physical condition which will make them feel better and allow them to participate in activities they enjoy (American Lung Association, 2011).

2. *Medications* may be prescribed to improve the breathing of people with COPD. While there are a variety of medications that are used, there is no one best for all people. Each person's COPD is different and therefore it is up to one's physician and health team to determine what medication is best. Often times, individuals with COPD are on multiple medicines designed to help them breathe better and/or reduce pain and discomfort often associated with COPD. Here is a list of different medications commonly prescribed for people with COPD:

   a. *Bronchodilators*—relax the muscles around the airways which help to keep the airways open and make it easier to breathe. They are often taken through an inhaler that can pass medicine directly to the lungs. There are two different types of bronco-dilators: short-acting and long-acting. Short-acting are designed to work quickly so that you feel fast relief from symptoms. Long-acting provide longer-lasting relief than short-acting, but they take longer to kick in.

   b. *Anti-Infammatories*—reduce swelling and mucus production inside the airways. When inflammation is reduced, it becomes easier to breathe. Most often, these are inhaled medications, yet some types of inflammatories come in pill form and are usually used for short periods of time in special situations such as when one's symptoms are getting worse. These medications can have serious side effects such as weight gain, diabetes, osteoporosis, cataracts and increased risk of infection.

   c. *Antibiotics*—people with COPD sometimes have flare-ups caused by bacterial or viral infections. Therefore, it may be important for your doctor to prescribe an antibiotic or an anti-viral medicine that you can have on hand if you get an infection.

   d. *Vaccinations*—with COPD one is at greater risk for serious complications from the flu and pneumonia. Therefore, it is important to protect oneself against the flu and be immunized every year.

3. *Supplemental Oxygen* (also known as oxygen therapy)—when lung function is reduced to the extent that a person's breathing becomes restricted and they cannot supply enough oxygen to survive normal daily functions (e.g., eating, digesting food, sitting, standing, walking) the body needs extra oxygen or supplemental oxygen. Often times, oxygen is delivered to one's home for use and stored in different sized steel or aluminum tanks allowing for transport either within or outside of one's home.

4. ***Surgery***—in severe cases, where medication and other treatments have been ineffective in helping people with COPD improve their breathing, surgery can become an option provided the individual is strong enough to withstand the stress of the surgery and the pulmonary rehabilitation program, thereafter. Two types of surgery for people with COPD are:

   a. ***Lung volume reduction surgery*** (LVRS): This is a surgery to remove diseased parts of the lung so healthier lung tissue can work better.

   b. ***Lung transplant***: This is a surgery to replace diseased lungs with one or two healthy lungs from an organ donor. This is a last resort.

5. ***Clinical Trials***—are regulated research studies that test how well new medical approaches work for people. Studies are designed to propose and answer research questions in order to find better ways to screen for, diagnose or treat a disease. Studies often answer specific questions about interventions-which can be new vaccines, drugs and devices-and measuring their effectiveness and safety for patients (American Lung Association, 2016). In order to participate in a clinical trial, you must qualify for the study by meeting certain criteria. These criteria can be based on age, gender, the type and stage of a disease, previous treatment history and other medical conditions.

6. ***Complimentary Therapies***—are therapies, philosophies and practices that are not considered conventional or standard in the United States. Some examples of complimentary therapy include massage, yoga, acupuncture and energy medicine. While these techniques are not designed to treat COPD, they may be able to improve symptoms by decreasing pain and discomfort and thus improving one's quality of life.

It is important to note that the therapies mentioned above are not mutually exclusive. In fact, it is quite common to combine multiple therapies in order to control pain, reduce anxiety, lessen side effect and improve quality of life. This process of combining two or more types of treatment is called integrated medicine.

In conclusion, there is no cure for COPD, however the above-mentioned lifestyle changes and treatments can help one to breathe easier, become more active, and slow the progress of the disease which can help to enhance the quality of life (National Heart, Lung, and Blood Institute, 2015).

Smoking and Cancer

Before explaining how smoking causes cancer, it is important to first understand exactly what cancer is and how it works and then discuss how smoking and cancer are related.

What is Cancer?

Cancer is a disease in which there is an uncontrolled growth of abnormal cells in the body. Abnormal cells divide out of control and are able to invade other tissues. Normally, human cells grow and divide to form new cells as the body needs them. When cells grow old or become damaged, they die and new cells take their place. When cancer develops, there is a breakdown in this process. Old or damaged cells survive when they should die and new cells form when they are not needed. These extra cells can divide without stopping and grow out of control, forming new, abnormal cells. These abnormal growths are called tumors and many cancers form solid tumors. Cancerous tumors are malignant, which means they can spread into or invade nearby tissues and as these tumors grow, some cancer cells can break off and travel to other parts of the body through the blood or the lymph system and form new tumors which are far from the original tumor. Unlike malignant tumors, benign tumors don't spread into or invade nearby tissues. When removed, benign tumors usually don't grow back, whereas malignant tumors sometimes do. It is important to note that not all cancers form tumors. Some cancers such as cancer of the blood known as leukemia, generally do not form solid tumors (National Cancer Institute, www.cancer.gov/about-cancer/understanding/what-is-cancer).

Out of all of different types of cancer, lung cancer is the leading cause of cancer death and the second most common cancer among men and women in the United States. Each year about 200,000 people in the U.S. are told they have lung cancer and about 150,000 die from this disease. According to the CDC, cigarette smoking is the #1 risk factor for lung cancer. In fact, in the U.S. cigarette smoking is linked to about 80%-90% of all lung cancers and smokers are 15-30X more likely to get lung cancer or die from lung cancer than people who do not smoke. If nobody smoked, one of every three cancer deaths in the United States would not happen (USDHHS, 2010).

Types of Cancer

There are more than 100 different types of cancer and most are named for the organs or tissues from where the cancer forms (e.g., lung cancer, pancreatic cancer, breast cancer).

Symptoms of cancer can include:

> A thickening or lump in any part of the body
> Weight loss or gain with no known reason
> A sore that does not heal
> Hoarseness or a cough that does not go away
> A difficult time swallowing
> Discomfort after eating
> Changes in bowel or bladder habits
> Unusual bleeding or discharge
> Feeling weak or very tired
> (National Institute on Aging, 2015).

It is alarming to think that smoking can cause cancer almost anywhere in the body (i.e., blood, bladder, breast, cervix, colon, esophagus, kidneys, larynx, lip, lungs, mouth, nasal cavity, breast, pancreas, skin, stomach, trachea) and then block the body from fighting it. The poisons in cigarette smoke can weaken the body's immune system and damage or change a cell's DNA. DNA is the cell's "instruction manual" and it controls a cell's normal growth and function. When DNA is damaged, a cell can begin growing out of control and create a cancerous tumor. When this occurs, cancer cells keep growing without being stopped, thus, interrupting the body's ability to function normally.

How Can Smoking-Related Cancers Be Prevented?

Obviously, the first and most important step is to not smoke, or if you do then stop. According to the USDHHS, quitting smoking will lower the risk for cancers of the lung, mouth, throat, esophagus, and larynx. Moreover, within 5 years of quitting, the chances of getting cancer of the mouth, throat, esophagus, and bladder are cut in half. In fact, ten years after quitting smoking, the risks of dying from lung cancer drops by half.

A second way to prevent cancer is through a cancer screening. A screening is when you check your body before you have symptoms. According to the U.S. Preventative Services Task Force (USPSTF) recommended screening tests for each of these cancers can reduce both morbidity and mortality (www.cdc.gov/cancer/dcpc/prevention/screening.htm). Moreover, screenings as recommended can help to detect these diseases at an early stage which can reduce the changes of cancer spreading and causing possible illness and/or death through proper treatment.

Smoking and the Circulatory System

While most people equate smoking deaths to cancer and lung disease, the fact is that more people will die from circulatory conditions from smoking than from cancer or other lung diseases. Moreover, they will die at a much younger age, too (Spitzer, 2001). The main cause of these problems stems from two chemicals found in cigarettes: nicotine and carbon monoxide.

Nicotine is a stimulant that speeds up the heart about 20 beats per minute with every cigarette. It raises blood pressure and it constricts the arteries in the body making it harder for the heart to pump through the constricted arteries. It also causes the body to release storages of fat into the bloodstream which can stick to and damage the vessel walls. This can harden and accelerate the narrowing and clogging of the arteries and veins. When coronary arteries become 100% clogged, they can no longer supply life giving oxygen and nutrients to the heart muscle and the end result is a heart attack. When the carotid arteries that supply life giving oxygen and nutrients to the brain become 100% clogged it's called a stroke.

Carbon Monoxide comes from tobacco smoke and it poisons the oxygen carrying capacity of the blood by damaging the coating layers of cells allowing fats and plaque to stick to vessel walls. This makes the heart have to work harder to get more blood to itself. Over time, the heart muscle will weaken and no longer be able to function at its normal capacity resulting in difficulty breathing, shortness of breath, chest discomfort and feeling tired often.

In addition to heart attack and stroke there is a third condition caused by circulatory problems due strictly to smoking and it is known as Buerger's Disease. Buerger's Disease is a condition where there is a complete cutoff of circulation to the fingers or toes, resulting in gangrene. Here is a breakdown of how Buerger's Disease can occur:

When you breathe tobacco smoke it can change your blood chemistry which can damage your blood vessels. Your heart rate and blood pressure will go up and your blood vessels will thicken and grow narrower – making it harder for blood to flow naturally in the body. This can cause a blood clot. While a clot is good when you get a cut because it helps to stop the bleeding, blood clots can cause trouble when they form inside your body. Clots can block blood flow to the heart, causing chest pain, weakness, and heart attack. Clots can block blood flow to the brain, causing strokes. Clots can also block blood flow to the limbs, causing skin ulcers and eventually tissue death and amputation. Completely blocked arteries can cause sudden death. Do you remember the picture of someone stepping on your garden hose? You turn up the water pressure and less water comes out. This is what happens when clotting occurs due to smoking.

Smoking and Asthma

Asthma is a chronic disease that affects the airways of the lungs. During an asthma attack, airways (tubes that carry air to your lungs) become swollen, making it hard to breathe (CDC, 2016). As the walls of the airways swell, they narrow, and less air gets in and out of the lungs. Cells in the airway can create a sticky thick liquid known as mucus which can make breathing even more difficult. An asthma attack can occur when something irritates the airways and "triggers" an attack (CDC, 2016). Smoking is one of the most common asthma triggers and the key to avoid an asthma attack is to stay far away from triggers like smoke.

Symptoms of an asthma attack include the following:

Shortness of breath and/or difficulty breathing
Coughing
Wheezing
Tightness or pain in the chest.

Smoking and Reproductive Health

Health professionals and research scientists have long known that cigarette smoking and exposure to tobacco smoke are harmful to reproductive health, affecting fertility and development of the fetus and reducing the chances or a healthy pregnancy and delivery. Research has concluded that smoking can make it more difficult for women to become pregnant with studies showing how smoking during pregnancy creates problems in the fallopian tubes that eggs travel through to reach the womb. Exposure to tobacco smoke reduces effective functioning of these tubes and could decrease fertility. Evidence suggests that smoking may lead to an increased risk of ectopic pregnancy, a condition in which the fertilized eggs attaches to the wall of the fallopian tube or elsewhere outside the womb and begins to develop, but cannot survive.

Ectopic pregnancy poses a serious risk to the health of the mother. Studies have also shown that tobacco smoke can deprive the fetus of oxygen. One in every five babies born to mothers who smoke during pregnancy has low birth weight and babies that are born too small or too early may not be as healthy. Babies whose mothers smoke are also about three times as likely to die from SIDS. Smoking can also affect men's sperm, which can reduce fertility and also increase risks for birth defects and miscarriage. (USDHHS, 2010).

Secondhand Smoke and Cardio Heart Disease

Even if you do not smoke, you can be at risk for smoking-related illness and disease just by being around people who smoke. This is a process known as secondhand smoke. Whether it is at home where family members smoke in your presence, at work with coworkers that smoke near you or friends that smoke when you are together, breathing secondhand smoke can harm your health and cause coronary heart disease, stroke and even cancer. Each year, in the United States alone, secondhand smoke causes nearly 34,000 early deaths from CHD, 8,000 deaths from stroke and 7,300 deaths from lung cancer. The fact is that nonsmokers who breathe secondhand smoke at home or in the workplace increase their risk of CHD by 25-30% and stroke by 20-30% (CDC, 2016). While most exposure to secondhand smoke occurs in homes and at work, secondhand smoke exposure continues to occur in public places such as restaurants, bars, casinos and in private vehicles.

The Effects of Smoking on Your Body

By this day and age, we all know that smoking is bad for you and that it causes a significant amount of harmful effects. While we may be aware of the deadly diseases that smoking causes (i.e., heart disease, cancer, stroke, etc.), we may not be aware of some of the other harmful effects that result from smoking. Table 13.4 includes a list of these other harmful effects created from smoking.

Table 13.4
Harmful Effects Created from Smoking

Smoking and your immune system—Smoking compromises the immune system, making smokers more likely to have respiratory infections and auto-immune deficiencies like Crohn's disease and rheumatoid arthritis.

Smoking and your bones—Smoking increases the risk of osteoporosis, a condition where the bones become weak and brittle and are more likely to break.

Smoking and your eyesight—Smoking is as bad for your eyes as it is for the rest of your body. Smokers are at a greater risk for diseases that can lead to blindness, including cataracts, optic nerve damage an age-related macular degeneration.

Smoking and aging—Smoking causes the skin to become inflamed which can damage the skin and accelerate the aging process.

Smoking and yellow teeth—Due to the nicotine and tar found in tobacco, smoking can cause teeth to become stained and yellow and increase the risk of cavities, gum disease, and eventually losing teeth.

Smoking and bad skin—Because smoking restricts blood vessels, it can prevent oxygen and nutrients from getting to the skin—which is why smokers often appear pale and unhealthy. Studies have also linked smoking to an increased risk of getting a type of skin rash called psoriasis.

Smoking and bad breath—Cigarettes can leave smokers with a condition called halitosis, or persistent bad breath. When the chemicals from smoking build up in the mouth they can stick to places like your teeth, gums, tongue and sides of your cheeks and dry out your mouth. This stops saliva from continuously flowing and cleansing the mouth resulting in certain types of bacteria forming and staying in your mouth for long periods of time. This creates a persistent bad odor in the mouth that can linger on for hours and develop what is known as "smoker's breath."

Smoking and bad-smelling clothes and hair—The smell of stale smoke tends to linger — not just on people's clothing, but on their hair, furniture, and cars and it's often hard to get the smell of smoke out.

Smoking and reduced athletic performance—People who smoke usually can't compete with non-smoking peers because the physical effects of smoking (like rapid heartbeat, decreased circulation, and shortness of breath) impair sports performance and cause a greater risk of injury and slower healing process once injured. One reason for this is because smoking affects the body's ability to produce collagen, a protein found in all connective tissue that provides strength and form to the skin. In sports, injuries and damage to tendons and ligaments are commonplace and when there is a low amount of collagen in the body due to smoking, the healing process will take longer.

Smoking and increased risk of illness—Studies show that smokers get more colds, flu, bronchitis, and pneumonia than nonsmokers and people with certain health conditions, like asthma become sicker if they smoke or if they're just around people who smoke). Since teens who smoke as a way to manage weight often light up instead of eating, their bodies also lack the nutrients they need to grow, develop, and fight off illness properly. This results in getting sicker more often.

Smoking and Death

In conclusion, cigarette smoking causes more than 480,000 deaths each year in the United States. This is nearly one in five deaths. This is more deaths each year than HIV, illegal drug use, alcohol use, motor vehicle and firearm-related injuries combined. More than 10 times as many U.S. citizens have died prematurely from cigarette smoking than died in all the wars fought by the United States during its history (USDHHS, 2016).

WHAT IT COSTS TO SMOKE

In the last section, the focus was on the health costs of being a smoker. In this section, the focus will be on the individual and governmental financial costs of smoking in the United States.

The Individual Costs of Being A Smoker

Over the years, there has been an extensive amount of research investigating the financial costs of being a smoker and it is estimated that it will cost a smoker between $1 million and $2 million in their lifetime. According to WalletHub, the average smoker starts smoking by age 18 and has a life expectancy of 69 years old and smokes between one and two packs of cigarettes per day for 51 years. At a price range of $7.00-$12.00 per pack it will cost the following over a lifetime: See Table 13.5 for a look at how much it will cost a smoker to smoke two packs of cigarettes a day for 51 years.

Table 13.5
How Much It Costs to Smoke Two Packs of Cigarettes Per Day

Price Per Pack	Daily Cost of 2 Packs Per Day	Weekly Cost of 2 Packs Per Day	Annual Cost of 2 Packs Per Day (365 days)	Cost of Smoking 2 Packs Per Day for 51 Years
$7.00	$14.00	$98.00	$5110	$260,610
$8.00	$16.00	$112.00	$5840	$297,840
$9.00	$18.00	$126.00	$6570	$335,070
$10.00	$20.00	$140.00	$7300	$372,300
$11.00	$22.00	$156.00	$8030	$409,530
$12.00	$24.00	$168.00	$8760	$446,760

It is important to note that the price of a pack of cigarettes will substantially increase over the course of 51 years resulting in the costs dramatically rising. (See Tables 13.6 & 13.7 to review the price of cigarettes by decade beginning in 1940 to 2009 and the actual and projected costs of cigarettes from 2010-2066).

Table 13.6
Actual Cost of Cigarettes from 1940-2009

Years by Decade	Annual Cost of a pack of Cigarettes	% Increase	Annual Cost based on 2 packs per day (365 days)	Cost of Smoking 2 packs per day over 51 years with annual cost increases included
1940-1949	.10 - .15	50	$73.00 - $109.50	$13,287.60
1950-1959	.15 - .20	25	$109.50 - $146.00	$26,522.00
1960-1969	.20 - .28	40	$146.00 - $204.40	$54,707.80
1970-1979	.28 - .46	64	$204.40 - $333.04	$100,821.50
1980-1989	.46 – 1.14	148	$333.04 - $832.20	$157,527.10
1990-1999	$1.14 – 2.47	117	$832.20 - $1803.10	$226,176.64
2000-2009	$2.47 - 5.08	106	$1803.10 - $3708.40	$290,780.50

Table 13.7
Actual and Projected Cost of Cigarettes from 2010-2066

Year	Cost of a pack of Cigarettes	% Increase	Annually (365 days)
2009-2010	$5.08-5.61	10.4	$3708.40 - $4095.30
2010-2011	$5.61-5.80	3.4	$4095.30 - $4234.00
2011-2012	$5.80-5.93	2.1	$4234.00 - $4328.90
2012-2013	$5.93-6.10	2.8	$4328.90 - $4453.00
2013-2014	$6.10-6.28	2.9	$4453.00 - $4584.40
2014-2015	$6.28-6.47	3.0	$4584.40 - $4723.10
2015-2016	$6.47-6.62	2.3	$4723.10 - $4832.60
2016-2017	$6.62-6.75	2.0	$4832.60 - $4927.50
2017-2018	$6.75-6.89	2.1	$4927.50 - $5029.70
2018-2019	$6.89-7.03	2.0	$5029.70 - $5131.90
2019-2020	$7.03-7.17	2.0	$5131.90 - $5234.10
2020-2029	$7.17-8.76	2.0	$5234.10 - $6394.80
2029-2039	$8.76-10.65	2.0	$6394.80 - $7774.50
2039-2049	$10.65-$13.10	2.0	$7774.50 - $9563.00
2049-2059	$13.10-$15.97	2.0	$9563.00 - $11,658.10
2059-2066	$15.97-18.35	2.0	$11,658.10 - $13,396.00

At a conservative increase of 2% annually the price of cigarettes will almost triple over the next 50 years from an average of $6.62 to $18.35 per pack. This will raise the annual cost from $4832 to $13,396. While the annual increases in the price of cigarettes may seem somewhat modest, the end result is that it will cost over $328,000 to smoke two packs of cigarettes over a 50-year period and that's just for cigarettes, alone. To further understand the overall financial costs of being a smoker, WalletHub devised the following formula to determine the true cost of smoking:

Financial Cost of Smoking = Out-of-Pocket Costs + Financial Opportunity Cost + Related Health-Care Costs + Income Loss Due to Smoking-Related Issues + Increase in Homeowner's Insurance Premium + Secondhand Smoke-Exposure Costs (Bernardo, 2016). They used one pack of cigarettes per day beginning at age 18 which is the legal age when a person can purchase tobacco products in the U.S. and a lifespan of 51 years taking into account that 69 years old is the average age when a smoker dies.

Out-of-Pocket Costs

Out-of-Pocket Costs were determined by taking the average cost of a pack of cigarettes in each state and multiplying that figure by the total number of days in 51 years.

Financial Opportunity Cost

To determine the per-person Financial Opportunity Cost, the amount of return a person would have earned by investing that exact same money in the stock market instead of buying cigarettes over the same period. The historical average market return rate for the S&P 500 minus the inflation rate during the same time period to reflect the return in present-value terms was used.

Health-Care Cost per Smoker

To calculate health-care costs, state-level data from the Centers for Disease Control and Prevention was used—namely the annual health care costs incurred from smoking being divided by the total number of adult smokers in each state.

Income Loss per Smoker

Previous studies have demonstrated that smoking can lead to loss of income—either because of absenteeism, workplace bias or lower productivity due to smoking-induced health problems—and create a wage gap between smokers and nonsmokers. To represent the negative relationship between earnings and smoking, an average 8 percent decrease in the median household income for each state was used. WalletHub arrived at this figure after accounting for the fact that, according to a recent study from the Federal Reserve Bank of Atlanta, smokers earn 20 percent less than nonsmokers, 8 percent of which is attributed to smoking and 12 percent to other factors (Bernardo, 2016).

Other Costs per Smoker

Nonsmokers are generally entitled to a homeowner's insurance credit of between 5 and 15 percent, according to the Independent Insurance Agents & Brokers of America. Therefore, an 11.1 percent increase (i.e. the inverse of a 10 percent credit, or the average between the two percentages) was used as a penalty cost for smokers. The results of the research from WalletHub are displayed in Table 13.8 The Cost to Smoke Over a Lifetime and Table 13.9 The Cost to Smoke Each Year (based on all 50 states and the District of Columbia).

As you can see, the numbers are quite staggering. Between the actual costs of a pack of cigarettes, the increased rates of health and medical costs, higher insurance premiums and lost productivity at work, smokers are paying between $1 million and $2 million dollars in their lifetime.

Table 13.8
The Cost to Smoke Over a Lifetime

Overall Rank	State	Total Cost per Smoker	Out-of-Pocket Cost (Rank)	Financial Opportunity Cost (Rank)	Health-Care Cost per Smoker (Rank)	Income Loss per Smoker (Rank)	Other Costs per Smoker (Rank)
1	Louisiana	$1,232,159	$87,937 (2)	$831,542 (2)	$115,351 (4)	$183,563 (8)	$13,765 (46)
2	Kentucky	$1,238,247	$90,022 (6)	$851,257 (6)	$111,475 (1)	$176,835 (4)	$8,658 (2)
3	Missouri	$1,254,421	$84,754 (1)	$801,442 (1)	$162,421 (28)	$194,877 (15)	$10,927 (29)
4	West Virginia	$1,255,852	$90,618 (7)	$856,890 (7)	$130,965 (10)	$169,630 (3)	$7,749 (1)
5	North Carolina	$1,263,332	$88,570 (4)	$837,527 (4)	$136,258 (13)	$190,507 (11)	$10,469 (23)
6	Georgia	$1,271,346	$89,222 (5)	$843,688 (5)	$125,750 (8)	$201,315 (20)	$11,371 (31)
7	Tennessee	$1,279,003	$93,131 (10)	$880,653 (10)	$113,598 (3)	$182,054 (6)	$9,567 (12)
8	South Carolina	$1,289,352	$92,833 (9)	$877,837 (9)	$124,027 (7)	$183,735 (9)	$10,920 (28)
9	Mississippi	$1,297,564	$95,886 (14)	$906,705 (14)	$122,394 (5)	$161,013 (1)	$11,565 (32)
10	Alabama	$1,305,465	$94,974 (13)	$898,080 (13)	$123,213 (6)	$177,525 (5)	$11,674 (33)
11	North Dakota	$1,311,675	$88,105 (3)	$833,127 (3)	$152,843 (23)	$226,762 (32)	$10,838 (27)
12	Idaho	$1,326,531	$94,173 (11)	$890,511 (11)	$139,159 (14)	$193,123 (14)	$9,565 (11)

Overall Rank	State	Total Cost per Smoker	Out-of-Pocket Cost (Rank)	Financial Opportunity Cost (Rank)	Health-Care Cost per Smoker (Rank)	Income Loss per Smoker (Rank)	Other Costs per Smoker (Rank)
13	Virginia	$1,358,856	$91,418 (8)	$864,459 (8)	$128,766 (9)	$264,351 (43)	$9,861 (16)
14	Arkansas	$1,362,519	$102,531 (22)	$969,546 (22)	$112,122 (2)	$168,357 (2)	$9,962 (19)
15	Indiana	$1,388,677	$100,335 (18)	$948,775 (18)	$131,814 (11)	$198,847 (16)	$8,905 (5)
16	Kansas	$1,392,642	$97,673 (15)	$923,603 (15)	$147,284 (19)	$211,638 (24)	$12,444 (36)
17	Wyoming	$1,393,990	$94,937 (12)	$897,728 (12)	$153,921 (24)	$237,668 (35)	$9,736 (13)
18	Oklahoma	$1,407,926	$102,327 (21)	$967,610 (21)	$136,245 (12)	$188,639 (10)	$13,106 (42)
19	Nevada	$1,413,733	$99,143 (16)	$937,509 (16)	$154,250 (25)	$212,996 (25)	$9,834 (14)
20	Nebraska	$1,430,473	$99,143 (16)	$937,509 (16)	$168,249 (33)	$213,792 (26)	$11,780 (34)
21	Florida	$1,453,333	$103,276 (23)	$976,587 (23)	$163,277 (31)	$192,625 (13)	$17,569 (51)
22	Ohio	$1,466,537	$105,603 (24)	$998,590 (24)	$154,322 (26)	$199,304 (18)	$8,719 (3)
23	Colorado	$1,467,140	$101,098 (19)	$955,992 (19)	$155,007 (27)	$242,548 (37)	$12,495 (38)
24	Oregon	$1,478,915	$106,236 (25)	$1,004,575 (25)	$152,750 (22)	$206,126 (23)	$9,228 (7)
25	Iowa	$1,502,649	$107,799 (27)	$1,019,361 (27)	$150,567 (21)	$215,081 (28)	$9,840 (15)
26	California	$1,512,519	$101,917 (20)	$963,737 (20)	$182,119 (38)	$250,875 (42)	$13,871 (47)
27	Texas	$1,515,958	$107,278 (26)	$1,014,432 (26)	$163,066 (30)	$214,510 (27)	$16,671 (50)
28	South Dakota	$1,532,326	$110,406 (29)	$1,044,005 (29)	$162,676 (29)	$205,379 (22)	$9,861 (17)
29	Montana	$1,570,221	$117,200 (31)	$1,108,254 (31)	$144,070 (16)	$190,805 (12)	$9,892 (18)
30	New Mexico	$1,570,517	$117,963 (32)	$1,115,471 (32)	$143,615 (15)	$183,469 (7)	$9,999 (20)
31	Delaware	$1,578,303	$108,302 (28)	$1,024,114 (28)	$191,345 (39)	$245,742 (39)	$8,800 (4)
32	Michigan	$1,618,008	$120,849 (36)	$1,142,755 (36)	$145,008 (18)	$200,275 (19)	$9,122 (6)
33	Utah	$1,639,415	$118,187 (33)	$1,117,583 (33)	$144,716 (17)	$244,172 (38)	$14,758 (49)

Overall Rank	State	Total Cost per Smoker	Out-of-Pocket Cost (Rank)	Financial Opportunity Cost (Rank)	Health-Care Cost per Smoker (Rank)	Income Loss per Smoker (Rank)	Other Costs per Smoker (Rank)
34	Pennsylvania	$1,647,463	$120,309 (34)	$1,137,650 (34)	$163,282 (32)	$216,709 (30)	$9,513 (10)
35	New Hampshire	$1,665,509	$113,086 (30)	$1,069,352 (30)	$203,236 (43)	$269,223 (44)	$10,612 (25)
36	Arizona	$1,677,137	$125,688 (38)	$1,188,521 (38)	$149,071 (20)	$203,706 (21)	$10,150 (21)
37	Maine	$1,680,849	$121,537 (37)	$1,149,268 (37)	$201,575 (42)	$199,120 (17)	$9,349 (8)
38	Maryland	$1,782,364	$120,439 (35)	$1,138,882 (35)	$208,567 (45)	$302,528 (51)	$11,948 (35)
39	Illinois	$1,828,314	$134,922 (39)	$1,275,830 (39)	$173,100 (34)	$233,237 (34)	$11,225 (30)
40	Wisconsin	$1,867,305	$140,171 (42)	$1,325,469 (42)	$177,071 (37)	$215,171 (29)	$9,424 (9)
41	Vermont	$1,945,299	$143,131 (43)	$1,353,457 (43)	$215,858 (46)	$222,144 (31)	$10,710 (26)
42	Dist Columbia	$1,949,488	$136,113 (40)	$1,287,095 (40)	$231,274 (47)	$282,479 (47)	$12,528 (39)
43	New Jersey	$1,953,106	$138,272 (41)	$1,307,514 (41)	$200,823 (41)	$294,013 (50)	$12,484 (37)
44	Washington	$1,954,162	$145,476 (45)	$1,375,636 (45)	$176,558 (36)	$246,000 (40)	$10,492 (24)
45	Minnesota	$1,973,941	$145,458 (44)	$1,375,460 (44)	$192,062 (40)	$248,178 (41)	$12,783 (40)
46	Rhode Island	$2,088,485	$153,537 (47)	$1,451,855 (47)	$239,578 (48)	$230,206 (33)	$13,310 (43)
47	Connecticut	$2,138,139	$152,848 (46)	$1,445,342 (46)	$241,423 (50)	$285,188 (48)	$13,338 (44)
48	Hawaii	$2,186,781	$164,538 (49)	$1,555,886 (49)	$175,171 (35)	$278,260 (46)	$12,927 (41)
49	Alaska	$2,243,640	$165,692 (50)	$1,566,799 (50)	$207,792 (44)	$293,062 (49)	$10,294 (22)
50	Massachusetts	$2,269,056	$163,458 (48)	$1,545,676 (48)	$269,447 (51)	$276,812 (45)	$13,663 (45)
51	New York	$2,452,735	$187,379 (51)	$1,771,868 (51)	$240,162 (49)	$239,443 (36)	$13,883 (48)

Table 13.9
The Cost to Smoke Per Year

Overall Rank	State	Total Cost per Smoker	Out-of-Pocket Cost (Rank)	Financial Opportunity Cost (Rank)	Health-Care Cost per Smoker (Rank)	Income Loss per Smoker (Rank)	Other Costs per Smoker (Rank)
1	Louisiana	$24,160	$1,724 (2)	$16,305 (2)	$2,262 (4)	$3,599 (8)	$270 (46)
2	Kentucky	$24,279	$1,765 (6)	$16,691 (6)	$2,186 (1)	$3,467 (4)	$170 (2)
3	Missouri	$24,596	$1,662 (1)	$15,715 (1)	$3,185 (28)	$3,821 (15)	$214 (29)
4	West Virginia	$24,625	$1,777 (7)	$16,802 (7)	$2,568 (10)	$3,326 (3)	$152 (1)
5	North Carolina	$24,771	$1,737 (4)	$16,422 (4)	$2,672 (13)	$3,735 (11)	$205 (23)
6	Georgia	$24,928	$1,749 (5)	$16,543 (5)	$2,466 (8)	$3,947 (20)	$223 (31)
7	Tennessee	$25,078	$1,826 (10)	$17,268 (10)	$2,227 (3)	$3,570 (6)	$188 (12)
8	South Carolina	$25,281	$1,820 (9)	$17,212 (9)	$2,432 (7)	$3,603 (9)	$214 (28)
9	Mississippi	$25,442	$1,880 (14)	$17,779 (14)	$2,400 (5)	$3,157 (1)	$227 (32)
10	Alabama	$25,597	$1,862 (13)	$17,609 (13)	$2,416 (6)	$3,481 (5)	$229 (33)
11	North Dakota	$25,719	$1,728 (3)	$16,336 (3)	$2,997 (23)	$4,446 (32)	$213 (27)
12	Idaho	$26,010	$1,847 (11)	$17,461 (11)	$2,729 (14)	$3,787 (14)	$188 (11)
13	Virginia	$26,644	$1,793 (8)	$16,950 (8)	$2,525 (9)	$5,183 (43)	$193 (16)
14	Arkansas	$26,716	$2,010 (22)	$19,011 (22)	$2,198 (2)	$3,301 (2)	$195 (19)
15	Indiana	$27,229	$1,967 (18)	$18,603 (18)	$2,585 (11)	$3,899 (16)	$175 (5)
16	Kansas	$27,307	$1,915 (15)	$18,110 (15)	$2,888 (19)	$4,150 (24)	$244 (36)
17	Wyoming	$27,333	$1,862 (12)	$17,603 (12)	$3,018 (24)	$4,660 (35)	$191 (13)
18	Oklahoma	$27,606	$2,006 (21)	$18,973 (21)	$2,671 (12)	$3,699 (10)	$257 (42)
19	Nevada	$27,720	$1,944 (16)	$18,383 (16)	$3,025 (25)	$4,176 (25)	$193 (14)

Overall Rank	State	Total Cost per Smoker	Out-of-Pocket Cost (Rank)	Financial Opportunity Cost (Rank)	Health-Care Cost per Smoker (Rank)	Income Loss per Smoker (Rank)	Other Costs per Smoker (Rank)
20	Nebraska	$28,048	$1,944 (16)	$18,383 (16)	$3,299 (33)	$4,192 (26)	$231 (34)
21	Florida	$28,497	$2,025 (23)	$19,149 (23)	$3,202 (31)	$3,777 (13)	$344 (51)
22	Ohio	$28,756	$2,071 (24)	$19,580 (24)	$3,026 (26)	$3,908 (18)	$171 (3)
23	Colorado	$28,767	$1,982 (19)	$18,745 (19)	$3,039 (27)	$4,756 (37)	$245 (38)
24	Oregon	$28,998	$2,083 (25)	$19,698 (25)	$2,995 (22)	$4,042 (23)	$181 (7)
25	Iowa	$29,464	$2,114 (27)	$19,987 (27)	$2,952 (21)	$4,217 (28)	$193 (15)
26	California	$29,657	$1,998 (20)	$18,897 (20)	$3,571 (38)	$4,919 (42)	$272 (47)
27	Texas	$29,725	$2,103 (26)	$19,891 (26)	$3,197 (30)	$4,206 (27)	$327 (50)
28	South Dakota	$30,046	$2,165 (29)	$20,471 (29)	$3,190 (29)	$4,027 (22)	$193 (17)
29	Montana	$30,789	$2,298 (31)	$21,730 (31)	$2,825 (16)	$3,741 (12)	$194 (18)
30	New Mexico	$30,794	$2,313 (32)	$21,872 (32)	$2,816 (15)	$3,597 (7)	$196 (20)
31	Delaware	$30,947	$2,124 (28)	$20,081 (28)	$3,752 (39)	$4,818 (39)	$173 (4)
32	Michigan	$31,726	$2,370 (36)	$22,407 (36)	$2,843 (18)	$3,927 (19)	$179 (6)
33	Utah	$32,145	$2,317 (33)	$21,913 (33)	$2,838 (17)	$4,788 (38)	$289 (49)
34	Pennsylvania	$32,303	$2,359 (34)	$22,307 (34)	$3,202 (32)	$4,249 (30)	$187 (10)
35	New Hampshire	$32,657	$2,217 (30)	$20,968 (30)	$3,985 (43)	$5,279 (44)	$208 (25)
36	Arizona	$32,885	$2,464 (38)	$23,304 (38)	$2,923 (20)	$3,994 (21)	$199 (21)
37	Maine	$32,958	$2,383 (37)	$22,535 (37)	$3,952 (42)	$3,904 (17)	$183 (8)
38	Maryland	$34,948	$2,362 (35)	$22,331 (35)	$4,090 (45)	$5,932 (51)	$234 (35)
39	Illinois	$35,849	$2,646 (39)	$25,016 (39)	$3,394 (34)	$4,573 (34)	$220 (30)
40	Wisconsin	$36,614	$2,748 (42)	$25,990 (42)	$3,472 (37)	$4,219 (29)	$185 (9)

Overall Rank	State	Total Cost per Smoker	Out-of-Pocket Cost (Rank)	Financial Opportunity Cost (Rank)	Health-Care Cost per Smoker (Rank)	Income Loss per Smoker (Rank)	Other Costs per Smoker (Rank)
41	Vermont	$38,143	$2,806 (43)	$26,538 (43)	$4,233 (46)	$4,356 (31)	$210 (26)
42	Dist Columbia	$38,225	$2,669 (40)	$25,237 (40)	$4,535 (47)	$5,539 (47)	$246 (39)
43	New Jersey	$38,296	$2,711 (41)	$25,638 (41)	$3,938 (41)	$5,765 (50)	$245 (37)
44	Washington	$38,317	$2,852 (45)	$26,973 (45)	$3,462 (36)	$4,824 (40)	$206 (24)
45	Minnesota	$38,705	$2,852 (44)	$26,970 (44)	$3,766 (40)	$4,866 (41)	$251 (40)
46	Rhode Island	$40,951	$3,011 (47)	$28,468 (47)	$4,698 (48)	$4,514 (33)	$261 (43)
47	Connecticut	$41,924	$2,997 (46)	$28,340 (46)	$4,734 (50)	$5,592 (48)	$262 (44)
48	Hawaii	$42,878	$3,226 (49)	$30,508 (49)	$3,435 (35)	$5,456 (46)	$253 (41)
49	Alaska	$43,993	$3,249 (50)	$30,722 (50)	$4,074 (44)	$5,746 (49)	$202 (22)
50	Massachusetts	$44,491	$3,205 (48)	$30,307 (48)	$5,283 (51)	$5,428 (45)	$268 (45)
51	New York	$48,093	$3,674 (51)	$34,743 (51)	$4,709 (49)	$4,695 (36)	$272 (48)

What Smoking Costs the United States

According to the American Lung Association, tobacco costs the United States of America $333 billion per year in health-care expenses and lost productivity (Tuttle, 2015). The Surgeon General reports that the estimated economic costs attributable to smoking and exposure to tobacco smoke continue to grow with direct medical costs of at least $130 billion and productivity loses of more than $150 billion per year (Surgeon General.Gov). According to the CDC, smoking costs employers approximately $193 billion annually in direct medical care costs (i.e., visits to the Dr., prescriptions for medications to treat illness related to smoking) and lost productivity (i.e., greater worker absenteeism, performance lower due to illness related to smoking) with studies estimating costs at $5816 per smoker per year for employers (Ting, 2015). Regardless of which source is the most accurate, the fact remains that it costs the United States hundreds of billions of dollars each because of smoking or does it?

All States Make a Profit from Smoking

Believe it or not, each of the 50 states actually makes a profit off of the tobacco industry. In fiscal year 2016, states will collect $25.8 billion from tobacco taxes and legal settlements. This is a dramatic increase from 2011, when state and local cigarette taxes brought in $17.1 billion. In 2009, the federal-per-pack tax soared from 39 cents to $1.01 raising an additional 15.5 billion in 2011. While each state makes a substantial profit on selling cigarettes and other tobacco-related products, they will only spend less than two percent on smoking prevention and cessation programs ($468 million). Currently, North Dakota is the only state that funds tobacco control programs at the CDC's recommended level. Only four other states (Alaska, Maine, Oklahoma and Wyoming) fund tobacco control programs at even half the recommended level.

Increase Cost, Decrease Smoking

As a result of the insufficiency of funds being used by each state to deter smoking, President Obama has raised excise tax on tobacco products to promote smoking cessation. As you know, smoking is a habit that tends to start early in life with four in five adult smokers starting before they were 18 years old. By exercising an increase in cigarette taxes, the cost of a pack of cigarettes increases, making it more difficult for young and lower income people to purchase. According to the Congressional Budget Office (CBO), a 10 percent increase in cigarette prices will lead people under the age of 18 to reduce their smoking by 5-15 percent. Among adults over 18, CBO concludes, the decline would be 3-7 percent. In 2015, President Obama proposed raising the federal cigarette tax from $1.01 to $1.95 per pack in 2015. The CBO estimated that a $1-per-pack increase would result in 8 percent (2.6 million) fewer smokers over age 18 in 2021. An examination of more than 100 international studies articulates the empirical consensus: "Significant increases in tobacco taxes are a highly effective tobacco control strategy and lead to significant improvements in public health (Chaloupka, F., Yurekli, A, & Fong, G.T., 2012).

Presently state surcharges on a pack of cigarettes vary widely, from 17 cents in Missouri to $4.35 in New York (CDC, 2012). See Table 13.10 for a State × State Comparison of the cost of a pack of cigarettes).

You can see, over the course of a lifetime, it costs millions of dollars to smoke. So is it really worth it to pay so much money for a product that increases sickness and medical expenses and decreases job productivity, longevity and quality of life? I think, not! Clearly, smokers are paying more to smoke in their lifetime then they could ever imagine. Moreover, these costs are increasing their frequency and severity of illness, thus depreciating their longevity and quality of life. It's time to stop smoking and in the next section several different strategies are presented to help smokers quit and become smoke-free for the rest of their lives.

Table 13.10
State × State Costs of a Pack of Cigarettes

State	Cost	State	Cost
Alabama	$5.51	Nebraska	$6.23
Alaska	$9.79	Nevada	$6.15
Arizona	$8.05	New Hampshire	$6.64
Arkansas	$6.07	New Jersey	$8.20
California	$5.89	New Mexico	$7.67
Colorado	$5.65	New York	$12.85
Connecticut	$9.52	North Carolina	$5.45
Delaware	$6.35	North Dakota	$5.33
Florida	$6.30	Ohio	$6.03
Georgia	$6.39	Oklahoma	$6.29
Hawaii	$9.55	Oregon	$5.69
Idaho	$5.41	Pennsylvania	$6.85
Illinois	$11.50	Rhode Island	$8.95
Indiana	$5.97	South Carolina	$5.85
Iowa	$6.29	South Dakota	$6.08
Kansas	$5.83	Tennessee	$5.30
Kentucky	$5.40	Texas	$6.69
Louisiana	$5.44	Utah	$6.89
Maine	$7.37	Vermont	$9.62
Maryland	$7.75	Virginia	$5.25
Massachusetts	$9.95	Washington	$9.30
Michigan	$8.00	Washington DC	$7.99
Minnesota	$8.10	West Virginia	$5.43
Mississippi	$6.34	Wisconsin	$8.82
Missouri	$5.25	Wyoming	$5.41
Montana	$5.46		

HOW TO QUIT SMOKING!!

This section will focus on a variety of strategies and interventions to help smokers quit and include the following:

1. Why it is so hard to quit smoking?
2. Focus on your health
3. Five ways to quit smoking
4. NRT
5. Behavior mod

Mark Twain once said, "Quitting smoking is easy. I've done it a thousand times." Well, contrary to Mr. Twain's thoughts, quitting smoking is not an easy process. While over 48 million people in the United States have quit smoking for good, there are still 36.5 million people today who continue to smoke (King, Neff, et al., 2016). The U.S. Surgeon General has said, "Smoking cessation (stopping smoking) represents the single most important step that smokers can take to enhance the length and quality of their lives." To have the best chance of quitting and staying quit, you need to know what you're up against, what your options are, and where to go for help.

Why is it so hard to quit smoking?

The answer is nicotine! Nicotine is a drug found naturally in tobacco that acts as a stimulant and causes a person to become physically dependent and emotionally addicted to it. The physical dependence causes unpleasant withdrawal symptoms when you try to quit and the emotional and mental dependence make it hard to stay away from nicotine after you quit. This level of dependence is referred to as an addiction (See Table 13.11 for a list of withdrawal symptoms commonly caused by smoking cessation). Interestingly, more people in the United States are addicted to nicotine than to any other drug (National Institute on Drug Abuse, 2012). In fact, research has inferred that nicotine may be as or even more addictive than heroin, cocaine, or alcohol.

Table 13.11
Withdrawal Symptoms Commonly Caused by Smoking Cessation

Feeling irritable, angry, or anxious	
Having difficulty thinking and trouble concentrating	Sleep disturbances, including having trouble falling asleep and staying asleep, and having bad dreams or even nightmares
Craving tobacco products	
Increased appetite and weight gain	Restlessness or boredom
Dizziness	Headaches
Depression	Tiredness
Feelings of frustration, impatience, and anger	Constipation and gas
Anxiety	Cough, dry mouth, sore throat, and nasal drip
	Chest tightness
	Lower heart rate

These symptoms can lead the smoker to start smoking again to boost blood levels of nicotine back to a level where there are no symptoms. (www.cancer.org)/ssLINK/guide-to-quitting-smoking-how-to-quit" \t "_top" How to quit.")

In most cases, regular smokers will still have nicotine or its by-products, such as cotinine, in their bodies for about 3 to 4 days after stopping. During this process, nicotine creates pleasant feelings and distracts the smoker from unpleasant feelings. This makes the smoker want to smoke again. Nicotine also acts as a kind of depressant by interfering with the flow of information between nerve cells. Smokers tend to smoke more cigarettes as the nervous system adapts to nicotine. This, in turn, increases the amount of nicotine in the smoker's blood. Over time, the smoker develops a tolerance to the drug. Tolerance means that it takes more nicotine to get the same effect that the smoker used to get from smaller amounts. This leads to an increase in smoking. At some point, the smoker reaches a certain nicotine level and then keeps smoking to keep the level of nicotine within a comfortable range.

There is some evidence that other chemicals in cigarette smoke may act with nicotine to make it harder to quit smoking. Research is still going on to learn more about the effects of smoking on monoamine oxidase (a brain chemical) and the substances called harman and norharman. For some people, withdrawal from smoking causes more severe mood problems, which can result in worse cravings and more trouble staying quit.

It is important to mention that smokers who are on medication for other pre-existing conditions or ailments put themselves at severe risk when they smoke because smoking can make the body get rid of some drugs faster than usual. When you quit smoking, it may change the levels of these drugs. Though it's not truly withdrawal, this change can cause problems and add to the discomfort of quitting. Therefore, it is important to ask your doctor if any medicines you take need to be checked or changed after you quit. (www.cancer.org/AboutUs/Honoring PeopleWhoAreMakingADifference/the-leo-rosen-family" 2012).

Focus on Your Health

One of the most powerful ways to enhance your motivation to quit smoking is to focus on your health. To put it simply, who does not want to live a healthy lifestyle? Who does not want to be able to breathe freely, without constant coughing, congestion and getting out of breath? Clearly, nobody wants to get sick and die from smoking and people who stop smoking significantly reduce their risk for disease and early death. Consequently, a key component of any tobacco cessation program is to encourage and help tobacco users to quit by emphasizing the immediate and long-term health benefits. Although quitting smoking at any age has its benefits, research has found that smokers who quit by the time they are 35 to 44 years of age avoid most of the risk of dying from a smoking-related disease (Ramasunarahettige, Landsman, Rostron, Thun, Anderson, McAfee, & Petro, 2013). Here is a list of the health benefits associated with smoking cessation:

- Reduced risk of developing some lung diseases (e.g., chronic obstructive pulmonary disease (COPD).

- Lowered risk for lung and many other types of cancer (mouth, throat, esophagus, and bladder).

- Reduced risk for heart disease, stroke, peripheral vascular disease (narrowing of the blood vessels outside your heart).

- Circulation improves and lung function increases.

- Reduced respiratory symptoms, such as coughing, wheezing, and shortness of breath.

- Reduced risk of diabetes.

- Reduced risk for infertility in woman of childbearing age.

- Women who stop smoking during pregnancy also reduce the risk of having a low birth weight baby.

- Ex-smokers live longer than people who keep smoking.

These are just a few of the health benefits of quitting smoking for good. The earlier you quit, the more you will reduce your health risks, however, quitting at any age can give back years of life that would be lost by continuing to smoke.

Five Ways to Quit Smoking

In many cases, smokers may recognize that it is time to stop smoking, yet not be sure of how to do so. Therefore, the very first step before a smoker selects a treatment should be to consult their physician and discuss the available treatments and what might be best for the smoker. Research has discovered a variety of different treatments to help people stop smoking. This section will introduce five different treatments that have been proven to be effective for smokers who want help to quit and they are: (1) Going Cold Turkey; (2) Mayo Clinic's 10 Step Process; (3) Reader's Digest 25 Strategies; (4) Rating The Importance of Your Smoking and (5) Nicotine Replacement Therapy (NRT).

1. *Going Cold Turkey*—One-way people try to quit smoking is by going "cold turkey." Cold turkey means relying solely on your willpower to quit. There are no drugs, no therapy and no replacement cigarettes to help you quit. Obviously, willpower is essential in quitting. You have to have the desire, both mentally and physically to quit and withstand the feelings, cravings and emotions that go along with smoking. Unfortunately, only 5% of the 15 million smokers who try to call it quits every year actually succeed (https://www.quit.com/considerong/cold-turkey.html). As alluded to in the previous section, the reason why this number is so low is because the nicotine in cigarettes is so addictive. People often underestimate how difficult it is to resist cravings using willpower alone. Without any help, overcoming smoking addiction can wind up being a lot tougher than it needs to be.

   Another very effective way to stop smoking is through behavior modification therapy. For quite some time, your behavior has revolved around smoking. As soon as you receive a craving to smoke the immediate thought is to satisfy that craving with a cigarette and while smoking may have started with a behavior for social acceptance, it soon became a powerful mental and physical addiction effecting your behavior multiple times per day. To put it simply, the way to quit is to change the behavior. Treatments 2, 3 and 4 are all behavioral modification therapies that you may find useful in quitting smoking.

2. ***Mayo Clinic's 10 Step Process***—The Mayo Clinic is a nonprofit organization that emphasizes research, education and clinical practice in caring for individuals who need healing. More than 45,000 people have used the services of the Mayo Clinic's Nicotine Dependence Center to learn to stop smoking or chewing tobacco. Here is just one of a variety of programs that the Mayo Clinic offers which is 10-step process to help smokers resist the urge to smoke and eventually quit.

   a. ***Delay***. Once you get the craving to smoke and you feel that tobacco craving, tell yourself that you must wait 10 more minutes and then do something to distract yourself for that period of time. This simple trick may be enough to derail your tobacco craving.

   b. ***Don't have "just one."*** Sometimes you might rationalize that you just want one cigarette to satisfy your tobacco craving. Don't fool yourself into believing that that you can stop at just one. More often than not, have "just one" leads to another and then another…

   c. ***Avoid triggers***. Your urges for tobacco are most likely the strongest in the situations and environments where you frequented smoking most often such as in your car, after a meal, with co-workers or friends who smoke, at parties or bars, etc. Identify your trigger situation and have a plan to replace smoking with something healthier like eating a fruit, chewing a piece of gum, talking to a friend, playing a game on your cell phone or drinking a bottle of water.

   d. ***Get physical***. Physical activity can help distract you from tobacco cravings and reduce the intensity of your cravings. So, when you get the urge to smoke, consider going for a walk or jog. If you are stuck at home or behind the desk at work, consider doing a few stretches, lunges, squats or even jogging in place for a minute or two. If physical activity doesn't interest you then how about doing some writing, crossword puzzles, playing card or board games on your cell phone or computer, meditating or praying, or even chores such as cleaning or organizing.

   e. ***Practice relaxation techniques***. While some individuals sought smoking as a way to relax, the chemicals in cigarettes have been found to create the opposite effect forcing the body to work harder to do basic functions like breathing. Nevertheless, people who want to quit smoking may find it a stressful process and therefore it can be helpful to engage in relaxation techniques such as deep breathing exercises, yoga, meditation, muscle relaxation, imagery, hypnosis and massage therapy.

   f. ***Call for reinforcements***. When you feel the struggle to resist smoking, touch base with a family member, friend of support group member for encouragement and moral support. Have a phone conversation that has nothing to do with smoking, go for a walk, share a good laugh or discuss your cravings.

g. ***Remember the benefits of quitting.*** When you get the urge to start smoking start writing down or verbally say out loud all the benefits of quitting and resisting tobacco cravings. Things like feeling better, living healthier, sparing your loved ones from secondhand smoke, breathing better, and saving countless dollars.

h. ***Go online.*** Go online and join a stop-smoking group or program. Read what others in your situation have gone through and how they succeeded.

i. ***Try nicotine replacements.*** Instead of smoking a cigarette, you can try a nicotine replacement. These include patches, gums, lozenges and nicotine replacement therapy which can be bought over the counter. You can also get nicotine nasal spray and the nicotine inhaler by prescription.

j. ***Chew on it.*** To fight your tobacco craving, you can give your mouth something else to do by chewing on sugarless gum or sucking on a hard candy. You can also eat vegetables like raw carrots or celery, nuts or sunflower seeds—something crunchy and satisfying (www.mayoclinic.org).

3. ***Reader's Digest 25 Ways to Stop Smoking*** Similar to the Mayo Clinic, Reader's Digest published a list of 25 Strategies to stop smoking cigarettes (www.rd.com/health/wellness/25-ways-to-stop-smoking-cigarettes?).

a. ***Make an honest list of all the things you like about smoking.*** Take a piece of paper and draw a line down the center of it and in column one create an honest list of all the things you like about smoking and in column two create a list of all the things you dislike about smoking. Get feedback from family, friends, co-workers about what they dislike about your use of cigarettes. When the negative side outweighs the positive side, you are ready to quit.

b. ***Create another list of why quitting won't be easy.*** Be thorough. Next to each of the items that you listed, list one or more options for overcoming that challenge. For example, you might write that "smoking helps me deal with stress." Then you write that you are going to start walking or jogging. The more you anticipate the challenges to quitting and provide yourself with a viable solution, the better your chances of success.

c. ***Set a quit date*** and write a "quit date contract" that includes your signature and that of a supportive witness.

d. ***Write down all of you reasons for quitting on an index card*** and keep it near you at all times. For example, live longer for my parents, my children, my friends, etc.

e. ***As you're getting ready to quit, stop buying cartons of cigarettes.*** Instead, buy one pack at a time and only carry two or three cigarettes with you at once. Eventually, you will find that when you want to smoke, you won't have any immediate cigarettes available and this will slowly wean you down to fewer cigarettes.

f. ***Keep a list of when you smoke,*** what you're doing at the time, and how bad the cravings are about a week before you decide to quit and see if specific times of the day or activities increase your cravings to smoke. Then plan to do fun, interesting things that you enjoy during those times to replace the craving to smoke (See Table 13.12 for a List of When You Smoke).

g. ***Prepare a list of things to do when a craving hits.*** For example, take a walk, drink a glass of water, hug your child, play fetch with your dog, wash your car, play a game on your cellphone, brush your teeth, chew a piece of gum, wash your face, practice deep breathing, praise yourself. Make copies of your list and keep one with you at all times so when the craving comes, you can whip out your list and quickly do something to take your mind off of smoking.

h. ***When your quit date arrives, throw out anything that reminds you of smoking.*** This includes all smoking paraphernalia-leftover cigarettes, matches, lighters, ashtrays, cigarette holders, and even the lighter in your car.

i. ***Instead of a cigarette break at work, play a game of solitaire on your computer*** or perhaps, a phone call, a stroll, a stretch at your desk, eating a piece of fruit can all serve to divert your attention away from the sensation to smoke and onto something else that occupies yourself for a few minutes. Plus, playing games is a lot more fun than smoking.

j. ***Switch to a cup of herbal tea whenever you usually have a cigarette.*** This might be at breakfast, midmorning, or after meals. The act of brewing the tea and slowly sipping it as it cools can provide the same stress relief as a hit of nicotine.

k. ***Switch your cigarette habit for a nut habit—four nuts in their shell for every cigarette you want to smoke.*** This way, you're using your hands and your mouth, getting the same physical and oral sensations you get from smoking.

l. ***Carry some cinnamon-flavored toothpicks with you—****Suck on the toothpick when a cigarette craving comes.*

m. ***Make an appointment with an acupuncturist.*** There is some evidence that auricular acupuncture (i.e., needles in the ears) curbs cigarette cravings quite successfully.

n. ***Go to the health food store for some Avena sativa (oat) extract.*** One study found that taken at 1 milliliter four times daily helped habitual tobacco smokers significantly decrease the number of cigarettes smoked.

0. ***Think of difficult things you have done in the past.*** Focus on the challenges that you faced and overcame successfully. Ask people who know you well to remind you of the challenges you faced in last and successfully overcame. This can increase your self-confidence to persevere not to smoke rather than give up.

p. ***To minimize cravings, you can change your routine.*** Sit in a different chair during meal time. Take a different route to work. Eat different foods. Plan to go for a walk during times when you plan to have a cigarette. Switch from coffee to tea.

q. ***Tell your friends, coworker, boss, partner, kids, etc., how you feel about situations instead of bottling up your emotions.*** Express your emotions rather than running for a cigarette. If you're angry, express it. If you're bored, express it and then find something energetic to do instead of lighting up (e.g., listening to music and dancing).

r. ***If you relapse, just start again.*** You haven't failed as long as you stay in action. Simply start again.

s. ***Put all the money you're saving on cigarettes in a large glass jar.*** You want to physically see how much you've been spending. Put a note on the jar for something you've always dreamed of doing, but couldn't afford like a cruise to Alaska or a new luxury car.

t. ***Switch to decaf until you've been cigarette free for two months.*** Two much caffeine while quitting can cause jitters.

u. ***Create a smoke-free zone.*** Do not allow anyone to use tobacco in your home and car. If you plan to go to a restaurant, make sure it is no smoking and if not, choose a restaurant that is smoke free. Create actual "No-Smoking" signs to hang in your house and your car.

v. ***Find a healthy snack food you*** and can keep it with you and use it in place of cigarettes to quench that urge for oral gratification. For example, try pistachio nuts, sunflower seeds, sugarless gum or lollipops, carrots or celery sticks.

w. ***Picture yourself playing sports.*** Researchers have found that people trying to quit smoking were better able to ignore their urges to smoke when they were told to visualize a tennis match. In case you don't play tennis, you can visualize many sports/activities that can decrease the urge to smoke like baseball, basketball, bowling, football, golf, hockey or soccer. Finally, how about taking up any one of these sports to replace smoking.

x. ***Quit when you're in a good mood.*** Studies have shown that you're less likely to be a successful quitter when you are depressed or under a great deal of stress.

y. ***Post this list in a visible location in your house.*** Whenever you're tempted to light up, take a look at all the ways smoking can damage your health:

Increases risk of lung, bladder, pancreatic, mouth, esophageal, and other cancers including leukemia

Reduces fertility

Contributes to think bones

Affects mental capacity and memory

Reduces levels of folate, low levels of which can increase the risk of heart disease, depression, and Alzheimer's disease

Increases likelihood of impotence

Affects ability to smell and taste

Results in low-birth-weight, premature babies

Increases risk of depression in adolescents

Increases risk of heart disease, stroke, high blood pressure

Increases risk of diabetes

Increases your child's risk of obesity and diabetes later in life if you smoked while pregnant

4. ***Rating the Importance of Your Smoking***—The next method to stop smoking is a four-step process that I created that involves rating the importance of each time you smoke on a daily basis. Most habitual smokers tend to smoke around the same times and/or places each and every day. Rating how important each cigarette is can help the smoker identify what specific times and/or places smoking is perceived to be more or less important and over time begin to replace smoking with healthy alternatives.

Step One—Quantifying Your Smoking—For one week, write down every cigarette that you smoke on a daily basis. Include the day, time, place and whom if anyone you smoked with. Jot down what you were doing while smoking (i.e., driving, walking, eating, etc.). At the end of the day, count the total number of cigarettes that you smoked and write it down at the bottom of the chart. This will help you to identify if there is a pattern to your smoking. Specifically, do you tend to smoke at the same times of the day, in the same places (car, home, work)? Do you smoke around the same people and if so, are they smokers, too?

Step Two—Rate the Importance of Each Cigarette Smoked—Just before you begin to smoke, rate how important it is for you to smoke at this time in this place from 1 (not important/didn't need it) to 9 (extremely important, had to have it). Once you have completed smoking, use the same scale to rate how important it was to smoke that cigarette. How many cigarettes did you rate 3 or lower? As time goes on, you may realize that your perception to smoke seemed more important than how you felt after you finished smoking.

Step Three—Consider a Healthy Alternative—Take all the cigarettes that you rated 1 to 3 (not important) and consider a healthy-alternative replacement for that cigarette. Since you rated these cigarettes as not important, then it is more than likely that you are smoking at these times simply due to the convenience of or simplicity of smoking more so that the physical or psychological need to smoke at that particular time. Therefore, look to replace smoking at this time with something that takes your mind off of smoking. For example, take a walk or jog in place, chew a piece of gum or suck on a candy, snack on a fruit or vegetable, have a cup of tea or glass of water, call or text a friend, play a game on your phone, create your to-do list and most important pat yourself on the back and praise yourself for the effort you are making to quit smoking. Continue to write down each time you smoke and when the week is up, go back and review your ratings of importance to smoke at the times and places you did. By planning out when not to smoke at certain times of the day and replacing smoking with a healthy alternative, you are taking a powerful step towards reducing the frequency and importance of smoking. Over time, the importance of each cigarette smoked should decrease and what was once considered a "must have" extremely important to smoke has now become a "not important" to smoke.

Step Four Results—Write down how many times you made the switch from smoking to a healthier alternative and how it made you feel to make that switch. When the week is up, simply repeat and keep doing so until you stop smoking.

If you are having difficulty stopping smoking using this method, then you should consider the environment that you frequent each day. If you are constantly surrounding yourself in places where smoking is popular it may be difficult for you to not smoke in these areas. Therefore, you may have to reduce the frequency of time you attend these places. Another important factor for you to consider is who are you spending most of your day with. If you spend lots of time with people that smoke either in your family, your friends or at work then you may have to request that these people do not smoke at certain times that you want to give

Table 13.12
Rating the Importance of My Smoking

# of Cigarettes Smoked	Day and Time When You Smoked	Place Where You Smoked & With Whom	What You Are Doing While Smoking	Importance of Smoking This Cigarette Before and After 1 (not important) to 9 (extremely important)	List Your Healthy Alternatives	How Many Times Did You Switch from Smoking to a Healthy Alternative
1				B 1 2 3 4 5 6 7 8 9 A 1 2 3 4 5 6 7 8 9		
2				B 1 2 3 4 5 6 7 8 9 A 1 2 3 4 5 6 7 8 9		
3				B 1 2 3 4 5 6 7 8 9 A 1 2 3 4 5 6 7 8 9		
4				B 1 2 3 4 5 6 7 8 9 A 1 2 3 4 5 6 7 8 9		

up smoking. If that does not work then you may need to reduce the times you spend with these people that smoke. Remember, stopping smoking is a process that takes times. You need to retrain your mind as well as your body to live without smoking. As you continue to reduce the number of cigarettes you smoke each day, the mental and physical sensation to smoke will decrease. (See Table 13.12 to review how to write down and rate the importance of smoking each and every cigarette over a week to week period.) (You can use Appendix 13A to rate the importance of your smoking and start your smoking cessation process.)

5. **Nicotine Replacement Therapy (NRT)**—NRT is a way of getting nicotine into the bloodstream without smoking so that the withdrawal symptoms can be reduced and eventually stopped. Here are six different types of NRT that are commonly used by smokers who want to quit, yet are addicted to nicotine. The first three (Nicotine Gum, Nicotine Lozenges, and Nicotine Patch) can all be purchased over the counter without a prescription while the Nicotine Inhaler and the Nicotine Nasal Spray are only available by prescription from one's physician.

   A. *Nicotine Gum*—a chewing gum specifically formulated with nicotine to help you kick the smoking habit one craving at a time. Nicotine gum gives you a steady release of nicotine through your mouth and it can help to relieve withdrawal symptoms and cravings to smoke while you are quitting or to help avoid urges to smoke months after quitting.

   How to use Nicotine Gum: Stop all tobacco use. Smoking an occasional cigarette can trigger a relapse and cause nicotine overdose. Chew very slowly until you feel a tingling or peppery taste in your mouth. Then hold the gum inside your cheek until the taste fades and once the peppery taste is gone then you can start to chew slowly. Each time the peppery taste returns, stop chewing and move the gum against a different place on your cheek or gum. Food and drink can affect how well the nicotine is absorbed, so do not eat or drink for at least 15 minutes before and during gum use. When choosing the proper dosage you should think about the following:
   - Do you smoke 25 or more cigarettes per day?
   - Do you smoke within 30 minutes of waking up?
   - Do you have trouble not smoking in restricted areas?

   If you answered yes to any of the 3 above-mentioned questions they you may need to start with a higher gum dose (4 mg). If you smoked fewer than 24 cigarettes per day then you can use the 2mg/piece of gum. It is recommended that you chew no more than 24 pieces if gum in one day. Nicotine gum is recommended for 6 to 12 weeks with the maximum being 6 months. An advantage of nicotine gum is that it allows you to control the nicotine doses. The gum can be used as needed or on a fixed schedule during the day. The most recent research has shown that scheduled dosing works better. A schedule of 1 to 2 pieces per hour is common. On the other hand, with an as-needed schedule, you can use it when you need it most—when you have cravings.

Side Effects and Reactions—Since nicotine has a peppery-like taste it may cause a bad taste in your mouth as well as a tingling sensation when chewed. During the first few days of treatment, you may experience throat irritation, mouth sores, jaw muscle aches, increased saliva production, indigestion, headaches and a rapid heartbeat. As you continue to chew the gum, these effects should disappear. Chewing the gum too fast can cause lightheadedness, dizziness, hiccups, nausea, vomiting or insomnia. If you experience these effects, then chew the gum more slowly. There is a low risk of an allergic reaction which can cause rash, itching, swelling, dizziness, trouble breathing. If you experience any of the symptoms or reactions, seek immediate medication attention.

The maximum recommended length of use is 6 months, but continuing to use the gum may be safer than going back to smoking if the cravings are still strong. Since there is little research on the health effects of long-term nicotine gum use, most health care providers still recommend limiting its use to 6 months. Talk to your doctor if you are having trouble stopping the gum.

Before using this medication, inform your doctor

- If you are taking any prescriptions for depression or asthma. Your dosage may need to be adjusted.
- If you are using non-nicotine stop smoking drugs like Chantix or Zyban.
- If you have heart disease or an irregular heart beat or if you have had a heart attack. Nicotine can increase your heart rate.
- If you have high blood pressure not controlled with medications. Nicotine can increase your blood pressure.
- If you are pregnant or nursing.
- If you experience nausea or vomiting while chewing nicotine gum it can be a sign of nicotine over-dose.

B. ***Nicotine Lozenges***—dissolve in the mouth to release a dose of nicotine to help smokers manage cravings as they occur. Nicotine-containing lozenges can be bought without a prescription. Like nicotine gum, the lozenge is available in 2 strengths: 2 mg and 4 mg. Smokers choose their dose based on how long after waking up they normally have their first cigarette. The lozenge makers recommend using them as part of a 12-week program. The recommended dose is:

- 1 lozenge every 1 to 2 hours for 6 weeks, then
- 1 lozenge every 2 to 4 hours for weeks 7 to 9, and finally,
- 1 lozenge every 4 to 8 hours for weeks 10 to 12.

How to Use the Nicotine Lozenge—When using the Nicotine Lozenge, the lozenge makers recommend:

- Stop all smoking.
- Place the lozenge in your mouth and suck on it until it slowly dissolves fully (about 20-30 minutes).
- Do not bite, chew or swallow the lozenge or pieces of the lozenge if broken since nicotine absorbs through the mucous membranes of the mouth.
- Move the lozenge from one side of the mouth to the other until completely dissolved.
- Do not eat or drink 15 minutes before using or while the lozenge is in the mouth since some drinks can reduce how well the lozenge works.
- It is recommended to use at least 9 lozenges per day for the first 6 weeks.
- Do not use more than one lozenge at a time or continuously use one lozenge after another since this may cause hiccups, heartburn, nausea or other side effects.
- Do not use more than 5 lozenges within a 6-hour time period or more than 20 lozenges per day.
- After 12 weeks, you should stop using the nicotine lozenge. If you still feel you need to use the lozenge, talk to your doctor.

Possible side effects of the nicotine lozenge include:

- Trouble sleeping
- Nausea
- Hiccups
- Coughing
- Heartburn
- Headache
- Flatulence (gas)

C. ***Nicotine Patch***—created to provide less nicotine over time to replace the cravings from cigarettes; The patch is placed on your body like a bandage where a measured dose of nicotine is slowly released into your body through the skin. You are weaned off nicotine by switching to lower-dose patches over a course of weeks. Patches can be bought with or without a prescription and come in a variety of types and strengths including both 16-hour and 24-hour patches. The 16-hour patch works well for light-to-average smokers and it is less likely to cause side effects like skin irritation, racing heartbeat, sleep problems, and headache. Since nicotine is not delivered during the night, it may not be right for those people with early morning withdrawal symptoms. The 24-hour patch provides a steady does of nicotine, avoiding peaks and valleys and it helps with early morning withdrawal. However, there may be more side effects like disrupted sleep patterns and skin irritation. The patch should only be used when you are not smoking and should not be used if you are pregnant. Before using the patch be sure to speak with your doctor especially if you have any of the following:

1. heart disease or irregular heart beat; nicotine can increase your heart rate;
2. high blood pressure that is not controlled with medications; Nicotine can increase your blood pressure.
3. if you are pregnant or nursing; Although NRT is believed to be safer than smoking, the risks to children are not fully known at this time.
4. If you are allergic to adhesives, patch ingredients or skin problems can cause rashes.
5. If you are using non-nicotine stop smoking drugs like Chantix or Zyban.
6. If you are experiencing nausea or vomiting while using the nicotine patch. This can be a sign of nicotine over-dose.
7. If you are taking prescriptions for depression or asthma, your dosage may need to be adjusted. (http://www.nysmokefree.com/Subpage.aspx?pn=PATCH).

It is important to be aware of the possible side effects and reactions to using the nicotine patch and they are:

1. Skin reactions like itching or burning which usually last from 15 to 60 minutes. If you continue to itch or feel a burning sensation, you can change the location of the patch which can reduce irritation.
2. Headache, dizziness, vertigo, insomnia, somnolence (drowsiness).
3. Sleeping problems or unusual dreams. You can remove the patch before you go to sleep if you are having difficulty sleeping with the patch on.
4. Muscle or joint pain, abdominal pain, nausea, diarrhea, and nervousness.
5. Anxiety, irritability, and depression may occur which are usually related more to nicotine withdrawal than the effects of the patch.
6. Racing heartbeat.

D. ***Using the Nicotine Inhaler***—The nicotine inhaler is a thin plastic tube that is shaped like a little cigarette with a nicotine cartridge inside. Unlike other inhalers, which deliver most of the medicine to the lungs, the nicotine inhaler delivers most of the nicotine vapor to the mouth. Nicotine inhalers are the FDA-approved nicotine replacement method that is most like smoking a cigarette, which some smokers find helpful. The nicotine inhaler is only available through prescription and it consists of a mouthpiece and cartridges that contain 10 mg of nicotine. The recommended dosage ranges between 4 and 20 cartridges per day, for up to 6 months.

It is important to note that this form of NRT poses an extra risk to small children and pets, since the used cartridges still have enough nicotine to cause harm if absorbed through the skin or mucous membranes (for instance, if licked or touched to the eyes, mouth, or other mucous membrane). Therefore, be sure to store and dispose the cartridges away from children and pets.

Guidelines for Taking this Medication:
1. Completely quit smoking before using the inhaler.
2. Puff frequently and follow your doctor's directions exactly.
3. Avoid soda, juices, and coffee 15 minutes before and after, as acid inhibits absorption of nicotine.
4. The recommended use is up to 6 months depending on the severity of the smoking addiction.
5. Reduce the frequency of dose over the last three to six months.
6. In temperatures below 40F, nicotine delivery from an inhaler is significantly reduced and therefore cartridges should be kept in an inside pocket or warm area.

Precautions—It is recommended that pregnant smokers should first be encouraged to quit without medicine treatment unless prescribed by their physician. Use caution for patients with cardiovascular conditions, asthma, vasospastic diseases (vascular spasm), over-active thyroid gland, insulin dependent diabetes, active peptic ulcer disease, or accelerated hypertension.

Side Effects
- Heartburn
- Sore throat/oral burning
- Irritation or soreness of the mouth
- Coughing after inhalation
- Rhinitis

E. *Nicotine Nasal Spray*—Nicotine is inhaled into the person's nose from a pump bottle, and absorbed through the nasal lining into the bloodstream. The nasal spray relieves withdrawal symptoms very quickly and lets you control your nicotine cravings. Smokers usually like the nasal spray because it's easy to use. Since Nicotine is addictive, and a person can transfer their dependence from cigarettes to the fast-delivering nasal spray, use it only as long as you need it, or as prescribed by your doctor. The FDA recommends that the spray be prescribed for 3-month periods and that it not be used for longer than 6 months.

One dose consists of 1 spray in each nostril for a total of 1.0 mg of nicotine. There are approximately 100 doses per bottle and you can use the spray up to five times an hour and up to 40 times per day. Initial dosing should be 12 doses per hour, increasing as needed for symptom relief. Eight to 40 doses per day is the recommended range. Generally, you should not use the nasal spray for longer than 6 months. The nasal spray is only available by prescription.

How do I take this medication?
- Stop smoking before using the nasal spray.
- Administer 1 spray to each nostril.
- Tilt your head slightly back when administering.
- To reduce irritating effects, avoid sniffing and swallowing;

Side Effects of Nasal Spray
- Nasal irritation, which should decrease in severity with continued use;
- Runny nose
- Throat irritation
- Coughing
- Watering Eyes
- Sneezing

There is also the danger of using more than is needed. If you have asthma, allergies, nasal polyps, or sinus problems, your doctor may suggest another form of NRT. This form of NRT poses a more serious risk to small children and pets, since even empty bottles of nasal spray contain enough nicotine to harm them. Nicotine absorbs through the skin as well as mucous membranes like the mouth or eyes, and can cause serious harm. If there is any skin contact, rinse thoroughly with plain water right away. If a bottle breaks or liquid leaks out, put on plastic or rubber gloves to clean it up. Call Poison Control and get emergency help if there is any question of overdose.

F. ***Combining Multiple Methods of NRT***—In some cases, combining more than one type of NRT has proven to be effective in helping those smokers who are having difficulty quitting with one type of NRT. There have been a few studies that have been done on combination NRT and they have found that it may work better than a single product. Still, more research is needed to prove this and find safe and effective doses. Presently, the combined use of NRT products has not yet been approved by the FDA. Therefore, if you are thinking about using more than one NRT product, be sure to talk it over with your doctor first.

Which type of nicotine replacement may be right for you?

There's no evidence that any one type of nicotine replacement therapy (NRT) is any better than another. When choosing which type of NRT you will use, think about which method will best fit your lifestyle and pattern of smoking. Do you need something in your mouth or something to keep your hands busy? Or you might be looking for a once-a-day convenience? Some important points to think about when choosing which method of NRT is best for you:

1. Nicotine gums, lozenges, and inhalers are substitutes you can put into your mouth that let you control your dosage to help keep cravings under better control.
2. Nicotine gums and lozenges are generally sugar-free, but if you are diabetic and have any doubts, check with the manufacturer.
3. Nicotine nasal spray works very quickly when you need it.
4. Nicotine inhalers allow you to mimic the use of cigarettes by puffing and holding the inhaler. It also works very quickly.
5. Nicotine patches are convenient and only have to be put on once a day.
6. Both inhalers and nasal sprays require a doctor's prescription.
7. Some people may not be able to use patches, inhalers, or nasal sprays because of allergies or other conditions.
8. Nicotine gum may stick to dentures or dental work making it hard to chew before "parking."

Whatever type you use, take your NRT at the recommended dose, and only for as long as it is recommended. If you use a different dose or stop taking it too soon, it can't be expected to work like it should. If you are a very heavy smoker or a very light smoker, you may want to talk with your doctor about whether your NRT dose should be changed to better suit your needs.

Stopping Nicotine Replacement Therapy

As mentioned earlier, most forms of NRT are meant to be used for limited periods of time. Use should be tapered down to a low dose before NRT is stopped. Research is still being done to refine the use of NRT. For example, even though the patch is usually used for 3 to 5 months, some studies have suggested that using it for 8 weeks or less works just as well. Other researchers, however, have noted that the risk of relapse goes up when nicotine replacement is stopped, even after it has been used for 5 months. These differences have not been fully explained. More studies are needed to learn which smokers are likely to be successful using shorter or longer NRT than usual. If you feel that you need NRT for a different length of time than is recommended, again, it is best to discuss this with your doctor.

In summary, NRT can be a viable method for quitting smoking. Since nicotine has such strong addictive properties, it can be easier to quit smoking by slowly reducing the inhalation/consumption over time instead of going cold turkey. Each of the above mention NRT's provides smokers with several options for quitting that focus on reducing the dependence of nicotine over time until the cravings cease and smoking is no longer a desire.

Counseling Services and Quit Smoking Programs

In addition to the above-mentioned treatments, there is a wide range of counseling services available to help smokers quit. As of 2009, all 50 states and the District of Columbia run some type of free telephone-based program that links callers with trained counselors. These specialists help plan a quit method that fits each person's unique smoking pattern. People who use telephone counseling have twice the success rate in quitting smoking as those who don't get this type of help. For many, telephone counseling is easier to use than some other support programs. It doesn't require driving, transportation, or child care, and it's available nights and weekends. Once treatment begins, counselors may suggest a combination of methods including medicines, local classes, self-help brochures, and/or a network of family and friends. To find counseling to quit smoking you can check with your local physician or insurance company as well as within your local community (i.e., hospitals, wellness centers) for credible counseling services specializing in smoking cessation.

In addition to counseling, there are an array of quit-smoking programs and support groups available for smokers. One long-standing peer help program is Nicotine Anonymous®, an open support group that offers a way to find others who are quitting tobacco and living smoke-free. It also offers a long-term approach to quitting. (www.cancer.org/ssLINK/guide-to-quitting-smoking). Again, some workplaces, hospitals, and wellness centers have stop-smoking programs, groups, or classes, too. They should be led by professionals with expertise in smoking cessation and focus on information and education centered around how to stop smoking.

In conclusion, smoking today has become less socially acceptable than ever. Almost all public workplaces have some type of smoking rules designed to prohibit smoking or designate it to certain areas generally outside of the facility. Some employers even prefer to hire non-smokers because of the increased costs accrued from smoking (out sick more, higher medical insurance premiums, greater maintenance costs). Landlords may choose not to rent to smokers since maintenance costs and insurance rates may rise when smokers live in buildings. Friends and relatives who do not smoke may ask you not to smoke in their homes or cars. Public buildings, concerts, and even sporting events are largely smoke-free and more and more communities are restricting smoking in all public places, including restaurants and bars. Like it or not, finding a place to smoke can be a hassle. Smokers may also find their prospects for dating or romantic involvement, including marriage, are largely limited to other smokers. The bottom line is this. There are far more incentives to quitting smoking than there is to smoke and at the top of the list are: (1) living a healthier lifestyle by reversing some of the harmful effects that smoking causes; (2) saving thousands of dollars per year and over a million dollars in a lifetime and (3) saving the lives of the people who are in your life; So the next time you think about smoking, think again. Choose one of the many behaviors and treatments listed throughout this chapter and enjoy your life.

REFERENCES AND RECOMMENDED READINGS

American Cancer Society. Cancer Facts & Figures 2012. Atlanta, Ga. 2012.

American Lung Association. Trends in Tobacco Use. 2011. Accessed at www.lungusa.org/ finding-cures/our-research/trend-reports/Tobacco-Trend- Report.pdf November 1, 2011.

Bernardo, R. (2016). The true cost of smoking by state. www.wallethub.com/edu/the-financial-costs-of-smoking-by-state/9520. January 18, 2016.

Centers for Disease Control and Prevention. Annual Smoking-Attributable Mortality, Years of Potential Life Lost, and Productivity Losses-United States, 1997-2001. Morbidity and Mortality Weekly Report. 2005; 54(250):625-628).

Centers for Disease Control and Prevention. Annual Smoking-Attributable Mortality, Years of Potential Life Lost, and Productivity Losses-United States, 2000-2004.http://www. cdc.gov/mmwr/preview/mmwrhtml/mm5745a3.htm). Morbidity and Mortality Weekly Report 2008; 57(45):1226-8.

Centers for Disease Control and Prevention. *Annual smoking-attributable mortality, years of potential life lost, and economic costs - United States, 2000-2004.* Morbidity and Mortality Weekly Report. 2008; 57:1226–1228. Accessed at www.cdc.gov/mmwr/preview/ mmwrhtml/mm5745a3.htm on October 26, 2011.

Centers for Disease Control and Prevention. *Asthma's Impact on the Nation: Data from the CDC National Asthma Control Program.* www.cdc.gov/asthma/impacts_nation/ AsthmaFactSheet.pdf.

Centers for Disease Control and Prevention. *Asthma: Back Information* (http://www.cdc.gov/ asthma/fags.htm).

Centers for Disease Control and Prevention. *Best Practices for Comprehensive Tobacco Control Programs-2014.* Atlanta: U.S. Department of Health and Human Services, Centers for Disease Control and Prevention, National Center for Chronic Disease Prevention and Health Promotion, Office on Smoking and Health, 2014.

Centers for Disease Control and Prevention. *Chronic Obstructive, Pulmonary Disease Among Adults-United States, 2011.* Morbidity and Mortality Weekly Report 2012; 61 (46):938-43).

Centers for Disease Control and Prevention. *Cigarette Smoking Among Adults and Trends in Smoking Cessation in the United States, 2008.* Morbidity and Mortality Weekly Report. 2009;58(44): 1227–1232. Accessed at www.cdc.gov/mmwr/preview/mmwrhtml/ mm5844a2.htm.

Centers for Disease Control and Prevention. *Combustible and Smokeless Tobacco Use Among High School Athletes-United States 2001-2013.* Morbidity and Mortality Weekly Report,

2015;   64(34):935-9.   Accessed   at   www.cdc.gov/mmwr/Preview/mmwrhtml. mm6434a2.htmJs cid=mm6434a2w.

Centers for Disease Control and Prevention. *Coronary Artery Disease (CAD),* August, 2015.

Centers for Disease Control and Prevention. QuickStats: Number of Deaths from 10 Leading Causes—National Vital Statistics System, United States, 2010. *Morbidity and Mortality Weekly Report 2013: 62*(08);155 [accessed 2015 Aug 17].

Centers for Disease Control and Prevention. *Quitting Smoking Among Adults-United States. 2001-2010*_____(http://www.cdc.giv/tobacco/datastatistics/mmwrs/byyear/2011 mm6044a2/intro.htm).

Centers for Disease Control and Prevention. *Secondhand Smoke (SHS) Facts.* http://www. cdc.gov/tobacco/data statistics/fact sheets/secondhand smoke/general facts/index.htm).

Centers for Disease Control and Prevention. *Smoking Cessation and Interventions Fact Sheet.* Accessed at www.cdc.gov/tobacco/data_statistics/fact_sheets/Cessation/quitting/index. htm. October 31, 2011.

Centers for Disease Control and Prevention. *Stroke, Nov, 2015.*

Centers for Disease Control and Prevention. Tobacco Use Among Middle and High School Students-United States 2011-2015. *Morbidity and Mortality Weekly Report, 2016; 65*(14):361-7.

Centers for Disease Control and Prevention. *24/7 Saving Lives, Protecting People.* www.cdc. gov/cancer/dcpc/resources/features/lungcancer/).

Centers for Disease Control and Prevention. Vital Signs: Current Cigarette Smoking Among Adults Aged >18 Years – United States, 2005-2010 www.cdc.gov/mmwrpreview/ mmwrhtml" www.cdc.gov/mmwrpreview/mmwrhtml *Morbidity and Mortality Weekly Report 2011; 60*(33):1207-12.

Chaloupka, F.J., Yurekli, A., & Fong, G.T. (2012). Tobacco taxes as a tobacco control strategy, Tobacco Control, 172-180, http://tobaccocontrol.bmj.com/content/21/2/172.full.

Choi, W.S., Ahluwalia, J.S., Harris, K.J. & Okuyemi, K. (2002). Progression to established smoking: The influence of tobacco marketing. *American Journal of Preventative Medicine, 22,* 4, 228-233.

Christen, Arden G. & Joan A. Christen, (1994). "Why is Cigarette Smoking So Addicting?" *Health Values, Vol. 18*, No.1, January/February.

Cobb, NK, Byron, MJ., Abrams, DB., Shields, P.G. (2010). Novel nicotine delivery systems and public health: the rise of the "e-cigarette." *American Journal of Public Health 2010*;100:2340-2.

Dewey, J.D. (1999). Reviewing the relationship between school factors and substance use for Elementary, middle and high school. *Journal of Primary Prevention, 19* (3): 177-225.

Dwyer, J.B., McQuown, S.C., & Leslie, F.M. (2009). The dynamic effects of nicotine on the developing brain. *Pharmacology & Theraputics, 122*, 2, 125-139.

Fibkins, William L., (1993), "Combating Student Tobacco Addiction in Secondary Schools," *NASSP Bulletin,* December.

Gilligan, K. (2015). Understanding Bronchitis Symptoms and Signs. www.knowzo.com

Guidelines for School Health Program to Prevent Tobacco Use and Addiction," (1994). *Journal of School Health, Vol. 64,* No. 9, November.

Howard, G., Burke, G.L., Szklo, M, Tell, G.S., Eckfledt, J. & Evans, G. (1994). Active and passive Smoking associated with increased carotid wall thickness. The atherosclerosis risk in community study. *Arch Inter Med, 154:* 1277-1282.

Institute of Medicine. Secondhand Smoke Exposure and Cardiovascular effects: Making Sense of the Evidence. Accessed at www.iom.edu/~?media/Files/Report%20Files/2009/Secondhand-Smoke-Exposure-and-Cardiovascular-Effects-Making-Sense-of-theEvidence/Second%20%Report%Brief%203.pdf. (PDF-747 KB) Washington:

King, B.A., Jama, A.O., MArynak, K.L., Promoff, G.R.. Attitudes Toward Raising the Minimum Age for Sale for Tobacco Among U.S. Adults. *American Journal of Preventive Medicine 2015.*

Lynch, Barbara S. & Richard J. Bonnie, (1994). *Growing Up Tobacco Free*. Washington D.C., National Academy Press.

Maxwell, J.C. (2016). The Maxwell Report: Year and Fourth Quarter 2015 Cigarette Industry. Richmond, VA:

Metzger, A., Dawes, N., Mermelstein, R., & Wakschlag, L. (2011). Longitudinal modeling of adolescents activity involvement, peer associations, and youth smoking. *Journal of Applied Developmental Psychology, 32,* (1): 1-9

Mokdad AH, Marks JS, Stroup DF, Gerberding JL. Actual Causes of Death in the United States. JAMA: *Journal of the American Medical Association 2004; 291* (10): 1238-45.

National Cancer Institute. Cigars: Health Effects and Trends [PDF–2.93 MB]. Smoking and Tobacco Control Monograph No. 9. Bethesda (MD): U.S. Department of Health and Human Services, National Institutes of Health, National Cancer Institute, 1998. [accessed 2015 Aug 17].

National Heart, Lung, and Blood Institute. How Does COPD Affect Breathing? www.nhlbi.nih.gov/health/public/lung/copd/what-is-copd/how-does-copd-affectbreathing.htm). (November 2015).

National Heart, Lung, and Blood Institute. *What Are the Signs and Symptoms of COPD?* www.nhlbi.nih.gov/health/health-topics/topics/copd/signs.html. July 31, 2015.

National Heart, Lung, and Blood Institute. How is COPD Treated? http://www.nhlbi.nih.gov/health/health-topics/topics/copd/treatment.html July 31, 2015. (National

Institute on Aging, 2016). *Cancer Facts for People Over 50.* (http://www.nia.nih.gov/health/publication/cancer-facts-people-over-50).

National Institute on Drug Abuse. *Research Report Series: Is Nicotine Addictive?* (http://www.drugabuse.gov/publications/research-reports/tobacco/nicotine-addictive). Bethesda, MD: National Institutes of Health, National Institute on Drug Abuse, 2012.

Ockene, IS, Miller NH. Cigarette Smoking, Cardiovascular Disease, and Stroke: A Statement for Healthcare Professionals from the American Heart Association (http://circ/ahajournals.org/content96/93243.full").

Orzechowski & Walker, 2014). *The Tax Burden on Tobacco* (http://www.taxadmin.org/fta/tobacco/papers/tax_burden_2014.pdf). Arlington, VA.

Pollay, R.W. (1964). "Promises, Promises: Self-Regulation of U.S. Cigarette Broadcast Advertising In the 1960's," *Tobacco Control, Vol 3*, (Summer, 1964), pp. 141-142.

Ramasundarahettige, J.P., Landsman, V, Rostron, B., Thun, M, Anderson, RN, McAfee, T, Petro, R. 21st century hazards of smoking and benefits of cessation in the United States. *New England Journal of Medicine, 2013; 368*(4):341-50.

Sargent, J.D., Beach, M.L., Adachi-Mejia, A.M., Gibson, J.J., Titus-Ernstoff, L.T., Carusi, J.P., Swain, S.D., Heatherton, T.F., & Dalton, M.A. (2005). Exposure to movie smoking: its relation to smoking initiation among US adolescents. Pediatrics, 116, (5), 1183-1191.

Sargent, J.D., Beach, M.L., Dalton, M.A., Mott, L.A., Tickler, J.J., Ahrens, M.B., Heatherton, T.F. (2001). Effect of seeing tobacco use in films trying smoking among adolescents: cross sectional study. BMJ (British Medical Journal), 323, (7326): 1394-7.

Shah, R.S. & Cole, J.W. (2010). Smoking and stroke: The more you smoke the more you stroke. Expert review of cardiovascular therapy, 8 7, 917-932.

Spitzer, J. (2001). Smoking and Circulation. Joel's Stop Smoking Library. www.WhyQuit.Com

Thrasher, J.F., Jackson, C., Arillo-Santillan, E., & Sargent, J.D. (2008). Exposure to smoking imagery in popular films and adolescent smoking in Mexico. American Journal of Preventative Medicine. 35 (2): 95-102.

Ting, D, April 1 2015 Smoking: How much does the habit really cost you? Healthplan.com, April, 2015.

Tobacco: The True Cost of Smoking from American Cancer Society http://www.cancer.org/research/infofraphicgallery/tobacco-related-health-care-costsmissing 4 so far!!!!

Tucker, J.S., Martinez, J.F., Ellickson, P.L., Edelen, M.O. (2008). Temporal associations of cigarette smoking with social influences, academic performance, and delinquency: a four-wave longitudinal study from ages 13-23. Psychology of ddictive Behaviors, 22(1), 1-11.

Tuttle, B. (2015). Smoking Can Cost You $1 Million to $2 Million in a Lifetime (www.time.com/money/3676521/smoking-costs-lifetime, January 21, 2015.

U.S. Department of Agriculture. *2012 Census of Agriculture: United States Summary and State Data, Volume 1, Part 51.* (http://agcensus.usda.gov/Publications/2012/ Full_Report/Volume 1, Chapter 1/US/usv1.pdf).

U.S. Department of Health and Human Services. *A Report of the Surgeon General. The Health Consequences of Smoking: What It Means to You.* Atlanta: U.S. Department of Health and Human Services, Centers for Disease Control and Prevention, National Center for Chronic Disease Prevention and Health Promotion, Office of Smoking and Health, 2004.

U.S. Department of Health and Human Services. *How Tobacco Smoke Causes Disease: What It Means to You* (http://www.cdc.gov/tobacco/datastatistics/sgr/2010 consumer booklet/ index.htm).

U.S. Department of Health and Human Services. *Let's Make the Next Generation Tobacco-Free: Your Guide to the 50th Anniversary Surgeon General's Report on Smoking and Health.* (http://www.cdc.gov/tobacco/data statistics/sgr/50th-anniversary/#booklet).

U.S. Department of Health and Human Services. *Million Hearts.* http://millionhearts.hhs.gov/ index.html) Nov/2015.

U.S. Department of Health and Human Services. *Preventing Tobacco Use Among Young People: A Report of the Surgeon General.* Atlanta: U.S. Department of Health and Human Services, Centers for Disease Control and Prevention, Office on Smoking and Health, 1994.

U.S. Department of Health and Human Services. *Preventing Tobacco Use Among Youth and Young Adults: A Report of the Surgeon General.* Atlanta: U.S. Department of Health and Human Services, Centers for Disease Control and Prevention, National Center for Chronic Disease Prevention and Health Promotion, Office on Smoking and Health, 2012.

U.S. Department of Health and Human Services. *Reducing the Health Consequences of Smoking: 25 Years of Progress A Report of the Surgeon* http://profiles.nlm. nih.gov/NN/B/BX/S. Rockville (MD). U.S. Department of Health and Human Services, Public Health Service, Centers for Disease Control, National Center for Chronic Disease Prevention and Health Promotion, Office on Smoking and Health.

U.S. Department of Health & Human Services. *The Health Benefits of Smoking Cessation: A Report of the Surgeon General. 1990.* Accessed at http://profiles.nlm.nih.gov/NN/B/C/T.

U.S. Department of Health and Human Services. *The Health Consequences of Involuntary Exposure to Tobacco Smoke: A Report of the Surgeon General. 2006.* www .surgeongeneral.gov/library/secondhandsmoke/report/

U.S. Department of Health and Human Services. *The Health Consequences of Smoking: A Report of the Surgeon General.* Atlanta: U.S. Department of Health and Human Services, Centers for Disease Control and Prevention, National Center for Chronic Disease

Prevention and Health Promotion, Office on Smoking and Health, 2004 [accessed 2015 Aug 17].

U.S. Department of Health and Human Services. *The Health Consequences of Smoking: A Report of the Surgeon General* (/tobacco/data statistics/sgr/sgr_2004/index.htm). Atlanta: U.S. Department of Health and Human Services, Centers for Disease Control and Prevention, National Center for Chronic Disease Prevention and health Promotion, Office on Smoking and Health.

U.S. Department of Health and Human Services. *The Health Consequences of Smoking-50 Years of Progress: A Report of the Surgeon General*: Atlanta: U.S. Department of Health and Human Services, Centers for Disease Control and Prevention, National Center for Chronic Disease Prevention & Health Promotion, Office on Smoking & Health, 2014.

U.S. Department of Health & Human Services. *The Health Consequences of Smoking: Nicotine Addiction: A Report of the Surgeon General. 1988.* Accessed at www.profiles.nlm.nih.gov/ NN/B/B/Z/D/.

U.S. Department of Health and Human Services. *Women and Smoking: A Report of the Surgeon General* (/tobacco/data statistics/sgr/sgr 2001/index.htm). Rockville (MD): U.S. Department of Health and Human Services, Public Health Service, Office of the Surgeon General, 2001.U.S. Department of Health and Human Services. U.S. Food and Drug Administration. Summary of Results: Laboratory Analysis of Electronic Cigarettes Conducted By FDA. Accessed at www.fda.gov/NewsEvents/PublicHealth Focus/ucm173146.htm.

Wannamathee, S.G., Shaper, A.G., Whincup, P.H. & Walker, M. (1995). Smoking cessation and the Risk of stroke in middle aged men. *JAMA, 274:* 155-160.

Wolf, P.A., D'Agostino, R.B., Kannel, W.B., Bonita, R., & Belanger, A.J. (1988). Cigarette smoking as a Risk factor for stroke. The Framingham Study. *JAMA, 259*, 1025-1029.

World Health Organization. *WHO Report on the Global Tobacco Epidemic, 2011.* Geneva: WHO, 2011.

World Health Organization. *Smokeless Tobacco and Some Tobacco-Specific N-Nitrosamines.* (PDF-3.18 MB). International Agency for Research on Cancer Monographs on the Evaluation of Carcinogenic Risks to Humans Vol. 89. Lyon, (France): World Health Organization, International Agency for Research on Cancer, 2007 [accessed 2015 Aug 17].

Websites

www.cancer.org/ssLINK/guide-to-quitting-smoking.

www.cancer.org/AboutUs/HonoringPeopleWhoAreMakingADifference/the-leo-rosen-family" 2012

www.cdc.gov/cancer/dcpc/prevention/screening.htm).

www.cdc.gov/cancer/dcpc/resources/features/lungcancer/.

www.cdc.gov/mmwr/preview/mmwrhtml/mm6235a6.htm?s_cid=mm6235a6_w

www.cdc.gov/tobacco/data_statistics/fact sheets/fast_facts/index.htm#toll.

www.lung.org/lung-health-and-diseases/lung-disease-lookup/copd/diagnosing, 2016.

www.mayoclinic.org/healthy-lifestyle/quit-smoking-in-depth/nicotine-craving/art…

www.medicinenet.com/smoking_and_heart_disease/article.htm

www.nysmokefree.com/Subpage.aspx?pn=PATCH.

www.quit.com/considering/cold-turkey.html.

www.quit.com/quit-smoking/understand/effects-of-smoking.html

www.rd.com/health/wellness/25-ways-to-stop-smoking-cigarettes?

www.webmd.com/lung/copd/what-is-emphysema).

APPENDIX 13A

RATING THE IMPORTANCE OF MY SMOKING

# of Cigarettes Smoked	Day and Time When You Smoked	Place Where You Smoked & With Whom	What You Are Doing While Smoking	Importance of Smoking This Cigarette Before and After 1 (not important) to 9 (extremely important)	List Your Healthy Alternatives	How Many Times Did You Switch from Smoking to a Healthy Alternative
1				B 1 2 3 4 5 6 7 8 9 A 1 2 3 4 5 6 7 8 9		
2				B 1 2 3 4 5 6 7 8 9 A 1 2 3 4 5 6 7 8 9		
3				B 1 2 3 4 5 6 7 8 9 A 1 2 3 4 5 6 7 8 9		
4				B 1 2 3 4 5 6 7 8 9 A 1 2 3 4 5 6 7 8 9		
5				B 1 2 3 4 5 6 7 8 9 A 1 2 3 4 5 6 7 8 9		
6				B 1 2 3 4 5 6 7 8 9 A 1 2 3 4 5 6 7 8 9		
7				B 1 2 3 4 5 6 7 8 9 A 1 2 3 4 5 6 7 8 9		
8				B 1 2 3 4 5 6 7 8 9 A 1 2 3 4 5 6 7 8 9		
9				B 1 2 3 4 5 6 7 8 9 A 1 2 3 4 5 6 7 8 9		
10				B 1 2 3 4 5 6 7 8 9 A 1 2 3 4 5 6 7 8 9		
11				B 1 2 3 4 5 6 7 8 9 A 1 2 3 4 5 6 7 8 9		
12				B 1 2 3 4 5 6 7 8 9 A 1 2 3 4 5 6 7 8 9		
13				B 1 2 3 4 5 6 7 8 9 A 1 2 3 4 5 6 7 8 9		
14				B 1 2 3 4 5 6 7 8 9 A 1 2 3 4 5 6 7 8 9		
15				B 1 2 3 4 5 6 7 8 9 A 1 2 3 4 5 6 7 8 9		
16				B 1 2 3 4 5 6 7 8 9 A 1 2 3 4 5 6 7 8 9		
17				B 1 2 3 4 5 6 7 8 9 A 1 2 3 4 5 6 7 8 9		
18				B 1 2 3 4 5 6 7 8 9 A 1 2 3 4 5 6 7 8 9		
19				B 1 2 3 4 5 6 7 8 9 A 1 2 3 4 5 6 7 8 9		
20				B 1 2 3 4 5 6 7 8 9 A 1 2 3 4 5 6 7 8 9		

# of Cigarettes Smoked	Day and Time When You Smoked	Place Where You Smoked & With Whom	What You Are Doing While Smoking	Importance of Smoking This Cigarette Before and After 1 (not important) to 9 (extremely important)	List Your Healthy Alternatives	How Many Times Did You Switch from Smoking to a Healthy Alternative
21				B 1 2 3 4 5 6 7 8 9 A 1 2 3 4 5 6 7 8 9		
22				B 1 2 3 4 5 6 7 8 9 A 1 2 3 4 5 6 7 8 9		
23				B 1 2 3 4 5 6 7 8 9 A 1 2 3 4 5 6 7 8 9		
24				B 1 2 3 4 5 6 7 8 9 A 1 2 3 4 5 6 7 8 9		
25				B 1 2 3 4 5 6 7 8 9 A 1 2 3 4 5 6 7 8 9		
26				B 1 2 3 4 5 6 7 8 9 A 1 2 3 4 5 6 7 8 9		
27				B 1 2 3 4 5 6 7 8 9 A 1 2 3 4 5 6 7 8 9		
28				B 1 2 3 4 5 6 7 8 9 A 1 2 3 4 5 6 7 8 9		
29				B 1 2 3 4 5 6 7 8 9 A 1 2 3 4 5 6 7 8 9		
30				B 1 2 3 4 5 6 7 8 9 A 1 2 3 4 5 6 7 8 9		
31				B 1 2 3 4 5 6 7 8 9 A 1 2 3 4 5 6 7 8 9		
32				B 1 2 3 4 5 6 7 8 9 A 1 2 3 4 5 6 7 8 9		
33				B 1 2 3 4 5 6 7 8 9 A 1 2 3 4 5 6 7 8 9		
34				B 1 2 3 4 5 6 7 8 9 A 1 2 3 4 5 6 7 8 9		
35				B 1 2 3 4 5 6 7 8 9 A 1 2 3 4 5 6 7 8 9		
36				B 1 2 3 4 5 6 7 8 9 A 1 2 3 4 5 6 7 8 9		
37				B 1 2 3 4 5 6 7 8 9 A 1 2 3 4 5 6 7 8 9		
38				B 1 2 3 4 5 6 7 8 9 A 1 2 3 4 5 6 7 8 9		
39				B 1 2 3 4 5 6 7 8 9 A 1 2 3 4 5 6 7 8 9		
40				B 1 2 3 4 5 6 7 8 9 A 1 2 3 4 5 6 7 8 9		